TRANSPLANTATION IMMUNOLOGY RESEARCH TRENDS

Transplantation Immunology Research Trends

Oliver N. Ulricker
Editor

Nova Biomedical Books
New York

Library of Congress Cataloging-in-Publication Data

Available upon request

ISBN: 978-1-60021-578-0

Published by Nova Science Publishers, Inc. ✦ New York

Contents

Preface

In recent years, transplantation immunology has evolved as a distinct field founded on the recognition that rejection of a transplanted organ or tissue is mediated by immune mechanisms in the host responding to antigens in the donor tissue. Included within the scope are T cell immunity ; Antigen presentation ; Alloreactivity ; Pancreas and islet cell transplantation ; Allogeneic bone marrow transplantation Models of tolerance induction ; Xenotransplantation and The swine leukocyte antigen (SLA) complex. This book gathers the latest research in the exciting new field of transplantation immunology.

Chapter I - The need for indefinite use of combinations of immunosuppressive drugs in organ transplantation may paradoxically impair long-term graft function. Tolerance induction may eliminate this need. One route for tolerance induction is to harness the power of dendritic cells (DCs) which are antigen presenting cells that have remarkable plasticity and the dichotomous function of directing immune responses toward either immunity or tolerance. It has also been recognized in recent years that a subtype regulatory T cells, the $CD4^+CD25^+$ T_{reg} cells, play a critical role in mediating allo-specific tolerance. More importantly, there appears to be bi-directional signaling between DCs and $CD4^+CD25^+$ T_{reg} cells. DCs mediate central as well as peripheral T_{reg} cell development and expansion. Conversely, T_{reg} cells may directly down-regulate the ability of DCs to stimulate effector T cells. Here we consider the specific characteristics of both DCs and $CD4^+CD25^+$ T_{reg} cells that are relevant to induction of transplant alloantigen-specific tolerance and discuss the therapeutic potential of DC or T_{reg} cell-based therapy in organ transplantation.

Chapter II - Chemokine receptors and their ligands control a wide variety of biological and pathological processes, ranging from immunosurveillance to inflammation, from viral infection to cancer, and from transplant rejection to transplant tolerance. It is not surprising that chemokine receptors and their ligands may be involved in rejection of allogeneic transplants because the chemokine receptor system plays an essential role in host defense. Allograft transplant rejection is mediated largely by circulating peripheral leukocytes induced to infiltrate the graft by various inflammatory factors. Of these, chemokine receptors and their ligands, which are expressed by early innate responding leukocytes, as well as by inflamed graft tissues, are responsible for the recruitment and infiltration of alloreactive leukocytes.

A complex process including both innate and acquired immune responses results in allograft rejection. Some chemokine receptors and their ligands play essential roles not only in leukocyte migration into the graft but also in facilitating dendritic and T cell trafficking between lymph nodes and the transplant in early and late stage of the allogeneic response. Analysis of gene knockout mice with targeted deletions of certain chemokine receptors and their ligands has gradually clarified their relative importance in allograft rejection. The present chapter focuses on the impact and mechanism of these chemoattractant proteins on transplant outcome and novel diagnostic and therapeutic approaches for antirejection therapy based on targeting chemokine receptors and/or their ligands.

Chapter III - The advent and successful evolution of human solid organ transplantation over the past 50 years has been a remarkable achievement that has provided thousands of patients with certain types of end stage organ disease an improved life with notably reduced morbidity and mortality. In order to achieve this success there has been the need for significant immunosuppression of the host to prevent recipient alloimmune responses from rejecting the genetically disparate donor organ. Unfortunately, the application of immunosuppression comes at a price and carries with it the potential for numerous life threatening and debilitating side effects. Since donor allograft tolerance has been extensively characterized and accomplished in animal models, transplant physicians have always attempted to achieve immunological tolerance in human transplant recipients in order to attain a state of specific nonreactivity to the donor transplant with little or no immunosuppression but without sacrificing graft function. To date, the realization of true immunological tolerance in human transplantation remains elusive; however, there have been many examples where a state of "operational" tolerance has been achieved. This chapter will describe these clinical occurrences and based upon animal models, an overview of some postulated mechanisms in immune tolerance.

Chapter IV - Lung transplantation has become established therapy in the treatment of selected patients with end stage lung diseases. However, five year survival after lung transplantation is little better than 50%, largely due to chronic graft failure. The basis of this failure is poorly understood but chronic rejection is probably a major factor. At the cellular level, graft rejection is associated with an increase in graft T-cell infiltration, alveolar macrophages, and pro-inflammatory cytokine expression. Although most effective transplantation immunosuppressive strategies are based on interruption of IL-2 signaling by calcineurin inhibitors, Cyclosporin A (CsA) and Tacrolimus (Tac), intensification of immuno-supressive therapies has not lead to any improvement in chronic graft failure. In addition, treatment with these drugs is associated with serious adverse side effects including specific organ toxicities, susceptibility to infections and an increased risk of developing a range of malignancies. Pharmacokinetic properties of both drugs show high inter- and intra-individual variability which may mean some patients do not require the high levels of drugs (that cause adverse side effects) for effective therapeutics. With the availability of novel flow cytometric techniques, recent research has focused on the measurement of inflammatory cytokines at the cellular level as a strategy to assess the physiological response to treatment. Importantly, cytokine levels in both peripheral blood and in the airways have been investigated, which has highlighted important differences in responses seen locally versus systemically. These techniques may complement or ultimately replace current standard approaches which rely on the measurement of plasma drug levels and monitoring by invasive biopsy. The application of these techniques has the potential to improve current immunosuppression protocols, optimise individual therapy and possibly provide new therapeutic options to improve the morbidity of lung transplant patients.

Chapter VI - Renal transplant recipients have benefited from short-term graft survival due to the introduction of new immunosuppressants. Despite this, long-term survival has improved only marginally during recent years. Chronic allograft nephropathy, cardiovascular disease, older donors, emerging new viruses and malignancies, among other factors, may be responsible for this situation. In addition, immunosuppression remains the cause of most morbidity following organ transplantation. Thus, minimization or, at least, tailoring of immunosuppression is an issue of great concern in this field. Minimization of immunosuppression is not itself a primary goal in organ transplantation, but it helps to reduce the risk of drug toxicity, as long as there is no compromise of immunosuppressive efficacy. In this respect, some strategies to achieve this goal may be: a) To minimize corticosteroid regimens, b) To minimize calcineurin inhibitor regimens, c) To tailor anticalcineuric drugs in order to optimize cardiovascular risk profile and renal function d) To use mammalian target-of-rapamycin inhibitors or purine synthesis inhibitors in order to prevent or reverse renal allograft dysfunction e) To establish therapeutic strategies against new viruses and malignancies, and f) To optimize immunosuppressive therapy in elderly patients. This review outlines several strategies for minimizing or tailoring the use of immunosuppressants in order to attain these objectives. The arguments for the various strategies are based on clinical trial data which suggest that most patients can be transplanted with less immunosuppression than is currently standard.

Chapter VII - Previous studies including those of our group have demonstrated that pre-transplant serum soluble HLA (sHLA-I) class I levels and the presence of HLA-DQB1*0302 allele in liver recipients are different factors implicated in acute rejection development. Indeed, this HLA allele is related to several autoimmune diseases and could be implicated in an increased alloreactivity state in determined individuals.

Our objective was to investigate the proliferation response of different HLA-DQB1 molecules with and without allogeneic sera sHLA depletion.

We examined the primary (MLR-I, mixed lymphocyte reaction) and secondary (MLR-II) proliferation response from individuals with different matching and mismatching HLA-DQ combinations in situations of sHLA molecules depletion in cellular cultures.

Sera soluble HLA class I molecules depletion was performed by ligation of the HLA class I antibody (IgG2a isotype, w6.32 clone) to Sepharose 4B gel and treatment of human sera samples, as previously published. Cellular cultures were performed by unidirectional primary MLR-I (5 days) and secondary MLR-II (re-stimulated at 5 days) by using allogeneic and autologous responder cells and irradiated stimulator cells (EBV-transformed lymphoblastoid lines) in allogeneic and autologous HLA-DQB1 specific combinations (presence or absence of HLA-DQB1*0302).

The relative response of HLA-DQB1*0302$^+$ lymphocytes in primary MLR-I, when the stimulator cells were semiallogeneic or incompatibles, did not show an increased proliferation, in situations of absence or presence of sHLA-I molecules.

However, in secondary MLR-II (primed responder cell against stimulator cell), we detected an increased relative response in situation of absence of allogeneic sHLA and using semiallogeneic HLA-DQB1*0302$^+$ cells. This result was not obtained with HLA-DQB1*0302$^-$ cells were used.

In conclusion, these data indicate that, in a primary response the different tested combinations show a similar manner to respond, but in the secondary response, when the responder cells have been primed and sensibilized, sHLA molecules plays a different role in proliferation response depending to specific HLA-DQ molecules constitution.

Chapter VIII - Research in pig-to-primate xenotransplantation aims to solve the great shortage of cells and organs for transplantation. Despite some great advances in the field, the main impediment to its clinical application is the strength of the immune response triggered by the xenograft. Cell-, tissue- and organ-based xenografts are subjected to distinct rejection processes that share humoral and cellular mechanisms. Rejection of vascularized organs is the best characterized and one of the most challenging. Various types of xenograft rejection have been described in solid organs that differ in the time of onset and the immune pathways involved. Hyperacute rejection (HAR) is the first to take place (within minutes to hours after transplantation). When HAR is averted, the xenograft succumbs to acute humoral xenograft rejection (AHXR) in a period of days to months. It is the main cause of rejection, as acute cellular xenograft rejection (ACXR, which is T cell-mediated and occurs in the same time frame) is presumably controlled by immunosuppression and is less severe than AHXR. Finally, chronic rejection is only observed in a few organs, those with the longest survival times.

The main triggers of HAR are well known: natural anti-Gal α1,3-Gal antibodies and complement. Consequently, the approaches developed to express human complement regulatory proteins or removal of the Gal α1,3-Gal antigen by genetic engineering of the donor pig have successfully averted HAR. On the contrary, the process of AHXR is more complex and key molecules that trigger AHXR remain to be identified. Both complement and the Gal α1,3-Gal antigen seem to exacerbate AHXR, but their inhibition does not prevent rejection. The presence of an innate cellular component (NK cells and macrophages) indicates these cells probably participate in AHXR. In vitro, human NK cells kill porcine cells by using two triggering receptors, NKG2D and NKp44, as well as the CD28 variant that binds the porcine costimulatory molecule CD86. Human monocytes also bind and activate porcine endothelial cells, but the molecular interactions remain to be fully characterized. In vivo, both NK cells and macrophages may have an effect on the B cell antibody response that ultimately leads to AHXR. Controlling the B cell response will be key to attain long-term xenograft survival. In summary, the elucidation of the mechanisms that contribute to acute xenograft rejection may allow the development of therapeutic solutions that result in successful clinical xenotransplantation.

Chapter IX - Increasing evidence suggests a role for viruses in allograft rejection in solid organ transplant recipients. Cytomegalovirus (CMV) disease is an independent risk factor for acute rejection in renal transplantation. CMV has also been described as a trigger for chronic rejection such as cardiac allograft vasculopathy in heart transplantation and chronic allograft nephropathy in renal transplantation. CMV may be involved in the pathology of acute rejection by several mechanisms, including up-regulation of adhesion molecules, increased expression of MHC class II antigens on allograft tissue, and release of variety of cytokines. Direct infection of arterial smooth muscle cells and endothelial cells accelerates the development of allograft vasculopathy. CMV-encoded chemokine receptor US28 has the ability to induce smooth muscle cell migration. Moreover, CMV abrogates the vascular protective effects of endothelium-derived nitric oxide system. Data on beneficial effects of antiviral prophylaxis on allograft rejection are inconsistent. Still, valacyclovir prophylaxis was associated with significant reduction of acute rejection in two randomized controlled trials in renal transplant recipients. In summary, viruses contribute importantly to the pathophysiology of acute and chronic allograft rejection. Further clinical trials are needed to determine favorable effects of antiviral prophylaxis on rejection rate.

In: Transplantation Immunology Research Trends   ISBN: 978-1-60021-578-0
Editor: Oliver N. Ulricker, pp. 1-35   © 2007 Nova Science Publishers, Inc.

Chapter I

Dendritic Cells and CD4⁺CD25⁺ T Reg Cells in Induction of Transplant Alloantigen-Specific Tolerance

Xunrong Luo[1,2], Joseph Leventhal[1] and Anat R. Tambur[1]
[1] Division of Organ Transplantation, Department of Surgery and
[2] Division of Nephrology and Hypertension, Department of Medicine
Northwestern University Feinberg School of Medicine, Chicago, IL

Abstract

The need for indefinite use of combinations of immunosuppressive drugs in organ transplantation may paradoxically impair long-term graft function. Tolerance induction may eliminate this need. One route for tolerance induction is to harness the power of dendritic cells (DCs) which are antigen presenting cells that have remarkable plasticity and the dichotomous function of directing immune responses toward either immunity or tolerance. It has also been recognized in recent years that a subtype regulatory T cells, the CD4⁺CD25⁺ T_{reg} cells, play a critical role in mediating allo-specific tolerance. More importantly, there appears to be bi-directional signaling between DCs and CD4⁺CD25⁺ T_{reg} cells. DCs mediate central as well as peripheral T_{reg} cell development and expansion. Conversely, T_{reg} cells may directly down-regulate the ability of DCs to stimulate effector T cells. Here we consider the specific characteristics of both DCs and CD4⁺CD25⁺ T_{reg} cells that are relevant to induction of transplant alloantigen-specific tolerance and discuss the therapeutic potential of DC or T_{reg} cell-based therapy in organ transplantation.

Introduction

The benefit of sustained and robust donor-specific tolerance would offer many benefits to transplant recipients. In the past half century, much effort has been devoted to understanding the cellular and molecular mechanisms of allograft rejection which has allowed the induction of tolerance possible in various animal models. The two cell types that have emerged to be critical players in tolerance induction are dendritic cells and regulatory T cells. Here, we will review recent advances in the understanding of the roles these two cell types play in transplant tolerance induction as well as their potentials as therapeutics in allogeneic transplant models.

Part I. Tolerogenic Dendritic Cells

Dendritic Cell Overview

Dendritic cells (DCs) were first discovered to derive from the bone marrow and share a common progenitor with macrophages and granulocytes[1]. They are uniquely equipped antigen presenting cells (APCs) whose primary function was originally thought to be initiation of innate and adaptive immunity in face of infectious organisms and other antigens such as allo-antigens from transplanted organs[2-5]. However, an expanding literature now suggests a critical role of DCs in induction of T cell tolerance[6, 7]. The dichotomy of DC functions is permitted possibly by the state of maturation DCs at which they are exposed to antigens, the type of DCs that encounter the antigen, and the context in which antigens are encountered.

State of Maturation

The conventional view states that DCs induce immunity or tolerance depending on their state of maturation, specifically, immature DCs induce T cell tolerance whereas mature DCs induce immunity. Many stimuli induce DC maturation. Ligands to Toll-like receptors (TLRs) are potent stimuli for DC maturation[8, 9]. These include microbial signals such as viral RNA and poly IC on TLR3, lipopolysaccharide (LPS) on TLR4, mycoplasma lipopeptide on TLR6, and CpG DNA (bacteria) on TLR9 among others. Several non-TLR pathway signals are also potent stimuli of DC maturation, such as TNF family members (TNF-α, FasL, CD40L) and type I interferons[10-12]. Upon maturation, DCs express higher levels of cell surface major histocompatibility complex (MHC) molecules as well as accessory molecules such as B7-family members (CD86, CD80, PD-L2/B7-DC, ICOS-L), TNF family members (CD137, CD124, CD70), and chemokine receptors (CCR5, CCR7)[13]. Matured DCs become potent stimulators of naïve $CD4^+$ and $CD8^+$ T cells. In contrast, immature DCs are poor stimulators of T cells at best. However, immature DCs are highly efficient in antigen uptake, processing, loading onto MHC class II molecules and transporting to cell surface, a feature that is to some degree dampened upon maturation[14]. The capacity for capturing and processing apoptotic cells by immature DCs is thought to be crucial in the maintenance of tolerance to self-antigens and non-inflammatory stimuli under steady-state conditions[6] It is therefore not surprising that experimental strategies for utilizing DCs to induce transplant tolerance center on blocking the DC maturation process. Approaches to "arrest" DC maturation can be broadly categorized into: 1) direct *in vivo* targeting of known cellular components of DC maturation pathway, and 2) *in vitro* generation of immature DCs under alternative culture conditions which result in alterations of accessory molecule expressions.

Targeting of Components of DC Maturation Pathway

Upregulation of costimulatory molecules upon DC maturation is in part dependent on NF-κB mediated gene transcription[15]. Strategies for blocking NF-κB signaling pathway have been studied to induce alloantigen specific tolerance. Lu *et al* described that bone marrow derived DCs treated with synthetic oligodexoynucleotides (ODN) containing consensus NF-κB binding sites showed decreased cell surface costimulatory molecules expression and induced allogeneic donor-specific hyporesponsiveness in mixed leukocyte reactions. When 2×10^6 NF-κB ODN treated DCs were injected into full MHC mismatched recipients, they were able to prolong allogeneic heart graft survival from a mean survival time (MST) of 10 days to 27 days[16, 17]. Similarly, Benigni *et al* used an adenoviral vector encoding for a kinase-defective dominant negative form of IKK2 to block NF-κB activation and observed similar prolongation of allogeneic graft survival in a rat kidney transplantation model[18]. Blocking TNF-α signaling in DCs using a recombinant adenoviral vector expressing soluble TNF-α receptor type 1 (sTNFR1) has also been shown to result in resistance to LPS induced maturation and further impairment of DC chemotaxis[19]. Pre-treatment with donor DC-sTNFR1 led to marked prolongation of allogeneic heart transplantation (MST from 12 to 87 days).

A signaling pathway proximal to NF-κB that has recently gained significant attention in studies of transplant rejection is the Toll-like receptor (TLR) pathway. TLRs are pattern recognition receptors expressed on surface of APCs that are critical in the host detection and defense against microbial pathogens. Various TLRs, upon ligation, initiate a signaling pathway via their common signal adaptor protein MyD88 which eventually leads to the translocation of NF-κB and the DC maturation. Using an HY-incompatible skin transplant model, Lakkis *et al* has demonstrated that activation of TLR signal adaptor protein MyD88 is crucial for rejection of allogeneic transplants[20]. Engagement of a single TLR using CpG injections at the time of allogeneic transplant was sufficient to abolish tolerance mediated by co-stimulation blockade[21]. TLR activation in this model is associated with prevention of intragraft recruitment of CD4$^+$Foxp3$^+$ regulatory T cells. Clinical studies in renal transplant recipients are beginning to reveal an association between TLR polymorphisms and the development of acute rejection post-transplant[22]. These data not only underscored the importance of innate immunity in allograft rejection, but more importantly provided basis for future therapeutic strategies that target the TLR signal transduction pathway for transplant tolerance induction.

A downstream effect of DC maturation, namely enhanced cell surface expression of the B7 costimulatory molecules CD80 and CD86, and subsequent augmented CD28-B7 interaction, can be blocked by the fusion protein cytotoxic T lymphocyte Ag-immunoglobulin (CTLA4-Ig)[23]. This protein competes with CD28 for B7 ligation thereby blocking B7-CD28 mediated T cell activation. DCs retrovirally transduced with CTLA-Ig have been shown to induce alloantigen-specific T cell hyporesponsiveness *in vitro* and *in vivo*[24]. Pretreatment with CTLA4-Ig transduced DCs significantly prolonged allograft survival in a murine model of cardiac transplantation which could be further augmented by additional costimulation blockade using anti-CD40L mAb. Systemic treatment of recipients with CTLA4-Ig-coding adenoviral vector also led to long term allograft survival[25]. The protective effects appeared to be at least in part mediated by DC secreted soluble factor(s). More recent data has shed light on a potential soluble factor, indoleamine 2,3-dioxygenase (IDO), a key enzyme in tryptophan catabolism[26]. It has been identified that CTLA4-Ig has a bidirectional signaling capacity: in addition to its negative effect on T cells (blocking CD28-mediated T cell activation), it also "reversely" signals the DCs through B7 molecules and promotes IDO production which in turn promotes T cell apoptosis[27]. This effect is paradoxically dependent on IFN-γ production[28]. This pathway provides an additional mechanism for DCs to maintain T cell homeostasis and self- tolerance by deletion.

In Vitro Generation of Immature DCs under Alternative Culture Conditions

Myeloid DCs can be derived from bone marrow progenitors in the presence of GM-CSF. Several natural cytokines have been exploited in altering DC differentiation and function. IL-10 is a multifunctional cytokine with diverse effects on many cell types. DCs that are exposed to IL-10 during differentiation or tranduced with viral vectors expressing IL-10 have been shown to display decreased levels of MHC II, CD80, and CD40, consistent with an immature state, and to induce antigen-specific T cell anergy *in vitro*[29]. *In vivo*, DCs engineered to express IL-10 alone did not significantly prolong allograft survival, but co-expression of another inhibitory cytokine TGF-β1[30] or the chemokine receptor CCR7[31] led to striking prolongation of allograft survival in heart transplant model.

Independent effects of TGF-β1 on DC differentiation and function have also been studied. DCs transduced to express TGF-β1 display a characteristic immature phenotype, exhibit poor allostimulaotry activity but enhance DC survival in allogeneic hosts[32]. Survival of allogeneic cardiac grafts could be prolonged in recipients injected with donor TGF-β1 transduced DCs prior to transplantation. TGF-β1 has also been shown to be crucial in $CD4^+CD25^+$ regulatory T cells induction and expansion[33], and a likely source of endogenous TGF-β1 is antigen presenting cells[34], the most efficient of which are the DCs. Most recently, it has been shown that DCs can be "licensed" by certain tumor cells to produce large quantities of TGF-β1 which then enable them to simulate $CD4^+CD25^+$ T_{reg} cell proliferation[35]. However, natural signals that stimulate DC TGF-β1 production remain to be determined.

DCs express high levels of vitamin D receptor (VDR)[36]. Results accumulated over the past two decades demonstrated that VDR ligands significantly modulate the phenotype and function of DCs (reviewed in[37]). Treatment of DCs with1,25-dihydroxyvitamin D₃, the active form of vitamin D, leads to downregulated expression of the costimulatory molecules and to decreased IL-12 and enhanced IL-10 production, resulting in decreased T cell activation[38, 39]. Interestingly, such VDR ligand treated DCs also seem to induce $CD4^+CD25^+$ T_{reg} cells, a mechanism that at least in part contribute to mediate transplant tolerance[40]. Direct *in vivo* tolerogenic effect of VDR ligand treated DCs has also been demonstrated by adoptive transfer of the treated DCs in allograft transplantation models[41]. Glucocorticoid is another agent that has been shown to arrest DC maturation with resulting down-regulation of costimulatory molecules and inflammatory cytokine secretions[42, 43]. Other pharmacological agents that have been studied in the process of DC maturation include

LF15-0195[44, 45] and nacystelyn[46] which also target the NF-κB pathway as discussed above.

Though significant effort from the past has focused on immature DCs, it has been recently recognized that immature DCs generated *in vitro* as such may not be the ideal candidate for tolerance induction *in vivo*. They may have inefficient migratory capacity from lacking appropriate chemokine receptor[47] and they may also mature *in vivo* upon encountering proinflammatory stimuli in host microenvironment. Effort in recent years has been made to study partially activated types of DCs for transplant tolerance and the terms "alternatively activated" or "semi-mature" DCs have been coined to distinguish such DCs from immature DCs. Several alternative maturation protocols have been studied[19, 42, 48], which include TNF-α stimulation, LPS or CD40 ligation in combination with dexamethasone, among others. Such "semi-mature" DCs have unique profiles of costimulation molecule and chemokine receptor expressions as well as cytokine secretion (IL12/IL-10 ratio, TGF-β1), such that they may be more resistant to further maturation *in vivo* and are more efficient in induce long term allograft survival.

Role of DC Subsets in Transplant Tolerance

DC populations with distinct phenotype and function have been described both in humans and rodents. In mice, one subset of DCs is characterized by CD8α$^+$CD11b^{low} cell surface markers and is remarkably efficient in taking up apoptotic cells compared to CD8α$^-$ DCs, the clearest differences in the functions of the CD8α$^+$ and CD8α$^-$ subsets[49-51]. The CD8α$^+$ DCs have been called lymphoid DCs because they were initially thought to develop from lymphoid rather than myeloid progenitors. Subsequent adoptive transfer studies suggested that the CD8α$^+$ DCs may also develop from myeloid progenitors[52]. Evidence emerged to indicate that constitutive presentation of antigens acquired from dying cells by DCs in steady state led to deletion of naïve peripheral T cells and systemic antigen-specific tolerance[51]. The first report of the role of CD8α$^+$ DCs in allogeneic transplant tolerance studied both freshly isolated immature and over-night GM-CSF matured CD8α$^+$ DCs, and found that both immature as well as matured CD8α$^+$ DCs markedly prolong allogeneic heart graft survival[53]. This effect was associated with specific impairment of anti-donor T cell proliferative responses, which was not reversed by exogenous IL-2. This finding contrasts that seen with CD8α$^-$ myeloid subset in that only the immature CD8α$^-$ DCs were able to prolong transplant graft survival. A more recent study demonstrated that the CD8α$^+$ DCs may be highly efficient in expanding antigen-specific CD4$^+$CD25$^+$ Tregs from a polyclonal repertoire comparing to whole splenic DCs or bone marrow-derived DCs[54]. This unique capacity of the CD8α$^+$ DCs was attributed to a lower background stimulation originating from T cell autoreactivity, possibly related to the resemblance between the CD8α$^+$ DCs and thymic DCs which are involved in negative selection of highly atuoreactive T cells in the thymus.

Another subset of DCs that has been increasingly recognized to play an important role in immune tolerance is the plasmacytoid DCs (pDCs), a term that portrays their resemblance to plasma cells. Mouse pDCs characteristically express B220 and Ly6C on their cell surface, and are CD11c^{dim}, secrete large amounts of type I interferons upon exposure to viruses, and are thought to play an essential role in protecting the host against inflammatory responses in setting of harmless antigens[55]. Their development from hematopoietic stem cells in humans as well as in mice is uniquely promoted by fms-like tyrosine kinase 3 ligand (Flt-3L)[56, 57]. They express TLR9 and respond to stimulation with TLR9 ligand CpG-oligonucleotide with upregulation of B7 molecules[58]. Initial suggestion of the pDCs as "tolerogenic" DCs came from murine allogeneic BM transplant models where the presence of these cells correlated with stem cell engraftment and decreased occurrence of GVHD[59, 60]. The same authors have also shown that pDCs were able to induce durable tolerance to skin allografts. Examination of pDCs in vascularized organ allograft survival revealed that a single preoperative infusion of pDC of donor origin prolong heart graft survival significantly compared with untreated mice (MST 22 vs. 9 days, respectively)[61]. Corroborating with *in vitro* data suggesting that immature pDCs can induce T$_{reg}$ cells, a recent study from Bromberg *et al* showed that alloantigen-presenting recipient pDCs home to local lymph nodes and induce generation of donor-specific CD4$^+$CD25$^+$Foxp3$^+$ regulatory T cells[62], a mechanism that at least in part contribute to tolerance induction by the well-characterized regimen using donor specific transfusion plus αCD40L. Depletion of pDCs in this model or prevention of pDC homing to LNs inhibit peripheral T$_{reg}$ cell development and tolerance induction, whereas adoptive transfer of tolerized pDCs induce T$_{reg}$ cell development and prolong cardiac graft survival. An alternative mechanism for pDC-induced tolerance has been proposed to be preferential induction of IDO expression upon ligation of a number of cell surface receptors[63]. As pointed out earlier, reverse signaling between CTLA4 and B7 upregulates IDO expression. This occurs with various degrees among different DC subsets, with the pDCs and the CD8α$^+$ DCs being predominantly the subsets that express IDO upon CTLA4-Ig treatment. Classic myeloid DCs (CD11c$^+$CD11b$^+$) have much fewer IDO$^+$ cells upon CTLA4-Ig treatment. More recently, another cell surface receptor, CD200R, which interacts with a broadly distributed cell surface glycoprotein CD200, has been identified to play an important role in the control of myeloid cellular activity and prevention of autoimmunity (reviewed in [64]). A fusion protein, CD200-Ig, has been shown to interact with CD200R expressed on murine pDCs. This can be further augmented by CpG oligodeoxynucleotide treatment. Ligation of CD200R on pDCs by CD200-Ig induces expression of IDO[65], which then initiates the tolerogenic pathway of tryptophan catabolism. As a result, pDCs are capable of suppressing antigen-specific responses *in vivo* when transferred into recipients after treatment with CD200-Ig. These studies underscore the novel functions and diverse mechanisms by which pDCs may be involved in host alloantigen-specific tolerance induction.

Indirect vs. Direct Pathway

In allogeneic transplantation, alloantigen directed immune responses are thought to be induced via two distinct pathways – the direct and the indirect pathways (reviewed in [66]). The direct pathway utilizes intact allogeneic MHC molecules on donor DCs to interact directly with recipient T cells, whereas the indirect pathway is driven by recipient DC-processed and self-MHC presented polymorphic sequences of allogeneic MHC molecules.

This concept has two immediate implications: 1. As donor DCs are derived from the transplanted organ, they are limited in numbers as well as life span. Following their elimination over time, it is conceivable that the strength of direct anti-alloantigen specific response would diminish accordingly; and 2. Among the normal T cell repertoire, there is a higher frequency of T cells with direct allo-specificity compared to that of T cells with indirect allo-specificity implying that the direct allo-response dominates the early post-transplantation phase whereas the indirect pathway plays a more important role during later stages post-transplantation[67-69]. As a consequence, a paradigm has evolved whereby the direct allo-specific response is thought to mediate acute allograft rejection whereas the indirect allo-specific response is considered the major mediator of chronic allograft rejection. The relative contribution of either pathway to allograft rejection in vivo remains a subject of intense studies over the past two decades. Direct visualization of DC trafficking and interactions between recipient CD4$^+$ T cells with donor (direct) or recipient (indirect) DCs using immunofluorescent technique demonstrated differential kinetics of homing and lymphoid tissue localization of donor vs. recipient DCs during acute rejection or tolerance induction[70], further differentiating the importance of either pathways in allograft transplantation.

Targeting the Direct Pathway of Alloantigen Presentation

Depletion of donor leukocytes prior to allograft transplantation could prolong allograft survival in certain experimental conditions. Early studies showed that in vitro culture of allografts prior to allograft transplantation depletes donor bone marrow derived "passenger" leukocytes and prolongs graft survival[71, 72]. Later studies demonstrated that spontaneous acceptance of allografts could be achieved by "parking" the graft in an intermediate recipient before transplantation which again serves to deplete donor leukocytes. Reconstitution in such recipients with donor DCs, even in small numbers, precipitates rapid graft rejection[73]. These data demonstrated a key role of donor DCs during the initial phase of allo-responses and therefore a potential target for allo-specific tolerance induction. For instance, chemokine-dependent homing of donor dendritic cells to secondary lymphoid tissues is essential for host sensitization and acute allograft rejection. Allografts transplanted into the plt (paucity of lymph node T cell) recipients that are deficient in secondary lymphoid expression of the CCR7 ligands, CCL21 and CCL19, enjoy indefinite graft survival in a kidney capsule islet transplant model[74]. Likewise, donor DCs that lack the adhesion molecule ICAM-1 show substantially decreased level of T cell priming and at least in part contribute to prolonged ICAM$^{-/-}$ cardiac graft survival in allogeneic transplant model[75].

Targeting donor DCs using immunosuppressive cytokines or agents that block the NF-κB pathway with a consequence of diminishing alloantigen presentation have also been widely used to prolong allograft survival. For instance transducing IL-10 in donor derived dendritic cells and injecting the modified DCs 7 days prior to transplantation moderately prolonged allograft survival in a small intestine transplant model[76]. Donor DCs generated in the presence of TGF-β1 or engineered to express TGF-β1 retain immature phenotype and with further costimulation blockade by anti-CD40L mAb induce long-term allograft survival[77, 78]. Likewise, donor DCs treated with double-strand NF-κB decoy oligodeoxynucleotides prolonged liver allograft survival and regeneration[79]. Furthermore, donor DCs engineered to express FasL have been used to deliver apoptotic signals to Fas$^+$ T cells thereby downregulating donor-specific T cell responses[80]. In addition to donor-specific anergy and deletion, tolerogenic donor DCs have also been shown to induce and expand regulatory CD4$^+$ T cells in both the central and peripheral compartments.

Targeting the Indirect Pathway of Alloantigen Presentation

In contrast to the diminishing direct allo-specific response over time, a series of clinical studies have demonstrated that indirect allo-reponse increases over time, with increased frequencies of T cells bearing indirect allo-specificities[81]. As previously discussed, recipient DCs are well-equipped with the capacity to uptake, process, and present allogeneic MHC peptides in the context of recipient MHC molecules, therefore are central to indirect allospecific T cell activation. Conditions likely exist that allow recipient DCs to tolerize, rather than activate, indirect allospecific T cells. Indeed, in a model of heart transplantation, tolerance could not be achieved in recipients that were incapable of mounting indirect anti-donor responses[82], suggesting that indirect allorecognition is necessary to induce stable tolerance. As such, strategies for tolerance induction have placed significant emphasis on targeting the recipient DCs.

Initial observation that targeting the indirect pathway leads to spontaneous allograft acceptance came from early studies by Lechler *et al.* In a rat kidney semiallogeneic transplant model, the authors showed that when an F1 (AS x AUG) kidney was re-transplanted from an immunosuppressed parent recipient one month later to a second parent recipient of the same strain, the grafts were spontaneously accepted without the need for any immunosuppression therapy, whereas a fully allogeneic kidney re-transplanted following the same protocol led to rejection[73]. The interpretation of the observation was that cells in the F1 graft co-expressing both AS and AUG MHC molecules developed the ability to silence AS T cells with indirect anti-AUG specificity. On the basis of these findings, the same authors tested the ability of F1 immature DCs to induce tolerance and regulation via the indirect pathway. Interestingly, injection of F1, but not donor, immature DCs was able to prolong allograft survival, confirming the privileged role of F1 DCs in the induction of indirect pathway regulation[83]. The protection was accompanied by donor-specific hyporesponsiveness by indirect presentation (tested with recipient DCs pulsed in vitro with allogeneic cell lysate). Furthermore, depletion of the CD25$^+$ T cell population unmasks a strong response to the donor antigen, suggesting the indirect regulation is in part mediated through development of regulatory T cells.

The above findings have obvious clinical relevance in tolerance induction in living related donor organ transplantations. However, other means for delivering donor antigens to recipient DCs are necessary to be investigated. Presentation of antigens from peripheral tissues by steady-state DCs in lymphoid organs has been shown to promote peripheral tolerance in mice. One strategy to deliver donor antigens to steady-state DCs with an inhibitory signal is by using donor cells undergoing apoptosis. Early studies using chemical cross-linking of soluble peptides to APCs by a chemical cross-linker 1-ethyl-3-(3'-dimethylaminopropyl)-carbodiimide (ECDI) have shown that such ECDI-coupled cells efficiently induce specific peptide tolerance and control autoimmunity[84]. Translating into alloantigen tolerance, subsequent studies using ECDI treated donor lymphocytes ("coupling" of cell surface MHC molecules to donor cells) have shown that i.v. injection of such cells prior to transplantation led to a transient but significant graft protection in full MHC-mismatched skin and heart transplant models[85, 86]. One possible mechanism underlying the protection of allografts may be induction of apoptosis by ECDI treatment and subsequent uptake of ECDI-fixed donor cells by host APCs[86]. *In vivo*, direct visualization by immunofluorescence revealed that recipient splenic CD8α$^+$ DCs are most efficient in uptaking i.v. injected apoptotic donor cells, and that capturing apoptotic donor cells does not mature recipient DCs (which have similar levels of MHC-I/II, CD40, CD80 and CD86 compared to DCs that have not internalized apoptotic cells)[87]. Instead, it allows the recipient DCs to delete alloreactive cells. *In vitro*, recipient DCs loaded with donor-derived apoptotic cells are able to cross-tolerize recipient T cells, and direct infusion of such DCs prior to transplantation prolongs allograft survival[88]. Evidence also exists that recipient macrophages may play a role in apoptotic cell induced donor specific regulation and that TGF-β1-dependent regulatory T cell expansion may partially contribute to the regulation[89].

Semi-Direct Pathway of Alloantigen Presentation

More recently, a third pathway for allo-recognition has been proposed: the semi-direct pathway. This model proposes that intact donor MHC molecules can be transferred *in toto* from donor cells (for instance, donor endothelial cells or donor DCs) to recipient DCs which then prime recipient alloreactive T cells with donor MHCs[90]. One way of recipient DCs acquiring intact donor MHC (class I and class II) molecules is through exosomes secreted by other DCs[91]. This pathway was initially proposed to explain the observation of "unlinked help" in which CD4$^+$ T helper cells with indirect allospecificity appeared to be able to amplify an effector CD8$^+$ T cell response with direct allospecificity[92]. With the semi-direct pathway, recipient DCs acquire and present intact donor MHC class I molecule to direct allospecific CD8$^+$ T cells on the one hand and present processed donor MHC molecules as polymorphic peptides to indirect allospecific CD4$^+$ T cells on the other. Therefore it solves the conundrum of the "unlinked help" and provides a mechanism for "linked help". Likewise, "linked suppression" describes indirect allospecific CD4$^+$ regulatory T cells regulating effector CD8$^+$ T cells with direct allospecificity[93].

Part II. The Role of DCs in Expansion and Induction of CD4$^+$CD25$^+$ T$_{reg}$ Cells

Regulatory T cells play a critical role in suppressing immune responses to a wide spectrum of antigens, therefore are emerging as key players in tolerance strategies in controlling autoimmune diseases and in allogeneic transplant rejections. Alloantigen-specific CD4$^+$CD25$^+$ cells are presumably generated in transplant recipients through multiple but not mutually exclusive pathways. There are several "types" of regulatory T cells. Tr1 and Th3 regulatory T cells depend on inhibitory cytokines IL-10 and TGF-β1 respectively for their function (reviewed in [94]). A different type referred to as the "natural" regulatory T cells (T$_{reg}$) develop in the thymus and are CD4$^+$ and CD25$^+$. They express the transcription factor Foxp3 which interacts with another calcium-regulated transcription factor NFAT to mediate their suppressive functions[95]. Recent data suggests a process of so-called "infectious tolerance", where CD4+CD25+ Treg in the periphery convert CD4+CD25- cells into T_{reg} cells [96] [97]. Foxp3 is upregulated in these "induced" T_{reg} cells. Whether these cells suppress in a cell-cell contact dependent or cytokine dependent manner remains to be determined. Both naturally and alloantigen-selected T_{reg} cells are expandable in the periphery by alloantigens and play important roles in controlling graft rejection and possibly lead to allograft tolerance. Numerous previously established tolerance protocols in rodents have focused upon generation and/or expansion of alloantigen-specific $CD4^+CD25^+$ cells using therapeutic manipulations in the transplant recipient. Examples of such tolerizing strategies include using monoclonal antibodies (mAb) specific for CD3, CD4 or CD154, a combination of 1,25-dihydroxyvitamin D3 with mycophenolate mofetil, pre-transplant donor blood transfusion, and administration of tolerogenic or regulatory dendritic cells [98-100]. Unfortunately, none of these approaches have been shown to expand $CD4^+CD25^+$ clones specifically and efficiently. Studies have shown that Treg can be effectively expanded *in vitro* (*ex vivo*) in the presence of immobilized anti-CD3 mAb plus IL-2 [101], or with antiCD3/CD28 coated microbeads and IL-2 [102]. This approach allows for expansion of the entire population of T_{reg} cells, while maintaining a diversified repertoire, so-called polyclonal regulatory cells. Infusion of *ex vivo* expanded polyclonal T_{reg} cells has been shown to delay or even prevent GVHD in mice [101, 103]. Alternatively, T_{reg} cells can be expanded and, at the same time, selected for their capacity to recognize allogeneic antigen, so that antigen specific T_{reg} cells can be obtained. Such antigen specific ex vivo expanded T_{reg} cells has also been shown to delay or prevent GVHD in mice [101, 104, 105]. In this section, we will focus on the role of DCs in peripheral expansion and generation of $CD4^+CD25^+$ $Foxp3^+$ T_{reg} cells.

The Role of DCs in In Vitro Expansion of $CD4^+CD25^+$ T_{reg} Cells

Initial studies of the $CD4^+CD25^+$ $Foxp3^+$ T_{reg} cells revealed that they are "anergic" to TCR stimulation in culture[106]. Combined with the small percentages (5-10%) of such cells in the periphery, it makes their experimental studies and application in clinical conditions difficult. In a pioneer study by Yamazaki *et al*, it was demonstrated that the *in vitro* relative anergic state of the $CD4^+CD25^+$ $Foxp3^+$ T_{reg} cells was in part due to the suboptimal antigen presenting cells used in those studies that were largely in an immature functional state[107]. In contrast, when mature DCs were used to present antigens, the T_{reg} cells broke their apparent anergic state and underwent vigorous proliferation. This proliferation could be further augmented with exogenous IL-2. The DC-dependent T_{reg} cell expansion is contingent upon B7-CD28 costimulation. The expanded T_{reg} cells maintained high levels of CTLA-4 and GITR expression, and were functionally suppressive, suggesting that the proliferation did not come at the expense of regulatory function.

Subsequently, mature DC expanded antigen-specific T_{reg} cells have been studied both in autoimmune models as well as allogeneic transplant models[108]. In models of autoimmune diabetes, it was shown that mature DCs presenting a single β cell autoantigen peptide were able to expand islet antigen specific $CD4^+CD25^+$ T_{reg} cells *in vitro*, and that the expanded $CD4^+CD25^+$ T_{reg} cells showed enhanced suppressive function compared to freshly isolated

T_{reg} cells and could effectively suppress diabetes in the NOD scid adoptive transfer model. Among the splenic CD11c⁺ DCs, the CD8α⁺ subset induces the least degree of basal activation when co-cultured with a polyclonal pool of T cells[54]. Therefore, when pulsed with peptide or tissue antigens, the CD11c⁺ CD8α⁺ DCs, among all DC subsets, allow the highest stimulation index of the co-cultured T cells compared to un-pulsed DCs. This feature makes the splenic CD11c⁺ CD8α⁺ DCs an ideal DC population for selective expansion of T_{reg} cells of rare autoantigen specificities as only the T cells with engaged TCRs would be stimulated to proliferate. Indeed, when present at as low as 0.01% among wild-type polyclonal T cells, transgenic T cells expressing a TCR specific for an HA epitope could be selectively expanded over 500 fold by HA peptide pulsed CD8α⁺ DCs. Furthermore, wild type T_{reg} cells with HA specificity could also be selectively expanded using CD11c⁺ CD8α⁺ DCs pulsed with either HA peptides or lysates of islet cells expressing HA as a neo-autoantigen. These selectively expanded HA-specific T_{reg} cells exert antigen-specific suppression *in vitro* after secondary stimulation, and more importantly suppress autoimmune diabetes in transgenic mice engineered to express HA in the pancreatic β cells.

With respect to alloantigen specific CD4⁺CD25⁺ T_{reg} cell expansion for transplant tolerance induction, allogeneic whole spleen APCs plus IL-2 was initially experimented by several groups, with the goal to increase the frequency of alloantigen-specific CD4⁺CD25⁺ T_{reg} cells from a polyclonal pool[104, 109-111]. Here, the initial frequency of alloreactive T cells is high in contrast to autoreactive T cells, presumably because of cross-reactivities between numerous allo-MHC peptide complexes and self-MHC molecules. These initial studies utilized skin graft transplantation or graft versus host disease (GVHD) models and demonstrate *in vivo* suppressive activity of the expanded T_{reg} cells. However, large numbers (10^6 to 10^7) of expanded T_{reg} cells were typically necessary to achieve alloantigen-specific suppression *in vivo*[104, 109, 110]. It was recently demonstrated that allogeneic mature DCs are much more efficient than whole splenic APCs at expanding alloantigen-specific CD4⁺CD25⁺ T_{reg} cells, with a three to five-fold expansion in cell numbers in 7-day mixed leukocyte reactions[112]. In addition, allogeneic DC expanded T_{reg} cells maintain higher levels of Foxp3 expression compared to whole spleen APCs, and can do so even in the absence of IL-2. The expanded T_{reg} cells show specific suppression of GVHD *in vivo*, whereas third party or syngeneic DC-expanded T_{reg} cells exhibit weaker suppression, indicating that an alloantigen-specific component of T_{reg} function has been induced following expansion with allogeneic DCs.

An alternative approach for expansion of the T_{reg} population is *de novo* induction CD4⁺CD25⁺Foxp3⁺ T cells from the non-regulatory naïve CD4⁺CD25⁻Foxp3⁻ T cells. This has been shown to be possible in the presence of nanomolar concentrations of TGF-β1[33]. Initial studies of *de novo* generation of CD4⁺CD25⁺Foxp3⁺ T cells again utilized non-specific stimulation with mitogenic antibodies or bulk splenic APCs. We have recently shown that in contrast to expanding existing CD4⁺CD25⁺ T_{reg} cells, mature DCs are much less efficient in converting naïve CD4⁺CD25⁻Foxp3⁻ T cells to CD4⁺CD25⁺Foxp3⁺ T cells in the presence of TGF-β1 (X Luo and KV Tarbell, unpublished). Rather, freshly isolated splenic CD11c⁺ DCs are able to induce Foxp3 expression in the presence of TGF-β1 in >90% of the resulting T cells that are initially Foxp3⁻. Functionally, these *in vitro* DC-generated CD4⁺CD25⁺Foxp3⁺

T cells show antigen-specific suppression *in vitro* and suppress autoimmune diabetes in NOD mice.

The Role of DCs in In Vivo Expansion of CD4$^+$CD25$^+$ T$_{reg}$ Cells

In vivo, several transplant tolerance protocols have been shown to generate alloantigen-specific T$_{reg}$ cells which might involve presentation of allogantigens by either donor or recipient DCs (reviewed in [96]). By using antigen conjugated to antibodies directed at the endocytic receptor DEC-205, which is expressed at high levels on DCs, Enk *et al* have shown that the targeted DCs were able to preferentially expand the number of CD4$^+$CD25$^+$ T$_{reg}$ cells in intact lymphoid tissue[113]. Furthermore, von Boehmer *et al* showed that DCs delivered with low dose antigen by DEC-205 targeting were able to differentiate non-regulatory CD4$^-$CD25$^+$ T cells into CD4$^+$CD25$^+$ Foxp3$^+$ T cells[114]. These observations suggest that *in vivo* renewal of CD4$^+$CD25$^+$ T$_{reg}$ cells can occur in response to antigens presented by steady state DCs.

Part III. Transplant Tolerance: From Mouse to Human

Human DC Subsets

Human DCs are all bone marrow-derived leukocytes and are comprised of at least four different sub-types. Human peripheral blood displays two subsets of DC precursors: monocytes, which differentiate into immature myeloid DC (mDC) upon exposure to GM-CSF and to IL-4; and plasmacytoid cells (pDC), which display features of the lymphoid lineage and require IL-3 for their development into plasmacytoid DC (pDC)[115, 116]. These two cell types are present also in lymphoid and non-lymphoid tissues. In addition, there are the dermal/interstitial DCs (DDC-IDCs) and the Langerhans cells (LCs)[117], which will not be discussed in this current review.

The most accessible human DC precursor is the CD14$^+$ monocytes from peripheral blood. These cells can be differentiated into mDC that are CD14$^-$, CD11c$^+$, CD83^{++}, HLA-DR^{++} following incubation with GM-CSF and IL-4. mDC maturation can be achieved by the addition of a variety of stimuli to the culture (e.g., TNF-α, LPS) and is usually measured functionally by the production of IL-12[118].

Human pDC can also be generated from peripheral blood by exposing lineage negative, HLA-DR^{++}, BDCA-2$^+$, BDCA-4$^+$ and CD123^{++} cells following FMS-like tyrosine kinase 3 ligand (Flt3-L) treatment[55, 119, 120]. Maturation of pDC is achieved by adding IL-3 in combination with CD154 (CD40L)[121]. Human pDC lack the mDC markers CD11c and CD33. For clinical vaccine trails the maturation cocktail usually contains a combination of IL-1, TNF-α, IL-6, and PGE$_2$[122]. pDC, upon exposure to viruses, produce very high levels of type I IFN, and are therefore considered the main link between the innate and adaptive immune systems[8]. Human mDC and pDC have been termed DC1 and DC2, respectively, due to their propensity to stimulate Th1 versus Th2 type responses. Current knowledge indicates that this is an oversimplification of the system, thus these terms will not be used in this review.

Effects of Pharmacological Agents on Human DCs

Many pharmacologic agents with known immunoregulatory effects, and specifically conventional immunosuppressant, have been investigated for their impact on human DC generation, maturation, and function. Immunosuppressive drugs can either indirectly target DC maturation and interfere with endocytosis developmentally or directly influence endocytosis irrespective of DC maturation.

Corticosteroids

Corticosteroids were shown to block *in vitro* differentiation of human monocytes into mDC[123]. *In vivo*, corticosteroids reduced the number and function of circulating human pDC as well as their numbers in tissues such as nasal and bronchial mucosae of atopic patients. Rozkova *et al*.[124] demonstrated that glucocorticoids dramatically impaired human monocyte differentiation, skewing the culture towards macrophage-like cells. The typical DC morphology was maintained, however, such that high levels of CD14 molecules were still present on the cell surface and costimulatory molecules were only mildly expressed. Glucocorticoid treated cells produced very low amounts of TNF and p70 IL-12 while producing higher amounts of IL-10 and retaining high endocytic activity. Interestingly, despite the fact that glucocorticoids increased the expression of Toll-like receptors TLR2, 3 and 4 on human DC, their stimulation with TLR-derived signals did not induce maturation[125, 126]. Hackstein *et al*.[127] studied the effect of immunosuppression, and in particular corticosteroid dosages, on DC precursor frequencies in peripheral blood of transplant recipients. Multivariate analysis revealed a significant negative impact that was dose dependent, mainly on the pDC sub-population. Functional studies performed by this group indicated a significant deficiency in IFN-α production after TLR7 and TLR9 stimulation, confirming the scarcity of pDCs in the circulation of these patients (Although TLR7 and TLR9 are expressed on cell types other than pDC, it is only the pDC that can secret IFN-α in response to their stimulation).

Calcineurin Inhibitors

FK506 (tacrolimus) inhibits the ability of human DC to allo-stimulate T-cells, but was reported to have heterogenous effects on DC maturation, depending on the stimuli used to trigger DC maturation[128]. The effects of Cyclosporine (CsA) however are rather controversial ranging from showing no effect on maturation or allostimulatory capacity of human mDC, to having a rather significant effect on DC maturation and function. Tajima *et al*.[129] presented data to support CsA inhibition on up-regulation of costimulatory molecules on both CD11c$^+$ mDC and CD11c$^-$ pDC subsets, with or without microbial stimuli and CD40L. They farther demonstrated that CsA negatively regulated the endocytic activity of mDCs during the immature state; and inhibited IL-12 production from mature mDC. CsA also reduced the IFN-α production from the pDCs. Schlichting *et al.*[130] investigated the impact of calcineurin inhibitors on DC binding and transmigration to allogeneic human microvascular endothelial cells (ECs) *in vitro*. Co-culture of DCs with ECs preincubated with CsA showed significant increased binding, whereas ECs preincubated with tacrolimus had minimal effect on DC binding. CsA effect was reversed using blocking antibodies to adhesion molecules such as VCAM-1. DC transmigration was also analyzed in this system demonstrating accelerated migration in the presence of CsA, as well as in the presence of high dose of tacrolimus. DC migration was significantly reduced in the tacrolimus treated group when PECAM-1 blocking antibodies were used. These data suggest different mechanisms associated with CsA and tacrolimus effects on DC binding and transmigration to allogeneic endothelial cells. This is in contrast to data from Szabo *et al.*[131] who showed that tacrolimus and CsA inhibit the allostimulatory capacity of *in vitro*-generated mDCs without significant effects on DC phenotypic maturation.

Sirolimus

Sirolimus (rapamycin; inhibits downstream signaling from the mammalian targets of rapamycin, mTOR) suppresses the generation of granulocyte–macrophage colony stimulating factor (GM-CSF) thus quantitatively reduces growth-factor-induced expansion of DC populations. Monti *et al.*[132] demonstrated that human DC in the presence of rapamycin express higher levels of CD1a, CD1b, and CD1c, and decreased levels of HLA class I, class II, CD40, CD80 and CD86. Consequently, CD40-ligand induced production of both IL-12 and IL-10 were reduced in rapamycin-treated DCs. Antigen uptake receptor expression (mannose receptor, CD32, CD46, CD91) was also reduced leading to impaired receptor-mediated and fluid phase endocytosis. Woltman *et al.*[133] have also shown that rapamycin induces apoptosis in monocyte-derived DCs while monocytes and macrophages are spared.

Aspirin

Hackstein *et al.*[134] reported that Aspirin, given in physiologic concentrations (1-3mM), was able to suppress the maturation and T cell-stimulatory function of human mDCs. It was speculated that the underlying molecular mechanism involves inhibitory effects on DCs maturation by inhibition of the p50 subunit of NF-κB. This pathway results in the inhibition of co-stimulatory molecules expression; e.g., CD40, CD80, CD83 and the MHC-II-complex [135]. Aspirin treated DCs retain their immature phenotype (round nucleus, prominent endocytic compartment compared) even if maturation is induced by lipopolysaccharide (LPS) stimulation; and exhibited decreased IL-12(p40) and IL10 secretion. In contrast TNF-α production was enhanced [136].

Vitamin D Receptor Analogues

DCs express the Vitamin D Receptor (VRD) on their cell surface, thereby becoming a key target to vitamin D and other VDR agonist [137]. The active metabolite of vitamin D, $1,25(OH)_2D3$, and its analogs have been found to inhibit the differentiation of human CD1a+ monocyte-derived DCs, leading to reduced expression of costimulatory molecules and alloreactive capacity [138, 139]. Adorini, and colleagues [140] reported that incubation with $1,25(OH)_2D3$ leads to a selective upregulation of ILT3 on immature as well as during maturation of DCs. pDCs, that express a priori high level of ILT3 obviously seems to be less affected than mDCs – which increase ILT3 expression considerably. Interestingly, ILT3 is selectively reduced by CD40 ligation on mDCs but not on pDCs. This selective responsiveness of ILT3 on the two DC cell populations suggests a novel mechanism for the immunomodulatory properties of this hormone that could play a role in the control of T-cell responses [141, 142].

Human Regulatory T Cells

During the last few years, researchers began to recognize the tolerizing function of the mDC and the pDC, as well as DCs in both immature and mature states. It has also become apparent that the tolerizing properties of DCs are likely linked to effects on regulatory T cells; and that the unique ability of DCs to capture and cross-present antigens can be used to induce donor-specific tolerance under noninflammatory conditions. Importantly, a dialogue between regulatory T cells and tolerogenic DCs is crucial for the regulation of alloimmune responses. Several subsets of regulatory T cells have been described in human.

CD4$^+$CD25^{bright} T$_{reg}$ Cells

Center stage in immunological research of regulatory T cells is currently focused on CD4$^+$CD25^{bright} T cells. Indeed, CD25 can be expressed also on recently activated non-regulatory T cells. Yet, such T cells usually express lower levels of CD25 on their cell surface compare with T$_{reg}$ cells. The simultaneous presence of dim and bright CD25 molecules on the cell surface complicate the identification of truly regulatory T cells in human studies. Naturally occurring CD4$^+$CD25^{bright} T$_{reg}$ cells were first described as actively engaged in maintaining immunological self-tolerance. Deficiency in these cells in human leads to the X-linked immunodeficiency syndrome IPEX (immune dysregulation, polyendocrinopathy, enteropathy, X-linked syndrome) that is associated with an autoimmune disease syndrome that involves multiple endocrine organs, severe allergy, inflammatory bowel disease and fatal infection [143]. The natural occurring T$_{reg}$ cells constitutively express GITR and CTLA-4 [144-147]. While they also express CD45RO, CD27, CD62L and CD122, these markers are also up-regulated upon T cell activation and therefore can not serve as specific markers to characterize T$_{reg}$ cells. FOXP3, which is considered a more specific marker for T$_{reg}$ cells in mouse, is also expressed by human T$_{reg}$ cells, although it is not exclusive to this population as is reported for mice. It is accepted to refer to the human molecule in capital letters (FOXP3) to distinguish it from the rodent counterpart – Foxp3. Similar to mouse T$_{reg}$ cells, human regulatory T cells do not proliferate when stimulated with anti-CD3 unless supplemented with high doses of IL-2 and are TLR ligation on DCs [148].

Costimulation of human naïve CD4$^+$ T cells with TGF-β induces the differentiation of CD4$^+$CD25$^+$ T$_{reg}$ cells that exhibit contact-dependent and antigen-nonspecific suppressive activity [149]. Importantly, the suppressor function of human CD4$^+$CD25$^+$ T$_{reg}$ cells is activation-dependent, requires protein synthesis; and can be inhibited by the presence of cycloheximide or monensin [150]. Furthermore, human CD25$^+$ T$_{reg}$ cells down-regulate the proliferation of conventional CD25$^-$ T cells while inducing suppressive activity in tolerized

CD4$^+$ T cells simultaneously - a phenomenon that has been termed infectious tolerance and is TGF-β dependent [150]. These studies have led to the speculation that the suppression of human CD25$^+$ T$_{reg}$ cells is "spread" into conventional CD4$^+$ T cells and that this might be the mechanism by which induction and maintenance of peripheral tolerance is achieved.

In addition to targeting effector T cells directly; T$_{reg}$ cells may also exert their suppressive activity by directly targeting DCs. For example, DCs may be rendered inefficient APCs following a cell-to-cell contact dependent interaction with CD4$^+$CD25$^+$ T$_{reg}$ cells, despite pre-stimulation with CD40L[151, 152]. DCs co-cultured with CD4$^+$CD25$^+$ T$_{reg}$ cells may also down-regulate the expression of costimulatory molecules, release high quantities of IL-10 and become unable to trigger T-cell activation properly [153, 154]. Houot and colleagues [155] studied the maturation of human mDC and pDC activated with TLR ligands in the presence of pre-activated T$_{reg}$ cells *in vitro*. They showed that CD4$^+$CD25$^+$ T$_{reg}$ cells modulate the expression of CCR7 and costimulatory molecules induced by TLR on mDC, but not on pDC. It was also the TLR-activated mDC, but not the pDC, that were inhibited from secretion of proinflammatory cytokines following incubation with activated T$_{reg}$ cells.

Another modulator of T$_{reg}$ cells is IL-7. In a study reported by Rosenberg and colleagues [156], IL-7 was administrated to patients with lymphopenia due to HIV infection or cancer-related chemotherapy treatment. These patients showed selective increase in CD4$^+$ and CD8$^+$ non-regulatory T cells. Interestingly, using microarray analysis, Liu *et al.* [157] demonstrated that the majority of T cells that down-regulated CD127 (IL-7 receptor) following activation - express FOXP3. FOXP3 expression, on the other hand, had no correlation to the level of CD25 expression on these cells membranes. More over, these CD4$^+$CD127$^{low/-}$ cells were anergic and were as suppressive as the "classical" CD4$^+$CD25^{bright} cells. In fact, the authors proposed the use of CD127 as a biomarker to selectively enrich human T$_{reg}$ cells. Seddiki and group [158] from Sydney, Australia corroborated this observation.

Human CD4$^+$CD25$^+$ T$_{reg}$ cells display a polyclonal TCR-Vβ repertoire, suggesting potential recognition of a broad variety of antigens. However, while most CD4$^+$CD25$^+$ T$_{reg}$ cells related publications discuss a suppressive effect of these cells in a non-antigen-specific manner, Levings and colleagues [159] showed that human non-proliferating CD4$^+$CD25$^+$ T$_{reg}$ cells that up-regulate CLTA-4 expression and secrete IL-10 upon stimulation, decrease the proliferative responses of CD4$^+$ T cell to specific alloantigens *in vitro*. Jiang and coworkers were also able to identify allopeptide-specific human CD4$^+$CD25$^+$ T$_{reg}$ cells [160, 161].

CD8$^+$CD28$^-$ Suppressor T Cells (Ts Cells)

A uniquely different family of human regulatory / suppressor T cells (Ts) was elegantly demonstrated by Suciu-Foca's group [162]. These cells express the CD3$^+$CD8$^+$CD28$^-$ FOXP3$^+$ phenotype, both *in vitro* and *in vivo*. In culture, Ts cells can be generated by multiple priming of responding T cells with irradiated APCs from an allogeneic donor during a 2 week time period [163]. Once these cells are incubated with endothelial cells (sharing at least one HLA class I antigen with the priming APCs), they cause inhibition of co-stimulation by down regulating CD40 and CD58 and induce the up-regulation of the inhibitory receptors ILT3 and ILT4 [164]. More importantly, down regulation of activation markers (CD40, CD54, CD62L, CD83, CD106, HLA-DR) and up-regulation of the inhibitory markers were observed even if endothelial cells were previously treated with IFN-γ or TNF-α. The specificity of the suppressive reaction was demonstrated when responses were tested using endothelial cells that share no HLA antigens with the priming APCs [165]. Similar effects were demonstrated when Ts were incubated with DCs. Thus, the Ts effect is HLA class I allo-restricted. It was further shown that the suppressive effect requires a direct interaction between CD8$^+$CD28$^-$ Ts cells and the APCs for priming. This contact leads to inhibition of the CD40-mediated up-regulation of costimulatory molecules such as CD80 and CD86 on the APC; and eventually translates into inhibitory signals transmitted by means of the inhibitory immunoglobulin-like transcript ILT3 and ILT4 up-regulation to the CD4$^+$ Th cells that bind the same APC [166]. The unresponsiveness induced by CD8$^+$CD28$^-$ Ts cells treated APCs on the CD4$^+$ Th cells is characteristic of T cell anergy, since the lost of CD4$^+$ cell proliferation capacity is reversed by the addition of exogenous IL-2.

ILT3 and ILT4 are novel cell surface molecules of the immunoglobulin superfamily, which are selectively expressed by monocytes, macrophages, mDC and endothelial cells. ILT4 is expressed predominantly on mDC and binds HLA-A, HLA-B, HLA-C and HLA-G molecules. The ligand for ILT3 is still unknown, however, it is mainly expressed on pDCs. Functional studies showed that ILT3 is efficiently internalized upon cross-linking, and delivers its ligand to an intracellular compartment. The ligand is then processed and presented to specific T cells. Thus, ILT3 is involved in antigen capture and presentation. The expression of ILT on DCs is tightly controlled by inflammatory stimuli, cytokines, and growth factors, and is down-regulated following DC activation.

Up-regulation of ILT3 and ILT4 has also been shown to render monocytes and DCs tolerogenic in vivo. CD8+CD28- Ts cells obtained from stable heart transplant recipients were able to induce the up-regulation of ILT3 or ILT4 and inhibit CD40-signaling by donor APCs, thus suggesting the presence of allospecific Ts cells that may inhibit the direct recognition pathway involved in allograft rejection [167]. Up-regulation of ILT3 and ILT4 molecules on the surface of human mDC can also be induced by treatment of the cells with IL-10, as reported by Manavalan et al.[168]. Importantly, IL-10 treated DC induced T cell anergy is blocked by antibodies specific for ILT3 and ILT4. Interestingly, LPS stimulation of DCs can elicit the production of soluble, rather than membrane-bound, ILT4 molecules. Soluble ILT4 may competitively block T lymphocyte binding to the DC-membrane-bound ILT4, thereby favoring a stimulatory DC phenotype. If LPS stimulation is applied to IL-10 treated DCs, soluble ILT4 is not expressed and the tolerogenic capacity of the IL-10 treated DCs is thus promoted.

Other Types of Regulator T Cells

Apart from the naturally occurring T$_{reg}$ cells and Ts cells, other distinct populations of regulatory T cells exist and are defined by their cytokine signature, such as secretion of high levels of IL-10 (Tr1) or TGF-β (Th3), depending on the route in which they encounter the antigen. For example, repeat stimulation of naïve T cells in vitro with immature DCs induced the generation of IL-10 producing Tr1 [169]. T-cell proliferation is not restored by the addition of IL-2. Tr1 cells inhibit the proliferation of Th$_1$ cells in a contact-dependent but antigen-nonspecific manner. In vivo, when human volunteers were immunized with a single subcutaneous injection of influenza peptide-pulsed immature DCs, as described by Dhodapkar et al.[170], a reduction of antigen-specific IFN-γ producing CD8$^+$ T cells was observed with a concomitant increase in IL-10 producing T cells. Th3 cells are inducible upon activation with an appropriate antigen or antibodies to CD3. These cells produce high levels of TGF-β and variable amounts of IL-4 and IL-10. Importantly, the loss of T-cell killing activity could not be attributed to deletion of effector cells but rather to modulation of the immune response.

A recent analysis revealed significant differences between the naturally occurring $CD4^+CD25^{bright}$ T_{reg} cells and IL-10-producing Tr1 cells. Specifically, suppressive $CD4^+CD25^{bright}$ T cell clones were shown to release TGF-β in the absence of IL-10 [171]. They inhibit the proliferation of bystander T cells irrespective of the presence of APCs, suggesting direct effects on effector T cells [172]. At variance with Tr1 cells, which expand in response to IL-2 and IL-15, $CD4^+CD25^{bright}$ T_{reg} cells failed to proliferate to these cytokines, either in combination or used alone. The observation that IL-15 can maintain Tr1 cell clones in culture for more than 30 days in the absence of TCR triggering suggests that IL-15, which is produced by several cell types during immune responses, might be involved in the long-term survival of Tr1 cells *in vivo* [173].

Effects of Pharmacological Agents on T_{reg} Cells

Valmori et al.[174] studied the effects of rapamycin in vitro on human circulating $CD4^+$ T cells, reporting that stimulation of these cells results in an increased suppressor activity in the cultures. Rapamycin delayed the differentiation of stimulated $CD4^+$ T cells, promoted an increase of $CD4^+CD25^{bright}$ T cells, and inhibited proliferation in cultures where suppressor cells were mixed with otherwise competent responder T cells. Interestingly, no increase in $FOXP3^+$ population correlated with rapamycin treatment in this study.

Over the last few years, the effect of immunosuppressive agents on the generation of Treg cells in vivo is extensively studied. San Segundo et al. [175] compared the effects of calcineurin inhibitors to those of rapamycin on T_{reg} cells in stable renal allograft recipients. T cells with the regulatory phenotype, $CD4^+CD25^{Bright}$, were decreased in stable renal transplant patients receiving calcineurin inhibitor immunosuppression compared with those receiving rapamycin therapy. Such differences were not observed with regard to $CD8^+CD28^-$ suppressor T cells. In this study only a modest association was observed between the presence of T_{reg} cells and renal function as measured by the delta serum creatinine.

A major concern was the potential effects of induction therapy with anti-CD25 (IL-2 receptor) monoclonal antibodies. Salama et al. [176] studied a cohort of 23 stable renal recipients and found a higher incidence of T_{reg} cells in patients with no history of acute rejection episodes compare to the group with history of rejection episodes. $CD4^+CD25^+$ regulatory cells were present in this study as early as 3 months post transplant, and the group concluded that induction treatment with anti-IL2R mAb did not prevent the development of T_{reg} cells. Game and colleagues [177] studied the effects of the rapamycin in combination with anti-CD25 monoclonal antibody basiliximab on the regulatory capacity of human $CD4^+CD25^+$ cells in vitro. They also concluded that $CD4^+CD25^+$ cells may still exert their effects in transplant recipients taking immunosuppression that interferes with IL-2 signaling.

Franske et al. [178], working with bone marrow transplant patients, have shown that G-CSF inhibit T-cell proliferative responses by eliciting the release of immunoregulatory soluble factors. Rutella and colleagues demonstrated that freshly isolated CD4$^+$ T cells, collected after clinical provision of G-CSF and challenged in vitro with alloantigens in the presence of autologous serum, were hyporesponsive in terms of proliferation and were polarized to a Tr1-like functional profile [179]. These cells acquired peculiar phenotypic features exhibiting reduced expression of CD62L and CD28, associated with high expression of the β chain (CD122) and γ chain (CD132) of the IL-2/IL-15 receptor complex, and were capable of suppressing bystander T cells through a mechanism that was largely cell contact-independent [179].

Ex-Vivo Expansion of Human T$_{reg}$ Cells

Naturally occurring CD4$^+$CD25$^+$ T$_{reg}$ cells are instrumental for immunoregulation. Their roles in numerous fields including transplant rejection, cancer, vaccine, allergy, and autoimmune diseases, are well recognized. However, harnessing these cells for large cohort clinical applications in human have been hampered by the paucity of CD4$^+$CD25$^+$ T$_{reg}$ cells in peripheral blood and the lack of appropriate ex-vivo expansion protocols. Only 1-2% or human peripheral blood lymphocytes are CD4$^+$CD25$^+$, translated to 3-5% of all CD4$^+$ T cells. Additionally, human CD25$^+$ cells are composed of two overlapping populations of CD25, one dimmer than the other, but an exact distinction between the two populations is difficult to assign. It is only the brighter population that matches the characteristics of regulatory cells.

As previously discussed, regulatory T cells do not proliferate in response to any of the normal physiologic stimuli ex vivo. The cells show a G1/G0 cell cycle arrest and no production of IL-2, IL-4, or IFN-γ at either protein or mRNA levels. The anergic state of CD4$^+$CD25$^+$ T cells is not reversible by the addition of anti-CD3, anti-CD28, anti–CTLA-4, anti–transforming growth factor ß, or anti–IL-10 antibody. Jonuleit et al. [150] demonstrated that the refractory state of CD4$^+$CD25$^+$ freshly isolated human T cells was partially reversible by the addition of IL-2 or IL-4. However, it could not be reversed by the addition of anti-CD3 or anti-CD28. Dieckmann and colleagues [180], using CD4$^+$CD25$^+$CD45RO$^+$ cells from healthy adult volunteers, presented data to support a synergistic effect between IL-2 and IL-15 for reversing the anergic state of the T$_{reg}$ cells, in the presence of an allogeneic stimulus, or a combination of immobilized anti-CD3 and anti-CD28. Following this protocol, Karakhanova and colleagues [181] used sorted CD4+CD25+ cells for further expansion. Activation was achieved by using paramagnetic beads coupled with anti-CD3 and anti-CD28. IL-2 and IL-15 were also added to the culture to farther augment the proliferation response to about 1000-fold after 2 cycles of re-stimulation.

Godfrey et al. [182] developed a method to propagate CD4$^+$CD25$^+$ T$_{reg}$ cells in culture up to 100-fold expansion over the initial culture. To this aim they used cleavable microbeads coated with low levels of anti-CD25 – thus allowing for better purification of CD25+ cells. Ligation of CD3 and addition of IL-2 resulted in only 5-10 fold expansion, prompting the researchers to look for additional co-stimulation – provided by the use of cell-sized Dynabeads with anti-CD3 and anti-CD28 mAbs covalently attached. Lastly, to provide the proper cytokine milieu, irradiated $CD4^+CD25^-$ feeder cells were added at the initiation of T_{reg} cultures (1:1 ratio) culminating in a 100-fold ex-vivo expansion of the original culture. Importantly, the cultured T_{reg} cells were shown to maintain the suppressive capabilities when co-cultured with either activated or matured dendritic cell-driven.

While ex-vivo expansion of T_{reg} cells facilitates more in-depth studies of the intracellular signaling and mechanisms associated with their unique function, a much larger ex-vivo expansion is required to accelerate clinical applications. Hoffmann et al. [183] achieved a significant milestone shortly thereafter. As in the previous protocol, the anergic state of pure $CD4^+CD25^{high}$ T cells was abrogated after simultaneous stimulation via TCRs and CD28 in the presence of IL-2. Unique to the Hoffman's protocol is the addition of $Fc\gamma RII$ (CD32)– bearing L cells in combination with stimulation via CD3 and CD28. Under these conditions T_{reg} cells expanded dramatically with an average 13 000-fold increase in cell numbers within 3 to 4 weeks. Using parallel cultures for several months, an ex-vivo expansion of up to 39,000 fold was established. Despite the long incubation, the expanded T_{reg} cells maintained high expression levels of both CD52L and CCR7, as well as their polycloncal repertoire of TCR $V\beta$.

The above-described methods for in vitro T_{reg} cell expansion have overcome the relative anergy of these cells. However, the expanded cells are polyclonal and antigen specificity has not been addressed. Evidence suggests that the in vivo efficacy of T_{reg}-based immuno-therapy is critically dependent on the specificity of the T_{reg} cells. Therefore the ability to expand T_{reg} cell populations with particular antigen specificities will allow using a lower number of cells to achieve the expected efficacy. By labeling freshly isolated $CD4^+CD25^+$ T_{reg} cells with CFSE and stimulating them with HLA mismatched gamma-irradiated alloantigen along with IL-2 plus IL-15, Koenen and colleagues [184] were able to focus on the alloantigen-reactive dividing T_{reg} cells in a short term culture – choosing cells characterized by diluted CFSE. Cells were also selected based on their CD27 expression, indicating a memory T_{reg} cell population. This robust ex-vivo technique allowed purification of highly potent human monoclonal alloantigen-specific T_{reg} cells. The authors went on to demonstrate that these cells have a high-effector-suppressor potential – 500:1 for the $CD27^+$ T_{reg} cells. The use of Antigen-specific T_{reg} cells, as opposed to polyclonal expanded regulatory cells, has the potential of increased efficacy required of a T_{reg} cell-based immunotherapy. However, much has still to be learned about additional qualities of these $CD27^+$ T_{reg} cells, for example their in vivo trafficking patterns, their interactions with B cells, etc.

HLA-G as Natural Inducer of Immuno-Tolerance

HLA-G expression was demonstrated in vivo on epithelial cells of an "accepted" allograft tissue as well as on infiltrating mononuclear cells [185]. In fact, HLA-G expression was documented on tumor cells that escaped immune surveillance [186]. HLA-G is a non-classical HLA class I antigen that has restricted expression in extravillous cytotrohpoblasts, thymic epithelium and cornea under non-pathologic conditions. Its expression was reported to be crucial for protection of fetal cytotrophoblast from destruction by the maternal immune system, and is probably associated with the "privileged" status of the eye. During inflammation or other pathologic conditions, however, HLA-G can be expressed by infiltrating mononuclear cells and can inhibit NK cell and cytotoxic T cell function; as well as CD4$^+$ T cell allo-proliferation. HLA-G can be expressed as one of multiple isoforms generated by alternative splicing of a single message, and give rise to four membrane-bound isoforms (HLA-G1 through -4) and three soluble isoforms (HLA-G5, -G6, and -G7). HLA-G appears to be recognized mainly by immunoglobulin-like transcript (ILT) receptors, which are expressed by T and B lymphocytes, as well as by NK cells, macrophages and DCs [187]. Convincing evidence for an ability of HLA-G to influence T cells was first presented by Sanders et al. who showed that HLA-G-expressing cells bind to CD8α-expressing cells [188]. HLA-G was also shown to modulate cytokine release from human allogeneic peripheral blood mononuclear cells in vitro [189] and to have a concentration-dependent effect on generation of an allogeneic CTL response [190]. As mentioned previously, an immune suppressive effect of HLA-G on APCs was documented by the finding that high levels of HLA-G proteins in the sera of heart transplant recipients with prolonged graft survival [191]. It has also been shown that HLA-G can be expressed by APCs themselves as a response inflammatory conditions during cytomegalovirus and other infections [192]. Since HLA-G exerts its effects via its interaction with the ILT-4 molecule on APCs [193, 194], it seems like HLA-G functions as a regulatory feed-back mechanism to control reactivity against noxious stimuli.

Concluding Remarks

A major goal in organ transplantation is to be able to harness tolerance processes so as to minimize the need for immunosuppressive drugs. Chronic immunosuppression is associated with increased risk of infection, malignancy, and aggregate impact of drug-specific toxicities. With respect to renal transplantation, the drugs cyclosporine and tacrolimus – current mainstays of most maintenance immunosuppressive protocols—are toxic to both native and transplanted kidneys. In addition, allografts are still at risk for development of chronic rejection, a process that currently limits the long-term survival of transplanted kidneys in many recipients. Transplantation tolerance is not only able to prevent acute or chronic rejection but also to avoid chronic immunosuppression and its associated complications. The clinical use of ex vivo expanded regulatory T cells to control GvHD and organ transplant rejection is a promising approach to modulate effector T cells, while preserving the beneficial effect mediated by other T cells. Results in preclinical models are promising, although efforts are required to optimize this procedure for clinical application regarding the number of T$_{reg}$ cells to be used to obtain long-lasting beneficial effect. Moreover, the impact of T$_{reg}$ cells on the reconstitution of the immune system still has to be completely unraveled. It still remains an open question, which is the most appropriate regulatory T-cell subset to be used. Although polyclonal CD4$^+$CD25$^+$ T$_{reg}$ cells can be easily isolated and their ex vivo expansion is feasible, their undefined antigen specificity and the possible contamination with non-suppressor cells in the ex vivo expanded population might represent limiting factors to the use of these subset of regulatory T cells. Conversely, ex vivo induced antigen specific cells ensure the antigen specificity, but their low frequency obtained by short-term manipulation could limit their in vivo efficacy. Advances in understanding the molecular basis for the activation and expansion of T$_{reg}$ cells together with the ongoing clinical trials will be crucial to dissect these issues and to unravel the therapeutic potential of regulatory T cells.

References

[1] Manz MG, Traver D, Miyamoto T, Weissman IL, Akashi K. 2001. Dendritic cell potentials of early lymphoid and myeloid progenitors. *Blood.* 97: 3333-41

[2] Guermonprez P, Valladeau J, Zitvogel L, Thery C, Amigorena S. 2002. Antigen presentation and T cell stimulation by dendritic cells. *Annu. Rev. Immunol.* 20: 621-67

[3] Pulendran B, Palucka K, Banchereau J. 2001. Sensing pathogens and tuning immune responses. *Science.* 293: 253-6

[4] Liu YJ. 2001. Dendritic cell subsets and lineages, and their functions in innate and adaptive immunity. *Cell.* 106: 259-62

[5] Rescigno M, Borrow P. 2001. The host-pathogen interaction: new themes from dendritic cell biology. *Cell.* 106: 267-70

[6] Steinman RM, Hawiger D, Nussenzweig MC. 2003. Tolerogenic dendritic cells. *Annu. Rev. Immunol.* 21: 685-711

[7] Barratt-Boyes B. 2003. The early history of cardiac surgery in New Zealand. *Heart Lung Circ.* 12 Suppl 1: S21-8

[8] Munz C, Steinman RM, Fujii S. 2005. Dendritic cell maturation by innate lymphocytes: coordinated stimulation of innate and adaptive immunity. *J. Exp. Med.* 202: 203-7

[9] Hemmi H, Akira S. 2005. TLR signalling and the function of dendritic cells. *Chem. Immunol. Allergy.* 86: 120-35

[10] Rescigno M, Piguet V, Valzasina B, Lens S, Zubler R, French L, Kindler V, Tschopp J, Ricciardi-Castagnoli P. 2000. Fas engagement induces the maturation of dendritic cells (DCs), the release of interleukin (IL)-1beta, and the production of interferon gamma in the absence of IL-12 during DC-T cell cognate interaction: a new role for Fas ligand in inflammatory responses. *J. Exp. Med.* 192: 1661-8

[11] Cella M, Scheidegger D, Palmer-Lehmann K, Lane P, Lanzavecchia A, Alber G. 1996. Ligation of CD40 on dendritic cells triggers production of high levels of interleukin-12 and enhances T cell stimulatory capacity: T-T help via APC activation. *J. Exp. Med.* 184: 747-52

[12] Luft T, Pang KC, Thomas E, Hertzog P, Hart DN, Trapani J, Cebon J. 1998. Type I IFNs enhance the terminal differentiation of dendritic cells. *J. Immunol.* 161: 1947-53

[13] Granucci F, Vizzardelli C, Virzi E, Rescigno M, Ricciardi-Castagnoli P. 2001. Transcriptional reprogramming of dendritic cells by differentiation stimuli. *Eur. J. Immunol.* 31: 2539-46

[14] Garrett WS, Chen LM, Kroschewski R, Ebersold M, Turley S, Trombetta S, Galan JE, Mellman I. 2000. Developmental control of endocytosis in dendritic cells by Cdc42. *Cell.* 102: 325-34

[15] Rescigno M, Martino M, Sutherland CL, Gold MR, Ricciardi-Castagnoli P. 1998. Dendritic cell survival and maturation are regulated by different signaling pathways. *J. Exp. Med.* 188: 2175-80

[16] Giannoukakis N, Bonham CA, Qian S, Chen Z, Peng L, Harnaha J, Li W, Thomson AW, Fung JJ, Robbins PD, Lu L. 2000. Prolongation of cardiac allograft survival using dendritic cells treated with NF-kB decoy oligodeoxyribonucleotides. *Mol. Ther.* 1: 430-7

[17] Chen Z, Lu L, Zhang H, Dean NM, Fung JJ, Qian S. 2003. Administration of antisense oligodeoxyribonucleotides targeting NF-kappaB prolongs allograft survival via suppression of cytotoxicity. *Microsurgery.* 23: 494-7

[18] Tomasoni S, Aiello S, Cassis L, Noris M, Longaretti L, Cavinato RA, Azzollini N, Pezzotta A, Remuzzi G, Benigni A. 2005. Dendritic cells genetically engineered with adenoviral vector encoding dnIKK2 induce the formation of potent CD4+ T-regulatory cells. *Transplantation.* 79: 1056-61

[19] Wang Q, Liu Y, Wang J, Ding G, Zhang W, Chen G, Zhang M, Zheng S, Cao X. 2006. Induction of allospecific tolerance by immature dendritic cells genetically modified to express soluble TNF receptor. *J. Immunol.* 177: 2175-85

[20] Goldstein DR, Tesar BM, Akira S, Lakkis FG. 2003. Critical role of the Toll-like receptor signal adaptor protein MyD88 in acute allograft rejection. *J. Clin. Invest.* 111: 1571-8

[21] Thornley TB, Brehm MA, Markees TG, Shultz LD, Mordes JP, Welsh RM, Rossini AA, Greiner DL. 2006. TLR agonists abrogate costimulation blockade-induced prolongation of skin allografts. *J. Immunol.* 176: 1561-70

[22] Ducloux D, Deschamps M, Yannaraki M, Ferrand C, Bamoulid J, Saas P, Kazory A, Chalopin JM, Tiberghien P. 2005. Relevance of Toll-like receptor-4 polymorphisms in renal transplantation. *Kidney Int.* 67: 2454-61

[23] Larsen CP, Ritchie SC, Hendrix R, Linsley PS, Hathcock KS, Hodes RJ, Lowry RP, Pearson TC. 1994. Regulation of immunostimulatory function and costimulatory molecule (B7-1 and B7-2) expression on murine dendritic cells. *J. Immunol.* 152: 5208-19

[24] Takayama T, Morelli AE, Robbins PD, Tahara H, Thomson AW. 2000. Feasibility of CTLA4Ig gene delivery and expression in vivo using retrovirally transduced myeloid dendritic cells that induce alloantigen-specific T cell anergy in vitro. *Gene Ther.* 7: 1265-73

[25] Laumonier T, Potiron N, Boeffard F, Chagneau C, Brouard S, Guillot C, Soulillou JP, Anegon I, Le Mauff B. 2003. CTLA4Ig adenoviral gene transfer induces long-term islet rat allograft survival, without tolerance, after systemic but not local intragraft expression. *Hum. Gene Ther.* 14: 561-75

[26] Fallarino F, Grohmann U, Vacca C, Bianchi R, Orabona C, Spreca A, Fioretti MC, Puccetti P. 2002. T cell apoptosis by tryptophan catabolism. *Cell Death Differ.* 9: 1069-77

[27] Munn DH, Sharma MD, Mellor AL. 2004. Ligation of B7-1/B7-2 by human CD4+ T cells triggers indoleamine 2,3-dioxygenase activity in dendritic cells. *J. Immunol.* 172: 4100-10

[28] Grohmann U, Orabona C, Fallarino F, Vacca C, Calcinaro F, Falorni A, Candeloro P, Belladonna ML, Bianchi R, Fioretti MC, Puccetti P. 2002. CTLA-4-Ig regulates tryptophan catabolism in vivo. *Nat. Immunol.* 3: 1097-101

[29] Zhang M, Wang Q, Liu Y, Sun Y, Ding G, Fu Z, Min Z, Zhu Y, Cao X. 2004. Effective induction of immune tolerance by portal venous infusion with IL-10 gene-modified immature dendritic cells leading to prolongation of allograft survival. *J. Mol. Med.* 82: 240-9

[30] Gorczynski RM, Bransom J, Cattral M, Huang X, Lei J, Xiaorong L, Min WP, Wan Y, Gauldie J. 2000. Synergy in induction of increased renal allograft survival after portal vein infusion of dendritic cells transduced to express TGFbeta and IL-10, along with administration of CHO cells expressing the regulatory molecule OX-2. *Clin. Immunol.* 95: 182-9

[31] Takayama T, Morelli AE, Onai N, Hirao M, Matsushima K, Tahara H, Thomson AW. 2001. Mammalian and viral IL-10 enhance C-C chemokine receptor 5 but down-regulate C-C chemokine receptor 7 expression by myeloid dendritic cells: impact on chemotactic responses and in vivo homing ability. *J. Immunol.* 166: 7136-43

[32] Lee WC, Zhong C, Qian S, Wan Y, Gauldie J, Mi Z, Robbins PD, Thomson AW, Lu L. 1998. Phenotype, function, and in vivo migration and survival of allogeneic dendritic cell progenitors genetically engineered to express TGF-beta. *Transplantation.* 66: 1810-7

[33] Chen W, Jin W, Hardegen N, Lei KJ, Li L, Marinos N, McGrady G, Wahl SM. 2003. Conversion of peripheral CD4+CD25- naive T cells to CD4+CD25+ regulatory T cells by TGF-beta induction of transcription factor Foxp3. *J. Exp. Med.* 198: 1875-86

[34] Marie JC, Letterio JJ, Gavin M, Rudensky AY. 2005. TGF-beta1 maintains suppressor function and Foxp3 expression in CD4+CD25+ regulatory T cells. *J. Exp. Med.* 201: 1061-7

[35] Ghiringhelli F, Puig PE, Roux S, Parcellier A, Schmitt E, Solary E, Kroemer G, Martin F, Chauffert B, Zitvogel L. 2005. Tumor cells convert immature myeloid dendritic cells into TGF-{beta}-secreting cells inducing CD4+CD25+ regulatory T cell proliferation. *J. Exp. Med.* 202: 919-29

[36] Griffin MD, Lutz W, Phan VA, Bachman LA, McKean DJ, Kumar R. 2001. Dendritic cell modulation by 1alpha,25 dihydroxyvitamin D3 and its analogs: a vitamin D receptor-dependent pathway that promotes a persistent state of immaturity in vitro and in vivo. *Proc. Natl. Acad. Sci. U S A.* 98: 6800-5

[37] Griffin MD, Kumar R. 2003. Effects of 1alpha,25(OH)2D3 and its analogs on dendritic cell function. *J. Cell Biochem.* 88: 323-6

[38] Penna G, Adorini L. 2000. 1 Alpha,25-dihydroxyvitamin D3 inhibits differentiation, maturation, activation, and survival of dendritic cells leading to impaired alloreactive T cell activation. *J. Immunol.* 164: 2405-11

[39] Adorini L, Penna G, Giarratana N, Roncari A, Amuchastegui S, Daniel KC, Uskokovic M. 2004. Dendritic cells as key targets for immunomodulation by Vitamin D receptor ligands. *J. Steroid Biochem. Mol. Biol.* 89-90: 437-41

[40] Adorini L, Penna G, Giarratana N, Uskokovic M. 2003. Tolerogenic dendritic cells induced by vitamin D receptor ligands enhance regulatory T cells inhibiting allograft rejection and autoimmune diseases. *J. Cell Biochem.* 88: 227-33

[41] Gregori S, Casorati M, Amuchastegui S, Smiroldo S, Davalli AM, Adorini L. 2001. Regulatory T cells induced by 1 alpha,25-dihydroxyvitamin D3 and mycophenolate mofetil treatment mediate transplantation tolerance. *J. Immunol.* 167: 1945-53

[42] Emmer PM, van der Vlag J, Adema GJ, Hilbrands LB. 2006. Dendritic cells activated by lipopolysaccharide after dexamethasone treatment induce donor-specific allograft hyporesponsiveness. *Transplantation.* 81: 1451-9

[43] Roelen DL, Schuurhuis DH, van den Boogaardt DE, Koekkoek K, van Miert PP, van Schip JJ, Laban S, Rea D, Melief CJ, Offringa R, Ossendorp F, Claas FH. 2003. Prolongation of skin graft survival by modulation of the alloimmune response with alternatively activated dendritic cells. *Transplantation.* 76: 1608-15

[44] Beriou G, Peche H, Guillonneau C, Merieau E, Cuturi MC. 2005. Donor-specific allograft tolerance by administration of recipient-derived immature dendritic cells and suboptimal immunosuppression. *Transplantation.* 79: 969-72

[45] Min WP, Zhou D, Ichim TE, Xia X, Zhang X, Yang J, Huang X, Garcia B, Dutartre P, Jevnikar AM, Strejan GH, Zhong R. 2003. Synergistic tolerance induced by LF15-0195 and anti-CD45RB monoclonal antibody through suppressive dendritic cells. *Transplantation.* 75: 1160-5

[46] Vosters O, Neve J, De Wit D, Willems F, Goldman M, Verhasselt V. 2003. Dendritic cells exposed to nacystelyn are refractory to maturation and promote the emergence of alloreactive regulatory t cells. *Transplantation.* 75: 383-9

[47] Emmanouilidis N, Guo Z, Dong Y, Newton-West M, Adams AB, Lee ED, Wang J, Pearson TC, Larsen CP, Newell KA. 2006. Immunosuppressive and trafficking properties of donor splenic and bone marrow dendritic cells. *Transplantation.* 81: 455-62

[48] Lan YY, Wang Z, Raimondi G, Wu W, Colvin BL, de Creus A, Thomson AW. 2006. "Alternatively activated" dendritic cells preferentially secrete IL-10, expand Foxp3+CD4+ T cells, and induce long-term organ allograft survival in combination with CTLA4-Ig. *J. Immunol.* 177: 5868-77

[49] Huang FP, Platt N, Wykes M, Major JR, Powell TJ, Jenkins CD, MacPherson GG. 2000. A discrete subpopulation of dendritic cells transports apoptotic intestinal epithelial cells to T cell areas of mesenteric lymph nodes. *J. Exp. Med.* 191: 435-44

[50] Iyoda T, Shimoyama S, Liu K, Omatsu Y, Akiyama Y, Maeda Y, Takahara K, Steinman RM, Inaba K. 2002. The CD8+ dendritic cell subset selectively endocytoses dying cells in culture and in vivo. *J. Exp. Med.* 195: 1289-302

[51] Liu K, Iyoda T, Saternus M, Kimura Y, Inaba K, Steinman RM. 2002. Immune tolerance after delivery of dying cells to dendritic cells in situ. *J. Exp. Med.* 196: 1091-7

[52] Traver D, Akashi K, Manz M, Merad M, Miyamoto T, Engleman EG, Weissman IL. 2000. Development of CD8alpha-positive dendritic cells from a common myeloid progenitor. *Science.* 290: 2152-4

[53] O'Connell PJ, Li W, Wang Z, Specht SM, Logar AJ, Thomson AW. 2002. Immature and mature CD8alpha+ dendritic cells prolong the survival of vascularized heart allografts. *J. Immunol.* 168: 143-54

[54] Fisson S, Djelti F, Trenado A, Billiard F, Liblau R, Klatzmann D, Cohen JL, Salomon BL. 2006. Therapeutic potential of self-antigen-specific CD4+ CD25+ regulatory T cells selected in vitro from a polyclonal repertoire. *Eur. J. Immunol.* 36: 817-27

[55] Liu YJ. 2005. IPC: professional type 1 interferon-producing cells and plasmacytoid dendritic cell precursors. *Annu. Rev. Immunol.* 23: 275-306

[56] Brawand P, Fitzpatrick DR, Greenfield BW, Brasel K, Maliszewski CR, De Smedt T. 2002. Murine plasmacytoid pre-dendritic cells generated from Flt3 ligand-supplemented bone marrow cultures are immature APCs. *J. Immunol.* 169: 6711-9

[57] Gilliet M, Boonstra A, Paturel C, Antonenko S, Xu XL, Trinchieri G, O'Garra A, Liu YJ. 2002. The development of murine plasmacytoid dendritic cell precursors is differentially regulated by FLT3-ligand and granulocyte/macrophage colony-stimulating factor. *J. Exp. Med.* 195: 953-8

[58] Boonstra A, Asselin-Paturel C, Gilliet M, Crain C, Trinchieri G, Liu YJ, O'Garra A. 2003. Flexibility of mouse classical and plasmacytoid-derived dendritic cells in directing T helper type 1 and 2 cell development: dependency on antigen dose and differential toll-like receptor ligation. *J. Exp. Med.* 197: 101-9

[59] Fugier-Vivier IJ, Rezzoug F, Huang Y, Graul-Layman AJ, Schanie CL, Xu H, Chilton PM, Ildstad ST. 2005. Plasmacytoid precursor dendritic cells facilitate allogeneic hematopoietic stem cell engraftment. *J. Exp. Med.* 201: 373-83

[60] Huang Y, Kucia M, Rezzoug F, Ratajczak J, Tanner MK, Ratajczak MZ, Schanie CL, Xu H, Fugier-Vivier I, Ildstad ST. 2006. Flt3-ligand-mobilized peripheral blood, but not Flt3-ligand-expanded bone marrow, facilitating cells promote establishment of chimerism and tolerance. *Stem Cells.* 24: 936-48

[61] Abe M, Wang Z, de Creus A, Thomson AW. 2005. Plasmacytoid dendritic cell precursors induce allogeneic T-cell hyporesponsiveness and prolong heart graft survival. *Am. J. Transplant.* 5: 1808-19

[62] Ochando JC, Homma C, Yang Y, Hidalgo A, Garin A, Tacke F, Angeli V, Li Y, Boros P, Ding Y, Jessberger R, Trinchieri G, Lira SA, Randolph GJ, Bromberg JS. 2006. Alloantigen-presenting plasmacytoid dendritic cells mediate tolerance to vascularized grafts. *Nat. Immunol.* 7: 652-62

[63] Munn DH, Sharma MD, Baban B, Harding HP, Zhang Y, Ron D, Mellor AL. 2005. GCN2 kinase in T cells mediates proliferative arrest and anergy induction in response to indoleamine 2,3-dioxygenase. *Immunity.* 22: 633-42

[64] Gorczynski RM. 2005. CD200 and its receptors as targets for immunoregulation. *Curr. Opin. Investig. Drugs.* 6: 483-8

[65] Fallarino F, Asselin-Paturel C, Vacca C, Bianchi R, Gizzi S, Fioretti MC, Trinchieri G, Grohmann U, Puccetti P. 2004. Murine plasmacytoid dendritic cells initiate the immunosuppressive pathway of tryptophan catabolism in response to CD200 receptor engagement. *J. Immunol.* 173: 3748-54

[66] Jiang S, Herrera O, Lechler RI. 2004. New spectrum of allorecognition pathways: implications for graft rejection and transplantation tolerance. *Curr. Opin. Immunol.* 16: 550-7

[67] Lindahl KF, Wilson DB. 1977. Histocompatibility antigen-activated cytotoxic T lymphocytes. I. Estimates of the absolute frequency of killer cells generated in vitro. *J. Exp. Med.* 145: 500-7

[68] Lindahl KF, Wilson DB. 1977. Histocompatibility antigen-activated cytotoxic T lymphocytes. II. Estimates of the frequency and specificity of precursors. *J. Exp. Med.* 145: 508-22

[69] Suchin EJ, Langmuir PB, Palmer E, Sayegh MH, Wells AD, Turka LA. 2001. Quantifying the frequency of alloreactive T cells in vivo: new answers to an old question. *J. Immunol.* 166: 973-81

[70] Ochando JC, Krieger NR, Bromberg JS. 2006. Direct versus indirect allorecognition: Visualization of dendritic cell distribution and interactions during rejection and tolerization. *Am. J. Transplant.* 6: 2488-96

[71] Talmage DW, Dart G, Radovich J, Lafferty KJ. 1976. Activation of transplant immunity: effect of donor leukocytes on thyroid allograft rejection. *Science.* 191: 385-8

[72] Bowen KM, Andrus L, Lafferty KJ. 1980. Successful allotransplantation of mouse pancreatic islets to nonimmunosuppressed recipients. *Diabetes.* 29 Suppl 1: 98-104

[73] Lechler RI, Batchelor JR. 1982. Restoration of immunogenicity to passenger cell-depleted kidney allografts by the addition of donor strain dendritic cells. *J. Exp. Med.* 155: 31-41

[74] Wang L, Han R, Lee I, Hancock AS, Xiong G, Gunn MD, Hancock WW. 2005. Permanent survival of fully MHC-mismatched islet allografts by targeting a single chemokine receptor pathway. *J. Immunol.* 175: 6311-8

[75] Zhang QW, Kish DD, Fairchild RL. 2003. Absence of allograft ICAM-1 attenuates alloantigen-specific T cell priming, but not primed T cell trafficking into the graft, to mediate acute rejection. *J. Immunol.* 170: 5530-7

[76] Zhu M, Wei MF, Liu F, Shi HF, Wang G. 2003. Interleukin-10 modified dendritic cells induce allo-hyporesponsiveness and prolong small intestine allograft survival. *World J. Gastroenterol.* 9: 2509-12

[77] Takayama T, Kaneko K, Morelli AE, Li W, Tahara H, Thomson AW. 2002. Retroviral delivery of transforming growth factor-beta1 to myeloid dendritic cells: inhibition of T-cell priming ability and influence on allograft survival. *Transplantation.* 74: 112-9

[78] Lu L, Li W, Fu F, Chambers FG, Qian S, Fung JJ, Thomson AW. 1997. Blockade of the CD40-CD40 ligand pathway potentiates the capacity of donor-derived dendritic cell progenitors to induce long-term cardiac allograft survival. *Transplantation.* 64: 1808-15

[79] Xu MQ, Suo YP, Gong JP, Zhang MM, Yan LN. 2004. Augmented regeneration of partial liver allograft induced by nuclear factor-kappaB decoy oligodeoxynucleotides-modified dendritic cells. *World J. Gastroenterol.* 10: 573-8

[80] Min WP, Gorczynski R, Huang XY, Kushida M, Kim P, Obataki M, Lei J, Suri RM, Cattral MS. 2000. Dendritic cells genetically engineered to express Fas ligand induce donor-specific hyporesponsiveness and prolong allograft survival. *J. Immunol.* 164: 161-7

[81] Hornick PI, Mason PD, Baker RJ, Hernandez-Fuentes M, Frasca L, Lombardi G, Taylor K, Weng L, Rose ML, Yacoub MH, Batchelor R, Lechler RI. 2000. Significant

frequencies of T cells with indirect anti-donor specificity in heart graft recipients with chronic rejection. *Circulation.* 101: 2405-10

[82] Yamada A, Chandraker A, Laufer TM, Gerth AJ, Sayegh MH, Auchincloss H, Jr. 2001. Recipient MHC class II expression is required to achieve long-term survival of murine cardiac allografts after costimulatory blockade. *J. Immunol.* 167: 5522-6

[83] Mirenda V, Berton I, Read J, Cook T, Smith J, Dorling A, Lechler RI. 2004. Modified dendritic cells coexpressing self and allogeneic major histocompatability complex molecules: an efficient way to induce indirect pathway regulation. *J. Am. Soc. Nephrol.* 15: 987-97

[84] Miller SD, Wetzig RP, Claman HN. 1979. The induction of cell-mediated immunity and tolerance with protein antigens coupled to syngeneic lymphoid cells. *J. Exp. Med.* 149: 758-73

[85] Elliott C, Wang K, Miller S, Melvold R. 1994. Ethylcarbodiimide as an agent for induction of specific transplant tolerance. *Transplantation.* 58: 966-8

[86] Kaneko K, Morelli AE, Wang Z, Thomson AW. 2003. Alloantigen presentation by ethylcarbodiimide-treated dendritic cells induces T cell hyporesponsiveness, and prolongs organ graft survival. *Clin. Immunol.* 108: 190-8

[87] Wang Z, Larregina AT, Shufesky WJ, Perone MJ, Montecalvo A, Zahorchak AF, Thomson AW, Morelli AE. 2006. Use of the inhibitory effect of apoptotic cells on dendritic cells for graft survival via T-cell deletion and regulatory T cells. *Am. J. Transplant.* 6: 1297-311

[88] Xu DL, Liu Y, Tan JM, Li B, Zhong CP, Zhang XH, Wu CQ, Tang XD. 2004. Marked prolongation of murine cardiac allograft survival using recipient immature dendritic cells loaded with donor-derived apoptotic cells. *Scand. J. Immunol.* 59: 536-44

[89] Kleinclauss F, Perruche S, Masson E, de Carvalho Bittencourt M, Biichle S, Remy-Martin JP, Ferrand C, Martin M, Bittard H, Chalopin JM, Seilles E, Tiberghien P, Saas P. 2006. Intravenous apoptotic spleen cell infusion induces a TGF-beta-dependent regulatory T-cell expansion. *Cell Death Differ.* 13: 41-52

[90] Huang JF, Yang Y, Sepulveda H, Shi W, Hwang I, Peterson PA, Jackson MR, Sprent J, Cai Z. 1999. TCR-Mediated internalization of peptide-MHC complexes acquired by T cells. *Science.* 286: 952-4

[91] Andre F, Chaput N, Schartz NE, Flament C, Aubert N, Bernard J, Lemonnier F, Raposo G, Escudier B, Hsu DH, Tursz T, Amigorena S, Angevin E, Zitvogel L. 2004. Exosomes as potent cell-free peptide-based vaccine. I. Dendritic cell-derived exosomes transfer functional MHC class I/peptide complexes to dendritic cells. *J. Immunol.* 172: 2126-36

[92] Lee RS, Grusby MJ, Glimcher LH, Winn HJ, Auchincloss H, Jr. 1994. Indirect recognition by helper cells can induce donor-specific cytotoxic T lymphocytes in vivo. *J. Exp. Med.* 179: 865-72

[93] Wise MP, Bemelman F, Cobbold SP, Waldmann H. 1998. Linked suppression of skin graft rejection can operate through indirect recognition. *J. Immunol.* 161: 5813-6

[94] Lan RY, Ansari AA, Lian ZX, Gershwin ME. 2005. Regulatory T cells: development, function and role in autoimmunity. *Autoimmun. Rev.* 4: 351-63

[95] Wu Y, Borde M, Heissmeyer V, Feuerer M, Lapan AD, Stroud JC, Bates DL, Guo L, Han A, Ziegler SF, Mathis D, Benoist C, Chen L, Rao A. 2006. FOXP3 controls regulatory T cell function through cooperation with NFAT. *Cell.* 126: 375-87

[96] Wood KJ, Sakaguchi S. 2003. Regulatory T cells in transplantation tolerance. *Nat. Rev. Immunol.* 3: 199-210

[97] Tarbell KV, Yamazaki S, Steinman RM. 2006. The interactions of dendritic cells with antigen-specific, regulatory T cells that suppress autoimmunity. *Semin. Immunol.* 18: 93-102

[98] van Maurik A, Herber M, Wood KJ, Jones ND. 2002. Cutting edge: CD4+CD25+ alloantigen-specific immunoregulatory cells that can prevent CD8+ T cell-mediated graft rejection: implications for anti-CD154 immunotherapy. *J. Immunol.* 169: 5401-4

[99] Sanchez-Fueyo A, Weber M, Domenig C, Strom TB, Zheng XX. 2002. Tracking the immunoregulatory mechanisms active during allograft tolerance. *J. Immunol.* 168: 2274-81

[100] Graca L, Thompson S, Lin CY, Adams E, Cobbold SP, Waldmann H. 2002. Both CD4(+)CD25(+) and CD4(+)CD25(-) regulatory cells mediate dominant transplantation tolerance. *J. Immunol.* 168: 5558-65

[101] Taylor PA, Lees CJ, Blazar BR. 2002. The infusion of ex vivo activated and expanded CD4(+)CD25(+) immune regulatory cells inhibits graft-versus-host disease lethality. *Blood.* 99: 3493-9

[102] Tang Q, Henriksen KJ, Bi M, Finger EB, Szot G, Ye J, Masteller EL, McDevitt H, Bonyhadi M, Bluestone JA. 2004. In vitro-expanded antigen-specific regulatory T cells suppress autoimmune diabetes. *J. Exp. Med.* 199: 1455-65

[103] Taylor PA, Panoskaltsis-Mortari A, Swedin JM, Lucas PJ, Gress RE, Levine BL, June CH, Serody JS, Blazar BR. 2004. L-Selectin(hi) but not the L-selectin(lo) CD4+25+ T-regulatory cells are potent inhibitors of GVHD and BM graft rejection. *Blood.* 104: 3804-12

[104] Cohen JL, Trenado A, Vasey D, Klatzmann D, Salomon BL. 2002. CD4(+)CD25(+) immunoregulatory T Cells: new therapeutics for graft-versus-host disease. *J. Exp. Med.* 196: 401-6

[105] Jones SC, Murphy GF, Korngold R. 2003. Post-hematopoietic cell transplantation control of graft-versus-host disease by donor CD425 T cells to allow an effective graft-versus-leukemia response. *Biol. Blood Marrow Transplant.* 9: 243-56

[106] Takahashi T, Kuniyasu Y, Toda M, Sakaguchi N, Itoh M, Iwata M, Shimizu J, Sakaguchi S. 1998. Immunologic self-tolerance maintained by CD25+CD4+ naturally anergic and suppressive T cells: induction of autoimmune disease by breaking their anergic/suppressive state. *Int. Immunol.* 10: 1969-80

[107] Yamazaki S, Iyoda T, Tarbell K, Olson K, Velinzon K, Inaba K, Steinman RM. 2003. Direct expansion of functional CD25+ CD4+ regulatory T cells by antigen-processing dendritic cells. *J. Exp. Med.* 198: 235-47

[108] Tarbell KV, Yamazaki S, Olson K, Toy P, Steinman RM. 2004. CD25+ CD4+ T cells, expanded with dendritic cells presenting a single autoantigenic peptide, suppress autoimmune diabetes. *J. Exp. Med.* 199: 1467-77

[109] Trenado A, Charlotte F, Fisson S, Yagello M, Klatzmann D, Salomon BL, Cohen JL. 2003. Recipient-type specific CD4+CD25+ regulatory T cells favor immune reconstitution and control graft-versus-host disease while maintaining graft-versus-leukemia. *J. Clin. Invest.* 112: 1688-96

[110] Nishimura E, Sakihama T, Setoguchi R, Tanaka K, Sakaguchi S. 2004. Induction of antigen-specific immunologic tolerance by in vivo and in vitro antigen-specific expansion of naturally arising Foxp3+CD25+CD4+ regulatory T cells. *Int. Immunol.* 16: 1189-201

[111] Joffre O, Gorsse N, Romagnoli P, Hudrisier D, van Meerwijk JP. 2004. Induction of antigen-specific tolerance to bone marrow allografts with CD4+CD25+ T lymphocytes. *Blood.* 103: 4216-21

[112] Yamazaki S, Patel M, Harper A, Bonito A, Fukuyama H, Pack M, Tarbell KV, Talmor M, Ravetch JV, Inaba K, Steinman RM. 2006. Effective expansion of alloantigen-specific Foxp3+ CD25+ CD4+ regulatory T cells by dendritic cells during the mixed leukocyte reaction. *Proc. Natl. Acad. Sci. U S A.* 103: 2758-63

[113] Mahnke K, Qian Y, Knop J, Enk AH. 2003. Induction of CD4+/CD25+ regulatory T cells by targeting of antigens to immature dendritic cells. *Blood.* 101: 4862-9

[114] Kretschmer K, Apostolou I, Hawiger D, Khazaie K, Nussenzweig MC, von Boehmer H. 2005. Inducing and expanding regulatory T cell populations by foreign antigen. *Nat. Immunol.* 6: 1219-27

[115] Robinson SP, Patterson S, English N, Davies D, Knight SC, Reid CD. 1999. Human peripheral blood contains two distinct lineages of dendritic cells. *Eur. J. Immunol.* 29: 2769-78

[116] MacDonald KP, Munster DJ, Clark GJ, Dzionek A, Schmitz J, Hart DN. 2002. Characterization of human blood dendritic cell subsets. *Blood.* 100: 4512-20

[117] Caux C, Massacrier C, Vanbervliet B, Dubois B, Durand I, Cella M, Lanzavecchia A, Banchereau J. 1997. CD34+ hematopoietic progenitors from human cord blood differentiate along two independent dendritic cell pathways in response to granulocyte-macrophage colony-stimulating factor plus tumor necrosis factor alpha: II. Functional analysis. *Blood.* 90: 1458-70

[118] Romani N, Reider D, Heuer M, Ebner S, Kampgen E, Eibl B, Niederwieser D, Schuler G. 1996. Generation of mature dendritic cells from human blood. An improved method with special regard to clinical applicability. *J. Immunol. Methods.* 196: 137-51

[119] Curti A, Fogli M, Ratta M, Biasco G, Tura S, Lemoli RM. 2001. Dendritic cell differentiation from hematopoietic CD34+ progenitor cells. *J. Biol. Regul. Homeost. Agents.* 15: 49-52

[120] McKenna HJ. 2001. Role of hematopoietic growth factors/flt3 ligand in expansion and regulation of dendritic cells. *Curr. Opin. Hematol.* 8: 149-54

[121] Dauer M, Obermaier B, Herten J, Haerle C, Pohl K, Rothenfusser S, Schnurr M, Endres S, Eigler A. 2003. Mature dendritic cells derived from human monocytes within 48 hours: a novel strategy for dendritic cell differentiation from blood precursors. *J. Immunol.* 170: 4069-76

[122] Lee AW, Truong T, Bickham K, Fontenau JF, Larsson M, Da Silva I, Somersan S, Thomas EK, Bhardwaj N. 2002. A clinical grade cocktail of cytokines and PGE2

results in uniform maturation of human monocyte-derived dendritic cells: implications for immunotherapy. *Vaccine*. 20 Suppl 4: A8-A22

[123] Matyszak MK, Citterio S, Rescigno M, Ricciardi-Castagnoli P. 2000. Differential effects of corticosteroids during different stages of dendritic cell maturation. *Eur. J. mmunol*. 30: 1233-42

[124] Rozkova D, Horvath R, Bartunkova J, Spisek R. 2006. Glucocorticoids severely impair differentiation and antigen presenting function of dendritic cells despite upregulation of Toll-like receptors. *Clin. Immunol*. 120: 260-71

[125] Mazzoni A, Segal DM. 2004. Controlling the Toll road to dendritic cell polarization. *J. Leukoc. Biol*. 75: 721-30

[126] Reis e Sousa C. 2006. Dendritic cells in a mature age. *Nat. Rev. Immunol*. 6: 476-83

[127] Hackstein H, Renner FC, Bohnert A, Nockher A, Frommer T, Bein G, Weimer R. 2005. Dendritic cell deficiency in the blood of kidney transplant patients on long-term immunosuppression: results of a prospective matched-cohort study. *Am. J. Transplant*. 5: 2945-53

[128] Schlichting CL, Schareck WD, Nickel T, Weis M. 2005. Dendritic cells as pharmacological targets for the generation of regulatory immunosuppressive effectors. New implications for allo-transplantation. *Curr. Med. Chem*. 12: 1921-30

[129] Tajima K, Amakawa R, Ito T, Miyaji M, Takebayashi M, Fukuhara S. 2003. Immunomodulatory effects of cyclosporin A on human peripheral blood dendritic cell subsets. *Immunology*. 108: 321-8

[130] Schlichting CL, Schareck WD, Weis M. 2005. Dendritic cell adhesion is enhanced on endothelial cells preexposed to calcineurin inhibitors. *J. Cardiovasc. Pharmacol*. 46: 250-4

[131] Szabo G, Gavala C, Mandrekar P. 2001. Tacrolimus and cyclosporine A inhibit allostimulatory capacity and cytokine production of human myeloid dendritic cells. *J. Investig. Med*. 49: 442-9

[132] Monti P, Mercalli A, Leone BE, Valerio DC, Allavena P, Piemonti L. 2003. Rapamycin impairs antigen uptake of human dendritic cells. *Transplantation*. 75: 137-45

[133] Woltman AM, van der Kooij SW, Coffer PJ, Offringa R, Daha MR, van Kooten C. 2003. Rapamycin specifically interferes with GM-CSF signaling in human dendritic cells, leading to apoptosis via increased p27KIP1 expression. *Blood*. 101: 1439-45

[134] Hackstein H, Morelli AE, Larregina AT, Ganster RW, Papworth GD, Logar AJ, Watkins SC, Falo LD, Thomson AW. 2001. Aspirin inhibits in vitro maturation and in vivo immunostimulatory function of murine myeloid dendritic cells. *J. Immunol*. 166: 7053-62

[135] Matasic R, Dietz AB, Vuk-Pavlovic S. 2001. Maturation of human dendritic cells as sulfasalazine target. *Croat. Med. J*. 42: 440-5

[136] Ho LJ, Chang DM, Shiau HY, Chen CH, Hsieh TY, Hsu YL, Wong CS, Lai JH. 2001. Aspirin differentially regulates endotoxin-induced IL-12 and TNF-alpha production in human dendritic cells. *Scand. J. Rheumatol*. 30: 346-52

[137] Piemonti L, Monti P, Sironi M, Fraticelli P, Leone BE, Dal Cin E, Allavena P, Di Carlo V. 2000. Vitamin D3 affects differentiation, maturation, and function of human monocyte-derived dendritic cells. *J. Immunol*. 164: 4443-51

[138] Adorini L. 2002. 1,25-Dihydroxyvitamin D3 analogs as potential therapies in transplantation. *Curr. Opin. Investig. Drugs.* 3: 1458-63

[139] Griffin MD, Xing N, Kumar R. 2003. Vitamin D and its analogs as regulators of immune activation and antigen presentation. *Annu. Rev. Nutr.* 23: 117-45

[140] Adorini L, Giarratana N, Penna G. 2004. Pharmacological induction of tolerogenic dendritic cells and regulatory T cells. *Semin. Immunol.* 16: 127-34

[141] Penna G, Vulcano M, Roncari A, Facchetti F, Sozzani S, Adorini L. 2002. Cutting edge: differential chemokine production by myeloid and plasmacytoid dendritic cells. *J. Immunol.* 169: 6673-6

[142] Penna G, Roncari A, Amuchastegui S, Daniel KC, Berti E, Colonna M, Adorini L. 2005. Expression of the inhibitory receptor ILT3 on dendritic cells is dispensable for induction of CD4+Foxp3+ regulatory T cells by 1,25-dihydroxyvitamin D3. *Blood.* 106: 3490-7

[143] Bennett CL, Ochs HD. 2001. IPEX is a unique X-linked syndrome characterized by immune dysfunction, polyendocrinopathy, enteropathy, and a variety of autoimmune phenomena. *Curr. Opin. Pediatr.* 13: 533-8

[144] Shevach EM, DiPaolo RA, Andersson J, Zhao DM, Stephens GL, Thornton AM. 2006. The lifestyle of naturally occurring CD4+ CD25+ Foxp3+ regulatory T cells. *Immunol. Rev.* 212: 60-73

[145] Lehmann J, Huehn J, de la Rosa M, Maszyna F, Kretschmer U, Krenn V, Brunner M, Scheffold A, Hamann A. 2002. Expression of the integrin alpha Ebeta 7 identifies unique subsets of CD25+ as well as CD25- regulatory T cells. *Proc. Natl. Acad. Sci. U S A.* 99: 13031-6

[146] Takahashi T, Tagami T, Yamazaki S, Uede T, Shimizu J, Sakaguchi N, Mak TW, Sakaguchi S. 2000. Immunologic self-tolerance maintained by CD25(+)CD4(+) regulatory T cells constitutively expressing cytotoxic T lymphocyte-associated antigen 4. *J. Exp. Med.* 192: 303-10

[147] Shimizu J, Yamazaki S, Takahashi T, Ishida Y, Sakaguchi S. 2002. Stimulation of CD25(+)CD4(+) regulatory T cells through GITR breaks immunological self-tolerance. *Nat. Immunol.* 3: 135-42

[148] Xu D, Liu H, Komai-Koma M. 2004. Direct and indirect role of Toll-like receptors in T cell mediated immunity. *Cell. Mol. Immunol.* 1: 239-46

[149] Yamagiwa S, Gray JD, Hashimoto S, Horwitz DA. 2001. A role for TGF-beta in the generation and expansion of CD4+CD25+ regulatory T cells from human peripheral blood. *J. Immunol.* 166: 7282-9

[150] Jonuleit H, Schmitt E, Stassen M, Tuettenberg A, Knop J, Enk AH. 2001. Identification and functional characterization of human CD4(+)CD25(+) T cells with regulatory properties isolated from peripheral blood. *J. Exp. Med.* 193: 1285-94

[151] Cobbold SP, Adams E, Graca L, Waldmann H. 2003. Serial analysis of gene expression provides new insights into regulatory T cells. *Semin. Immunol.* 15: 209-14

[152] Cobbold SP, Nolan KF, Graca L, Castejon R, Le Moine A, Frewin M, Humm S, Adams E, Thompson S, Zelenika D, Paterson A, Yates S, Fairchild PJ, Waldmann H. 2003. Regulatory T cells and dendritic cells in transplantation tolerance: molecular markers and mechanisms. *Immunol. Rev.* 196: 109-24

[153] Misra N, Bayry J, Lacroix-Desmazes S, Kazatchkine MD, Kaveri SV. 2004. Cutting edge: human CD4+CD25+ T cells restrain the maturation and antigen-presenting function of dendritic cells. *J. Immunol.*172: 4676-80

[154] Cederbom L, Hall H, Ivars F. 2000. CD4+CD25+ regulatory T cells down-regulate co-stimulatory molecules on antigen-presenting cells. *Eur. J. Immunol.* 30: 1538-43

[155] Houot R, Perrot I, Garcia E, Durand I, Lebecque S. 2006. Human CD4+CD25high regulatory T cells modulate myeloid but not plasmacytoid dendritic cells activation. *J. Immunol.* 176: 5293-8

[156] Rosenberg SA, Sportes C, Ahmadzadeh M, Fry TJ, Ngo LT, Schwarz SL, Stetler-Stevenson M, Morton KE, Mavroukakis SA, Morre M, Buffet R, Mackall CL, Gress RE. 2006. IL-7 administration to humans leads to expansion of CD8+ and CD4+ cells but a relative decrease of CD4+ T-regulatory cells. *J. Immunother.* 29: 313-9

[157] Liu W, Putnam AL, Xu-Yu Z, Szot GL, Lee MR, Zhu S, Gottlieb PA, Kapranov P, Gingeras TR, Fazekas de St Groth B, Clayberger C, Soper DM, Ziegler SF, Bluestone JA. 2006. CD127 expression inversely correlates with FoxP3 and suppressive function of human CD4+ T reg cells. *J. Exp. Med.* 203: 1701-11

[158] Seddiki N, Santner-Nanan B, Martinson J, Zaunders J, Sasson S, Landay A, Solomon M, Selby W, Alexander SI, Nanan R, Kelleher A, Fazekas de St Groth B. 2006. Expression of interleukin (IL)-2 and IL-7 receptors discriminates between human regulatory and activated T cells. *J. Exp. Med.* 203: 1693-700

[159] Levings MK, Sangregorio R, Roncarolo MG. 2001. Human cd25(+)cd4(+) t regulatory cells suppress naive and memory T cell proliferation and can be expanded in vitro without loss of function. *J. Exp. Med.* 193: 1295-302

[160] Jiang S, Camara N, Lombardi G, Lechler RI. 2003. Induction of allopeptide-specific human CD4+CD25+ regulatory T cells ex vivo. *Blood.* 102: 2180-6

[161] Jiang S, Lechler RI. 2003. Regulatory T cells in the control of transplantation tolerance and autoimmunity. *Am. J. Transplant.* 3: 516-24

[162] Vlad G, Cortesini R, Suciu-Foca N. 2005. License to heal: bidirectional interaction of antigen-specific regulatory T cells and tolerogenic APC. *J. Immunol.* 174: 5907-14

[163] Suciu-Foca N, Manavalan JS, Cortesini R. 2003. Generation and function of antigen-specific suppressor and regulatory T cells. *Transpl. Immunol.* 11: 235-44

[164] Chang CC, Ciubotariu R, Manavalan JS, Yuan J, Colovai AI, Piazza F, Lederman S, Colonna M, Cortesini R, Dalla-Favera R, Suciu-Foca N. 2002. Tolerization of dendritic cells by T(S) cells: the crucial role of inhibitory receptors ILT3 and ILT4. *Nat. Immunol.* 3: 237-43

[165] Manavalan JS, Kim-Schulze S, Scotto L, Naiyer AJ, Vlad G, Colombo PC, Marboe C, Mancini D, Cortesini R, Suciu-Foca N. 2004. Alloantigen specific CD8+CD28-FOXP3+ T suppressor cells induce ILT3+ ILT4+ tolerogenic endothelial cells, inhibiting alloreactivity. *Int. Immunol.* 16: 1055-68

[166] Suciu-Foca N, Manavalan JS, Scotto L, Kim-Schulze S, Galluzzo S, Naiyer AJ, Fan J, Vlad G, Cortesini R. 2005. Molecular characterization of allospecific T suppressor and tolerogenic dendritic cells: review. *Int. Immunopharmacol.* 5: 7-11

[167] Colovai AI, Mirza M, Vlad G, Wang S, Ho E, Cortesini R, Suciu-Foca N. 2003. Regulatory CD8+CD28- T cells in heart transplant recipients. *Hum. Immunol.* 64: 31-7

[168] Manavalan JS, Rossi PC, Vlad G, Piazza F, Yarilina A, Cortesini R, Mancini D, Suciu-Foca N. 2003. High expression of ILT3 and ILT4 is a general feature of tolerogenic dendritic cells. *Transpl. Immunol.* 11: 245-58

[169] Jonuleit H, Schmitt E, Schuler G, Knop J, Enk AH. 2000. Induction of interleukin 10-producing, nonproliferating CD4(+) T cells with regulatory properties by repetitive stimulation with allogeneic immature human dendritic cells. *J. Exp. Med.* 192: 1213-22

[170] Dhodapkar MV, Steinman RM, Krasovsky J, Munz C, Bhardwaj N. 2001. Antigen-specific inhibition of effector T cell function in humans after injection of immature dendritic cells. *J. Exp. Med.* 193: 233-8

[171] Levings MK, Bacchetta R, Schulz U, Roncarolo MG. 2002. The role of IL-10 and TGF-beta in the differentiation and effector function of T regulatory cells. *Int. Arch. Allergy Immunol.* 129: 263-76

[172] Levings MK, Sangregorio R, Sartirana C, Moschin AL, Battaglia M, Orban PC, Roncarolo MG. 2002. Human CD25+CD4+ T suppressor cell clones produce transforming growth factor beta, but not interleukin 10, and are distinct from type 1 T regulatory cells. *J. Exp. Med.* 196: 1335-46

[173] Bacchetta R, Sartirana C, Levings MK, Bordignon C, Narula S, Roncarolo MG. 2002. Growth and expansion of human T regulatory type 1 cells are independent from TCR activation but require exogenous cytokines. *Eur. J. Immunol.* 32: 2237-45

[174] Valmori D, Tosello V, Souleimanian NE, Godefroy E, Scotto L, Wang Y, Ayyoub M. 2006. Rapamycin-mediated enrichment of T cells with regulatory activity in stimulated CD4+ T cell cultures is not due to the selective expansion of naturally occurring regulatory T cells but to the induction of regulatory functions in conventional CD4+ T cells. *J. Immunol.* 177: 944-9

[175] Segundo DS, Ruiz JC, Fernandez-Fresnedo G, Izquierdo M, Gomez-Alamillo C, Cacho E, Benito MJ, Rodrigo E, Palomar R, Lopez-Hoyos M, Arias M. 2006. Calcineurin Inhibitors Affect Circulating Regulatory T Cells in Stable Renal Transplant Recipients. *Transplant. Proc.* 38: 2391-3

[176] Salama AD, Najafian N, Clarkson MR, Harmon WE, Sayegh MH. 2003. Regulatory CD25+ T cells in human kidney transplant recipients. *J. Am. Soc. Nephrol.* 14: 1643-51

[177] Game DS, Hernandez-Fuentes MP, Lechler RI. 2005. Everolimus and basiliximab permit suppression by human CD4+CD25+ cells in vitro. *Am. J. Transplant.* 5: 454-64

[178] Franzke A, Piao W, Lauber J, Gatzlaff P, Konecke C, Hansen W, Schmitt-Thomsen A, Hertenstein B, Buer J, Ganser A. 2003. G-CSF as immune regulator in T cells expressing the G-CSF receptor: implications for transplantation and autoimmune diseases. *Blood.* 102: 734-9

[179] Rutella S, Pierelli L, Bonanno G, Sica S, Ameglio F, Capoluongo E, Mariotti A, Scambia G, d'Onofrio G, Leone G. 2002. Role for granulocyte colony-stimulating factor in the generation of human T regulatory type 1 cells. *Blood.* 100: 2562-71

[180] Dieckmann D, Plottner H, Berchtold S, Berger T, Schuler G. 2001. Ex vivo isolation and characterization of CD4(+)CD25(+) T cells with regulatory properties from human blood. *J. Exp. Med.* 193: 1303-10

[181] Karakhanova S, Munder M, Schneider M, Bonyhadi M, Ho AD, Goerner M. 2006. Highly efficient expansion of human CD4+CD25+ regulatory T cells for cellular immunotherapy in patients with graft-versus-host disease. *J. Immunother.* 29: 336-49

[182] Godfrey WR, Ge YG, Spoden DJ, Levine BL, June CH, Blazar BR, Porter SB. 2004. In vitro-expanded human CD4(+)CD25(+) T-regulatory cells can markedly inhibit allogeneic dendritic cell-stimulated MLR cultures. *Blood.* 104: 453-61

[183] Hoffmann P, Eder R, Kunz-Schughart LA, Andreesen R, Edinger M. 2004. Large-scale in vitro expansion of polyclonal human CD4(+)CD25high regulatory T cells. *Blood.* 104: 895-903

[184] Koenen HJ, Fasse E, Joosten I. 2005. CD27/CFSE-based ex vivo selection of highly suppressive alloantigen-specific human regulatory T cells. *J. Immunol.* 174: 7573-83

[185] Creput C, Durrbach A, Menier C, Guettier C, Samuel D, Dausset J, Charpentier B, Carosella ED, Rouas-Freiss N. 2003. Human leukocyte antigen-G (HLA-G) expression in biliary epithelial cells is associated with allograft acceptance in liver-kidney transplantation. *J. Hepatol.* 39: 587-94

[186] Lefebvre S, Antoine M, Uzan S, McMaster M, Dausset J, Carosella ED, Paul P. 2002. Specific activation of the non-classical class I histocompatibility HLA-G antigen and expression of the ILT2 inhibitory receptor in human breast cancer. *J. Pathol.* 196: 266-74

[187] Allan DS, McMichael AJ, Braud VM. 2000. The ILT family of leukocyte receptors. *Immunobiology.* 202: 34-41

[188] Sanders SK, Giblin PA, Kavathas P. 1991. Cell-cell adhesion mediated by CD8 and human histocompatibility leukocyte antigen G, a nonclassical major histocompatibility complex class I molecule on cytotrophoblasts. *J. Exp. Med.* 174: 737-40

[189] Kanai T, Fujii T, Kozuma S, Yamashita T, Miki A, Kikuchi A, Taketani Y. 2001. Soluble HLA-G influences the release of cytokines from allogeneic peripheral blood mononuclear cells in culture. *Mol. Hum. Reprod.* 7: 195-200

[190] Kapasi K, Albert SE, Yie S, Zavazava N, Librach CL. 2000. HLA-G has a concentration-dependent effect on the generation of an allo-CTL response. *Immunology.* 101: 191-200

[191] Lila N, Amrein C, Guillemain R, Chevalier P, Latremouille C, Fabiani JN, Dausset J, Carosella ED, Carpentier A. 2002. Human leukocyte antigen-G expression after heart transplantation is associated with a reduced incidence of rejection. *Circulation.* 105: 1949-54

[192] Onno M, Pangault C, Le Friec G, Guilloux V, Andre P, Fauchet R. 2000. Modulation of HLA-G antigens expression by human cytomegalovirus: specific induction in activated macrophages harboring human cytomegalovirus infection. *J. Immunol.* 164: 6426-34

[193] Colonna M, Navarro F, Bellon T, Llano M, Garcia P, Samaridis J, Angman L, Cella M, Lopez-Botet M. 1997. A common inhibitory receptor for major histocompatibility complex class I molecules on human lymphoid and myelomonocytic cells. *J. Exp. Med.* 186: 1809-18

[194] LeMaoult J, Rouas-Freiss N, Carosella ED. 2005. Immuno-tolerogenic functions of HLA-G: relevance in transplantation and oncology. *Autoimmun. Rev.* 4: 503-9

In: Transplantation Immunology Research Trends
Editor: Oliver N. Ulricker, pp. 37-86

ISBN: 978-1-60021-578-0
© 2007 Nova Science Publishers, Inc.

Chapter II

Chemokine Receptors and Transplantation

Tan Jinquan, *Zhou Gang, Xie Luokun,*
Wang Li, Chen Lang and He Yuling
Department of Immunology, Wuhan University School of
Basic Medical Sciences, Wuhan University, Wuhan 430071, P. R. China

I. Abstract

Chemokine receptors and their ligands control a wide variety of biological and pathological processes, ranging from immunosurveillance to inflammation, from viral infection to cancer, and from transplant rejection to transplant tolerance [1]. It is not surprising that chemokine receptors and their ligands may be involved in rejection of allogeneic transplants because the chemokine receptor system plays an essential role in host defense [2]. Allograft transplant rejection is mediated largely by circulating peripheral leukocytes induced to infiltrate the graft by various inflammatory factors. Of these, chemokine receptors and their ligands, which are expressed by early innate responding leukocytes, as well as by inflamed graft tissues, are responsible for the recruitment and infiltration of alloreactive leukocytes.

A complex process including both innate and acquired immune responses results in allograft rejection. Some chemokine receptors and their ligands play essential roles not only in leukocyte migration into the graft but also in facilitating dendritic and T cell trafficking between lymph nodes and the transplant in early and late stage of the allogeneic response. Analysis of gene knockout mice with targeted deletions of certain chemokine receptors and their ligands has gradually clarified their relative importance in allograft rejection. The present chapter focuses on the impact and mechanism of these chemoattractant proteins on transplant outcome and novel diagnostic and therapeutic

---

* Corresponding and reprint require to Tan Jinquan, M. D., Ph. D.; Wuhan University School of Basic Medical Sciences; Donghu Road No. 115, Wuchang; Wuhan 430071, P. R. China; Tel: 0086 27 68759039; Fax: 0086 27 68759039; Email: jinquan_tan@hotmail.com

approaches for antirejection therapy based on targeting chemokine receptors and/or their ligands.

II. Introduction of Chemokine and Chemokine Receptor Family

A. The Chemokine Family

Cellular migration, known as chemotaxis under a certain circumstance, is a biological phenomenon which has been studied over the past century. In 1884, Pfeffer first assigned the term *chemotaxis* in his paper about the migration of plant sperm [3]. Four years later, it was Leber who first pose the definition of chemotaxis as leukocytes migrating along a gradient in a directional manner [4]. Later on, he further defined that chemotaxis is a biological process of directed cell migration along a concentration gradient of a proper stimulus known as chemoattractant [5]. During the same period, the relevance of chemotaxis in biology was observed by Merchnikoff, who first demonstrated how primary defense mechanisms rely on the migration of inflammatory cells to areas of injury.

The real milestone was made by Boyden in 1962 since his invention of Boyden chamber assay which is able to examine the chemotactic behavior of cells and to quantitatively define and characterize chemoattractant [6]. In 1980, Falk and his colleagues developed a reproducible, accurate and sensitive assay, that is, 48-well microchamber chemotaxis technique [7]. Currently, this assay is widely adopted for analysis of chemotaxis of various cells including lymphocytes, monocytes, basophils and eosinophils. Another milestone was the Oppenheim's work based on many discoveries of new chemoattractant cytokines defined two major subfamilies according to their structure and biological functions [8]. This area has largely expanded since. The finding that CCR5 is a co-receptor of HIV to infect CD4+ T cells induced a passionate interest in the research fields of chemokine receptors and their ligands [9].

In the strict sense, chemokine is a kind of chemoattractants with special structure and being cytokine [8, 10]. The term "chemokines", which is an abbreviation of "chemoattractant cytokines", was created by the Third International Symposium of Chemotactic Cytokines in 1992 to describe a family of around 50 related proteins that have roles in leukocyte activation, selectin/integrin up-regulation, hematopoiesis, angiogenesis, and adaptive immunity both during development and in the adult. Chemokines were originally discovered for their ability to function as chemoattractants [11-13]. This family of chemotactic proteins appears to be conserved evolutionarily, as evidenced by its high degree of homology (20 to 70% in amino acid sequences) across species from mammals to fish. Chemokines are low molecular weight proteins (8–15 kDa), which usually contain four cysteine residues and are subdivided into four different families in terms of the arrangement of the first two N-terminal cysteine residues: the CXC (α), CC (β), C (γ) and CX3C (δ) families of chemokines (table 1). Most chemokines belong to the CC and CXC families and they have received the greatest attention in experimental models of disease and inflammation [14, 15]. In addition, the CXC subfamily has been divided into two groups depending on the presence of the ELR motif preceding the first cysteine: the ELR-CXC chemokines and the non-ELR-CXC chemokines [16].

Many chemokines have more than one name. To avoid possible confusion, a new nomenclature for these special chemotactic cytokines was established at the 1999 Chemokine Keystone Symposium [17]. The chemokines are numbered following the order they are discovered and an L (ligand) is added. All chemokines are listed in table 1 according to the suggested new nomenclature.

B. The Chemokine Receptor Family

The chemokine receptor researching area is fully developing and extending insight into other areas of medium as the importance of chemokine receptor expression and function is now documented for malignant diseases and rejection of transplanted organ [18, 19]. Many researchers consider that several chemokine receptors are markers of Th1 and Th2 cells [20]. As one after one new finding appears, the number of important biological aspects of chemotaxis and related areas seems almost endless. Today, this research area deals not only with cellular migration, trafficking, adhesion, accumulation, differentiation, maturation, activation, but also with receptor expression, signal transduction, viral infection, ect..

All known chemokines bind to seven-transmembrane G-protein-coupled receptors, that signal through heterotrimeric GTP-binding proteins. G-proteins are composed of three subunits, α, β, and γ. The ability of any particular chemokine to activate a given leukocyte is via the expression of corresponding receptors on the surface of the cell. Upon ligand binding, chemokine receptor activates G-protein, particularly the *Bordetella pertussis* toxin-sensitive receptor which is a subfamily of G proteins (Gi/Go). Although they have structural similarity and couple to the same type of G protein, chemokine receptors can activate specific signal transduction pathways leading to diverse physiological and pathophysiological responses in different cells or organs [21]. The specificity and complexity of the chemokine system stem from the regulated expression of their receptors.

In general, the genes encoding chemokine receptors are clustered on chromosome 2 and chromosome 3. Chemokine receptors range from 340 to 370 amino acids in length, with a relatively short extracellular acidic N-terminus as well as numerous serines and threonines in the short intracellular C-terminal tail that become phosphorylated upon ligand binding to the receptor. The seven-transmembrane domains are α-helical, and three intracellular and three extracellular loops exist between the transmembrane domains [22]. Some chemokine receptors form homodimers that may be involved in receptor signal transduction [23, 24]. Ligation of chemokines to corresponding receptors initiates signaling cascades that are involved in cytoskeletal reorganization, integrin activation, and other biochemical processes that result in enhanced cellular adhesion, migration and activation. The C and CX3C chemokines bind to only one receptor, whereas the CC and CXC chemokines are promiscuous, with most binding to two or more receptors each, for instance CCL5 binds to CCR1, CCR3, and CCR5. Even in the case of a particular chemokine binding to only a single receptor, chemokine receptors also can bind more than one ligand, for example only CCR6 and CCR9 from CCR1-11 bind only one CC chemokine. Chemokine receptors are named after their specific chemokine preferences (table 1): CCR1–11, CXCR1–6, XCR1, CX3CR1 and chemokine-binding proteins Duffy, D6 [25, 26].

Table 1. Classification of chemokines and chemokine receptors [27-30]

Ligands	Synonyms	Receptors
CXC (α)		
CXCL1	Groα, MGSA-α, GRO-1, NAP-3	CXCR2>CXCR1, Duffy
CXCL2	Groβ, MGSA-β, MIP-2α, GRO-2	CXCR2>CXCR1
CXCL3	Groγ, MGSA-γ, MIP-2β, GRO-3	CXCR2>CXCR1
CXCL4	PF4	CXCR1,2
CXCL5	ENA-78, AMCF-II	CXCR1,2
CXCL6	GCP-2, CKα3	CXCR1,2
CXCL7	NAP-2, MDGF	CXCR2, Duffy
CXCL8	IL-8, NCF, NAP-1, MDNCF, LUCT, AMCF-1, MONAP	CXCR1,2, Duffy
CXCL9	Mig	CXCR3
CXCL10	IP-10, CRG-2	CXCR3
CXCL11	I-TAC, b-R1, H174, IP-9	CXCR3
CXCL12	SDF-1α/β, PBSF, hIRH, TLSR-α/β, TPAR1	CXCR4
CXCL13	BLC/BCA-1, CXC-X, BLR1L, Angie	CXCR5
CXCL14	BRAK, CXC-X3, Bolekine, NJAC, BMAC	Unknown
CXCL15	CINC-2β-like, Lungkine, Weche	Unknown
CXCL16	SR-PSOX	CXCR6
CC (β)		
CCL1	I-309, TCA-3, P500	CCR8, Duffy
CCL2	MCP-1, MCAF, LDGF, GDCF, TDCF, SMC-CF, HC11, TSG8	CCR2, D6
CCL3	MIP-1α, LD78α, LD78β, GOS19, Pat464	CCR1,5
CCL4	MIP-1β, pAT744, ACT-2, G-26, HC21, H400, MAD-5, LAG-1	CCR5, D6
CCL5	RANTES	CCR1,3,5, Duffy, D6
CCL6	MRP-1, C10	Unknown
CCL7	MCP-3, NC28, FIC, MARC	CCR1,2,3
CCL8	MCP-2, HC-14	CCR1,2,3,5, D6
CCL9	MRP-2, MIP-1γ	CCR1
CCL10	CCF18, C10-like	CCR1
CCL11	Eotaxin	CCR3>CCR5
CCL12	MCP-5	CCR2
CCL13	MCP-4, Ckβ10, NCC-1	CCR1,2,3, D6
CCL14	HCC-1, MCIF, Ckβ1, NCC-2, HCC-3	CCR1,3,5, D6
CCL15	HCC-2, MIP-1δ, Lkn-1, CC-2, MIP-5, CCF-18, NCC-3	CCR1,3, D6
CCL16	HCC-4, LEC, LCC-1, ILINK, NCC-4, LMC, CKβ12	CCR1,2,5,8
CCL17	TARC, Dendrokine, ABCD-2	CCR4,8
CCL18	DC-CK1, PARC, AMAC-1, MIP-4, Dctactin	Unknown
CCL19	ELC, MIP-3β, Exodus-3, Ckβ11	CCR7,11
CCL20	LARC, MIP-3α, Exodus-1, Mexikine, ST38, CKβ4	CCR6
CCL21	SLC, 6Ckine, Exodus-2, TCA4, CKβ9	CCR7,11
CCL22	MDC, STCP-1, DCtactin β, ABCD-1, DC/B-CK	CCR4
CCL23	MPIF-1, Ckβ8, MIP-3	CCR1
CCL24	Eotaxin-2, MPIF-2, Ckβ6	CCR3
CCL25	TECK	CCR9,11
CCL26	Eotaxin-3, Finetaxin, TMkine, IMAC	CCR3

Table 1. (Continued).

Ligands	Synonyms	Receptors
CCL27	Eskine, CTACK, ILC, PESKY, ALP, skinkine	CCR10
CCL28	MEC, CCK1	CCR3,10
C (γ)		
XCL1	Lymphotactin, SCM-1α, ATAC	XCR1
XCL2	SCM-1β	XCR1
CX3C (δ)		
CX3CL1	Fractalkine, ABCD-3, Neurotactin	CX3CR1

III. The Status of Historical and Current Research on Chemokine Receptor Effects in Allograft Transplant

The early history of transplantation is linked with the earliest attempts at plastic surgery. Tagliacozzi did classic work of attaching a skin flap from the forearm to the nose and then severing its original connections some weeks later, which started the modern era of transplantation. In the early 1960s, the course of clinical transplantation was changed by three events. The first was the emergence and improvement of tissue typing and these early methods gave the hope that close matching could eventually be obtained. The second was the development of methods for regular dialysis treatment, a therapy which could be integrated with transplantation. The third and most important was the occurrence of new, potent, immunosuppressive drugs [31].

However, the use of immunosuppressive agents can facilitate the development of cancer in allograft recipients. Allograft recipients are usually treated with immunosuppressive agents, such as azathioprine, corticosteroids, cyclosporine A, cyclophosphamide, antilymphocyte globulin, chlorambucil, the actinomycins and local radiotherapy. Other drugs often used include a wide variety of antibiotic, antihypertensive, antidiabetic, antiepileptic and sedative. Some of these agents which can immunosuppress certain types of lymphocytes and impair immune surveillance have shown to have carcinogenic effects. For instance, azathioprine is known to cause chromosome breaks and nuclear abnormalities in human and animals, and potentiate the actions of other oncogenic stimuli [32, 33].

Since the early 1990s, more and more attention have been concentrated on chemokine receptors and their ligands in experimental models of transplant rejection, primitively like CXCL8 and CCL2, because the study on target chemokine receptor may contribute to develop a novel satisfactory therapeutic agent in controlling allograft rejection [34, 35]. Transplant rejection usually links to the infiltration of immune cells, largely composed of monocytes, macrophages, T-lymphocytes and natural killer cells. Therefore, it is convinced that chemokine receptors may be involved in allogeneic rejection because the chemokine receptor system plays an essential role in leukocyte activation and migration.

Organ transplantation is often the only option of irreversible organ failure. An understanding of the immune processes leading to injury of grafted organs is essential for extending organ lifespan in addition to allowing transplants from poorly matching individuals and animal sources. Currently, graft injury is believed to proceed in three overlapping stages: transplantation injury, acute rejection and chronic rejection [36].

Transplant injury is due to the transplantation process itself and includes both physical traumas from the surgery as well as cellular damage including ischemia reperfusion injury (IR). IR is a period of oxygen deprivation followed by oxygen restoration, and is one of the major causes of graft dysfunction as well [37]. Neutrophil accumulation is one of the hallmarks of IR and is thought to be responsible for much of the tissue injury [38]. Given the importance of leukocyte trafficking in IR, it is not surprising that chemokine receptors and their ligands have been shown to play a role. For instance, CXCL8 which is a potent neutrophil chemoattractant and activator has been shown in many cases to be upregulated after reperfusion as early as one hour [39, 40].

Acute rejection remains a major problem in solid organ transplantation, because rejection may lead to either acute or chronic loss of graft function. In the early stage of the allogenic response, chemokine receptors, chemokines, and adhesion molecules play important roles not only in leukocyte migration into the graft but also in facilitating dendritic and T cell trafficking between lymph nodes and the transplant [2, 28, 41, 42]. Several recent studies indicate the importance of the chemokine receptors and their ligands in the allograft rejection process. For instance, CXCR3-/- mice display a substantial prolongation of vascularized heart allograft survival [43]. CCR1-/- mice either will not or will only slowly reject cardiac allografts bearing isolated MHC class II or combined MHC class I and II disparities, respectively [44]. The activation of donor T cells after small bowel allotransplantation induces production of a Th1 profile of cytokines and CXCL10, and then increases infiltration of host T cells and NK cells in small bowel allografts. Blocking this pathway may be of therapeutic value in controlling small bowel allograft rejection [45].

Chronic rejection is the main cause of most long-term organ failures but its mechanisms are still poorly understood. It is characterized and diagnosed by progressive function and structural deterioration including occlusive vasculopathy usually with occurrence of infiltrates of T helper cells, cytotoxic T cells, natural killer cells, and particularly monocytes and macrophages [46]. Risk factors include both alloantigen-dependent and independent factors, such as the number of acute episodes and the length of cold-ischemic time. The importance of antigen-independent factors is particularly emphasized by the development of structural changes resembling those of chronically rejecting allografts in syngeneic transplants, although the process is slower and less severe [47-49]. Chemokine expression has also received enough attention in chronically rejecting organs. In human heart transplantation, CCL5 mRNA and protein expression are detected in lymphocytes, macrophages, myofibroblasts and endothelial cells of arteries undergoing accelerated atherosclerosis. But this does not happen in normal coronary arteries [50]. In rat renal allograft model, CCL5 expression peaked at 2 weeks as reported [49]. Similarly, increased levels of CCL2 expression occur in rat cardiac and renal transplantation models and persist for several months after transplantation. This result is consistent with the idea that chronic rejection is an ongoing immune process [34, 49, 51, 52]. However, causative roles must be assigned cautiously because a little knowledge about the exact mechanisms of chronic rejection is obtained so far. Indeed, recent application of IFN-γ knockout mice suggests that the observed arteriosclerosis, one of the hallmarks of chronic rejection, may only be symptomatic of organ failure [53].

Regulation of chemokine expression is important in controlling leukocyte trafficking under both normal and inflammatory circumstances. Destructive infiltration and tissue damage are usually caused by inappropriate expression of these molecules. This phenomenon is clearly demonstrated and confirmed in the pathogenesis of graft rejection, which probably depend on chemokine expression [36].

IV. The Functions of Chemokine Receptors in Various Organ/Tissue Allograft Transplants

A. Chemokine Receptors and Transplantation Rejection

With several models of allograft transplantation (heart, lung, kidney, liver, pancreatic islet, bone marrow, and skin), recent data all suggest that recruitment of host leukocytes into the allograft involves chemokine receptors mediated pathways. Following will discuss the correlation between some particular chemokine receptors and various tissue transplant rejection.

Heart Transplantation

CXCR3 exert potent biological effects on both immune and vascular cells. The dual targets suggest their important roles in cardiac allograft vasculopathy (CAV) and rejection. In experimental model, CXCR3 play a key role in the development of transplant rejection through inducing T cell activation, recruitment, and human cardiac allograft destruction [43, 54]. Interestingly, CXCR3 show a unique pattern of expression by immunohistochemical staining: it is observed that expressing weakly on cells in the outer layer of the neointima and adventitia and the strongest staining in the innermost layer of the neointima [55]. In some patients, there is a trend for persistent expression of CD3+ and CXCR3+ expressing infiltrates in the later phase of the first posttransplant year. The CXCL9, CXCL10, CXCL11, ligands of CXCR3, which are rarely expressed in normal biopsies, are markedly induced in acute rejection [56]. Persistent elevation of CXCL10 and CXCL11 is associated with CAV. Double immunohistochemistry reveal differential cellular distribution of CXCR3 chemokines. Intragraft vascular cells express high levels of CXCL10 and CXCL11, while CXCL9 is localized predominantly in infiltrating macrophages [57]. In addition, the adenovirus mediated gene transfer and expression of viral IL-10 (vIL-10) are reported to be able to prolong cardiac allograft survival, through the inhibition of the immune response to both alloantigen and adenoviral antigens. Most of the Th1 related chemokine genes, such as CXCL9 and CXCL10, are inhibited or down regulated by vIL-10 administration, which may help to decrease leukocyte infiltration and prolong graft survival. The vIL-10 administration also induced the expression of the Th2 associated chemokines CCL24 and CCL9, suggesting Th1 to Th2 immune deviation [58]. CXCR3 is localized in vascular and infiltrating cells, while CXCR3 chemokines are induced in cardiac allografts and differentially associated with CAV and rejection. Differential cellular distribution of these chemokines in allografts indicates their central roles in multiple pathways involving CAV and rejection. This chemokine pathway may serve as a monitor and target for novel therapies to prevent CAV and rejection [57].

The inbred mice with a targeted deletion of the CCR1 show significant prolongation of cardiac allograft survival in experimental models [44]. Another study examines the effect of BX471, the CCR1 antagonist, in a rat heterotopic heart transplant rejection model. Treatment of animals with BX471 and a subtherapeutic dose of cyclosporin are much more efficacious in postponing transplant rejection than animals treated with either cyclosporin or BX471 alone [59]. The mechanism of action of the CCR1 antagonist is that the antagonist blocks the firm adhesion of monocytes triggered by CCL5 and/or CCL3 on inflamed endothelium [60]. These findings provide evidence that in vivo blockade of CCR1/ligand interactions is of therapeutic significance in preventing acute and chronic rejection clinically.

The CCR2 pathways associated with macrophage activation are upregulated in hearts undergoing chronic rejection. CCL2 gene transcript and gene product in rat cardiac allografts increase significantly (8-12 fold) on day 7 and remain high levels on days 14 and 28 posttransplantation. This induction is not observed with naive hearts, syngeneic transplants, and paired host hearts. For the inducible gene CCL2, high transcript level in cardiac allograft is in contrast with low level in host spleen [51]. CCL2 positive cells represent a subpopulation of activated macrophages. The persistent expression of CCL2 in association with increased macrophage localization suggests that CCL2, binding its receptor CCR2, contributes to the chronic inflammatory response following cardiac transplantation and that it may play a role in the pathogenesis of transplant arteriosclerosis [34].

Chronic graft rejection mediated by cellular immune responses still poses a serious clinical problem in transplant surgery. Allogeneic hearts are transplanted into CCR4 deficient (CCR4-/-) and control recipients. Compared to wild-type controls, acute allograft rejection in CCR4-/- recipients is only slightly prolonged. In contrast, cardiac graft survival is significantly prolonged in CCR4-/- recipients in chronic cardiac allograft rejection model. It is observed that the percentage of graft-infiltrating CD8+ T cells increase relatively in CCR4-/- recipients within 30 days after transplantation and CD4+ T cells decrease simultaneously. Moreover, the percentage of NK1.1+CD3+ graft-infiltrating cells is significantly reduced on day 5 and day 30 posttransplantation. These findings suggest that CCR4 is responsible for the recruitment of NK1.1+CD3+ cells into cardiac allograft and plays an important novel role in chronic graft rejection [61].

CCR5 play a crucial role in the development of acute and chronic allograft rejection. The induction of CCR5 expression in endomyocardial biopsy tissue is known to correlate with leukocyte graft infiltration. CCR5 ligands are upregulated during allograft rejection aiding infiltration of leukocytes. Using wild type and CCR5-/- mice as recipients of fully MHC mismatched heart and carotid-artery allografts seek to identify potential pathophysiologic mechanisms leading to allograft damage. In spite of no change in histologic rejection grade status, CCR5 expresses higher level in heart allograft biopsies during later rejection than episodes occurring shortly after transplantation [60, 62]. Four metalloproteinase genes, that are matrix metalloproteinase (Mmp) 3, Mmp12, Mmp13 and a disintegrin and metalloprotease domain (Adam) 8, significantly diminish intragraft mRNA expression in CCR5-/- mice on day 6 after transplantation. Accordingly, less tissue remodeling and thus better preservation of the myocardial architecture are observed in allografts from CCR5-/- mice, compared with allografts from wild type recipients. Moreover, survival of cardiac allografts prolong significantly in CCR5-/- mice. Carotid artery allografts from CCR5-/- recipients show better tissue preservation, and significant reduction of neointima formation and CD3+ T cell infiltration. CCR5 exhibits an essential role in transplant associated arteriosclerosis that may involve metalloproteinase mediated vessel wall remodeling. It is concluded that early tissue remodeling may be a critical feature in the predisposition of allografts to the development of chronic dysfunction [63]. Another research investigates the impact of CCR5 gene polymorphism on cardiac transplant. Individuals homozygous for a 32 base pair deletion in the CCR5 gene (CCR5Delta32) have an inactive receptor. There is no correlation between CCR5Delta32 polymorphism of recipient and outcome following human cardiac transplantation. However, a significant correlation is observed between donor genotype and mortality of transplant recipients in a nonischemic condition. It suggests that donor CCR5 may be more important for leukocyte trafficking during rejection than recipient CCR5 expression [64]. The analysis of a cohort of heart transplant patients show that the interaction of functional genetic variants links with the outcomes of acute rejection episodes. For example, subjects carrying the allele-allele CX3CR1 249I and CCR5 No-E are at significant lower risk of suffering early acute rejection (0-3 months after transplantation). In contrast subjects carrying both the CCR5 E and CCL5 403A allele were at significant higher risk of experiencing late acute rejection (4-12 months after transplantation) [65]. It suggests that increased intensity of inflammation in rejection occurring at later times posttransplant can be revealed by molecular analyses of the graft.

Alloantigen presentation to antigen specific T lymphocytes by donor or recipient dendritic cells (DCs) induces acute rejection after solid organ transplantation. DCs can be divided into two subsets, myeloid (mDC) and plasmacytoid (pDC) dendritic cell, which circulate differentially between bone marrow, heart and lymphoid tissues after cardiac transplantation. Subsets are further characterized for maturation marker CD83 and lymphoid homing chemokine receptor CCR7. Although the number of both DC subsets remain low in the whole post cardiac transplantation period, it is observed that a negative association of mDCs with rejection grade. The investigation shows that only mDCs decreased during acute rejection episodes. Rejectors have lower mDC numbers after a 3-month follow-up compared to nonrejectors. Furthermore, patients during acute rejection exhibit low proportions of mDCs positive for CD83 or CCR7. These findings suggest peripheral blood mDC depletion in association with selective lymphoid homing of this subset during acute rejection after clinical cardiac transplantation [66].

CX3CL1 is a structurally unusual member of the chemokine family. The mice with a targeted disruption of CX3CR1 are generated to determine the role of CX3CL1 in vivo. Heterotopic MHC class I / II cardiac transplants are performed from BALB/c mice into C57BL/6 mice. In the absence of cyclosporin A (CsA), there is no difference in graft survival time between CX3CR1-/- and wild type recipient mice. However, in the presence of subtherapeutic levels of CsA, graft survival time is significantly increased in the CX3CR1-/- mice. Characterization of cells infiltrating into the grafts revealed a selective reduction in natural killer cells in the CX3CR1-/- recipients in the absence of CsA and a reduction in macrophages, natural killer cells, and other leukocytes in the presence of CsA. It is concluded that the development of CX3CR1 antagonists may allow reductions in the doses of immunosuppressive drugs used in transplantation [67].

Allogeneic transplantation presents several challenges to the innate and adaptive immune systems including leukocyte recruitment, activation, and effector function. The chemokine receptors and their ligands are induced by the transplant procedure, alloantigen and gene transfer vector administration in murine cardiac grafts. For instance, CXCR3, CCR5, CCR2, CCR3 genes and those of their corresponding ligands are selectively and strongly induced in grafts that develop transplant vasculopathy. The expression patterns of these receptors are similar in both cardiac and aortic allografts, although their induction and absolute expression levels are amplified several folds in the grafted aorta compared with heart grafts. The genes which are induced before morphologic changes became apparent, and then expression is sustained during the whole period of neointimal formation [55, 56]. It is observed an induction of a programmed, time-dependent cascade of chemokines after transplantation. Antagonists to chemokine receptors and their ligands have the potential to become important therapeutics in treatment of acute and chronic rejection. However, the therapeutic options will likely have to differ depending on the stage of rejection because of the complexity of the chemokine cascade. For example, a reasonable strategy might be to target CXCR1 and CXCR2 to decrease the innate immune response induced by the transplant procedure at the earliest stages; later on, targeting CCR7 will interfere with APC homing to lymphoid organs. Once rejection begins, multiple potent Th1 type chemokines CXCL8, CXCL9, CXCL10, CCL2, CCL3, and CCL5 may have to be ablated simultaneously, as almost all the inflammatory chemokines have been shown to be involved in this period [68, 69].

Lung Transplantation

Lung transplantation remains the only effective therapy for patients with end stage lung disease, but survival is limited by the development of bronchiolitis obliterans syndrome (BOS). BOS is characterized by persistent peribronchiolar leukocyte recruitment leading to airway fibrosis and obliteration. The ELR+ CXC chemokines can mediate neutrophil recruitment and promote angiogenesis. CXCR2 is their shared endothelial cell receptor, that is, CXCR2 play a role in the regulation of angiogenesis-mediated airway fibroproliferation [70]. The elevated levels of multiple ELR+ CXC chemokines correlate with the presence of BOS. A murine model of BOS can not only demonstrate an early neutrophil infiltration but also mark vascular remodeling in the tracheal allografts. In addition, tracheal allograft ELR+ CXC chemokines are persistently expressed even in the absence of significant neutrophil infiltration and are temporally associated with vascular remodeling during fibro-obliteration of the tracheal allograft. Furthermore, treatment with anti-CXCR2 antibodies inhibits early neutrophil infiltration and later vascular remodeling, which result in the attenuation of murine BOS. A more profound attenuation of fibro-obliteration is seen when CXCR2-/- mice received cyclosporin A. This supports the notion that the CXCR2/CXCR2 ligand biological axis has a bimodal function during the course of BOS: it is important for neutrophil recruitment in early stage; and during fibro-obliteration, it is important for vascular remodeling independent of neutrophil recruitment in late stage. By integrating an understanding of neovascularization into the study of events that occur between inflammation and fibrosis, it becomes increasingly possible to rationally design therapies that can halt conditions of maladaptive fibrosis [71].

Acute lung transplant rejection is characterized by a perivascular/bronchiolar leukocyte infiltration. The ELR- CXC chemokines CXCL9, CXCL10, and CXCL11 are potent chemoattractants for leukocytes and act through their common receptor CXCR3. Increased expression levels of these chemokines in bronchoalveolar lavage fluid are linked with human continuum from acute to chronic lung allograft rejection. In a rat orthotopic lung allograft acute rejection transplantation model, it is observed that increased expression of CXCL9 and CXCL10 parallels the recruitment of mononuclear cells and cells expressing CXCR3 to the allograft. CXCL9 and CXCL10 are up-regulated in unique patterns following tracheal transplantation in mice. CXCL9 expression peaks on day 7 posttransplant, while CXCL10 expression peaks on day 1 and then again day 7 posttransplant. The expression of CXCL10 increases in bronchoalveolar lavage fluid taken from human lungs 24 hours after lung transplantation. Further analysis find that 3 hours after transplantation CXCL10 is donor tissue derived and not dependent on IFN-γ or STAT1, while 24 hours after transplantation CXCL10 is from recipient tissue and regulated by IFN-γ and STAT1. Expression of both CXCL9 and CXCL10 7 days posttransplant is regulated by IFN-γ and STAT1 [72]. In vivo neutralization of CXCR3 or its ligands CXCL9 and CXCL10 decrease intragraft recruitment of CXCR3+ mononuclear cells and attenuated BOS. However, deletion of either CXCL9 or CXCL10 did not affect airway obliteration. These data show that in this murine model of obliterative bronchiolitis, these chemokines are differentially regulated following transplantation, and that deletion of either chemokine alone does not affect the development of airway obliteration. Furthermore, the combination of low dose cyclosporin A with anti-CXCL9 therapy had more profound effects on intragraft leukocyte infiltration and in reducing acute allograft rejection. This supports the notion that ligand/CXCR3 plays an important role in the recruitment of mononuclear cells, a pivotal event in the pathogenesis of BOS [73, 74].

The early epithelial marker of progenitor epithelial cells which exists in the bone marrow and the circulation are cytokeratin 5 (CK5) and CXCR4. In a mouse model of sex-mismatched tracheal transplantation, it is found that CK5+ circulating progenitor epithelial cells contribute to re-epithelialization of the airway and re-establishment of the pseudostratified epithelium. The presence of CXCL12 in tracheal transplants provides a mechanism for CXCR4+ circulating progenitor epithelial cell recruitment to the airway. Depletion of CXCL12 results in the epithelium defaulting to squamous metaplasia, which is derived solely from the resident tissue progenitor epithelial cells. These findings demonstrate that CXCR4/CXCL12 mediated recruitment of circulating progenitor epithelial cells is necessary for the re-establishment of a normal pseudostratified epithelium after airway injury posttransplant [75].

CCL2 is a potent mononuclear cell chemoattractant. The expression of CCL2/CCR2 during an allogeneic-response promotes persistent recruitment of leukocytes and ultimately leads to rejection. The elevated levels of biologically active CCL2 in human bronchial lavage fluid are associated with the continuum from acute to chronic allograft rejection. Increased CCL2 expression parallels mononuclear cell recruitment and CCR2 expression in a murine model of BOS. In CCR2-/- mice or in wild type mice treated with neutralizing antibodies to

CCL2, loss of CCL2/CCR2 signaling significantly reduce recruitment of mononuclear phagocytes following tracheal transplantation and lead to attenuation of BOS. But lymphocyte infiltration is not reduced under these conditions [76]. In addition, CCL5 is also a potent mononuclear cell chemoattractant. Patients with allograft rejection have a significant increase in CCL5 in their bronchoalveolar lavages compared with healthy allograft recipients. Rat lung allografts demonstrate a marked time-dependent increase in levels of CCL5 compared with syngeneic control lungs. CCL5 levels correlate with the temporal recruitment of mononuclear cells and the expression of corresponding receptors CCR1 and CCR5. In vivo neutralization of CCL5 attenuated acute lung allograft rejection and reduced allospecific responsiveness by markedly decreasing mononuclear cell recruitment [77]. Other studies demonstrate that the concentration of human β-defensin-2, which can elicit adaptive immune response by means of recruitment of immature CD34+ dendritic cells and CD4+CD45RO+ memory T cells through interactions with its receptor CCR6, is significantly elevated in bronchoalveolar lavage fluid with BOS [78]. These results support the idea that CCR1, CCR2, CCR5, and CCR6 have an important role in the pathogenesis of acute lung allograft rejection.

Kidney Transplantation

Some chemokine receptors have been shown to play important roles in acute renal transplant rejection and chronic allograft nephropathy. Infiltration of renal allografts by leukocytes is a hallmark of acute transplant rejection [79]. Ischemia/reperfusion injury is an inherent consequence of solid organ transplantation that increases tissue inflammation and negatively impacts organ transplant function and survival. Following ischemia/reperfusion, CXCR2 produced in graft attract and activate granulocytes in a rat model, which in turn promote graft damage. It is effective that using repertaxin, a CXCR2 inhibitor, to treat the recipient animal can prevent granulocyte infiltration and renal function impairment in allogeneic transplantation. The possibility to modulate ischemia/reperfusion injury in this rat model opens new perspectives for preventing posttransplant delayed graft function in humans [80]. Another research investigates the expression levels of CXCL8, one of CXCR2 ligands, gene in living versus cadaver donor renal allografts before and after reperfusion. CXCL8 expression increase 50% from ischemia to reperfusion in living donor grafts but increase more than 13 folds during reperfusion of cadaver donor grafts. Increased total ischemia time induce greater CXCL8 expression during reperfusion. Expression levels of CXCL8 correlate with the ischemic time imposed on the renal graft [81]. In biopsy-proven acute rejections, which occur less than 2 months after transplantation, urinary CXCL8 concentrations are elevated markedly, preceding clinical diagnosis of rejection. After treatment, the CXCL8 concentration in urine decrease back to normal. The highest urinary CXCL8 concentrations are seen in patients with biopsy-proven rejection in combination with acute tubular necrosis. CXCL8 positive staining is found within interstitial mononuclear cells, arteriolar smooth muscle, and tubular cells of all biopsy specimens showing rejection. It is necessary to further determine the clinical value of urinary CXCL8 determinations in the diagnosis of rejection and to evaluate the role of CXCL8 in the pathogenesis of acute allograft rejection [82].

CXCR3 also plays pivotal roles in the recruitment and activation of inflammatory cells during renal allograft injury. CXCR3 is expressed by infiltrating inflammatory cells, but not by intrinsic renal structures. CXCR3 positive cells are found to be involved in tubulitis and vascular rejection. The area of CXCR3 positive staining is significantly larger in biopsies with acute interstitial rejection and acute vascular rejection as compared with normal renal graft biopsies. There is a strong morphological and numerical correlation between CXCR3 and CD4+ and CD8+ T cells, respectively. During renal allograft rejection, the number of CD4+ and CD8+ T cells expressing CXCR3 increase significantly at the site of injury and might be targeted by CXCR3 blocking agents [83]. The levels of CXCL10, a CXCR3 ligand, in pretransplant serum represent a clinically useful parameter for the identification of subjects exhibiting high risk of acute rejection, chronic allograft nephropathy and graft failure [84]. These results might be used to individualize immunosuppressive therapies.

B cells also play a crucial role in acute renal allograft rejection. The partial patients with acute rejection show a substantial infiltration of cluster forming B cells into transplants. CXCL13 and its receptor CXCR5 are exclusively detected in areas of B cell clusters. Intrarenal CXCL13 mRNA expression is 27 folds higher in transplants with B cell clusters than rejecting allografts without B cell accumulation. It is suggested that a striking colocalization of CXCL13 expression with CXCR5+ and CD20+ B cells in renal transplants undergoing rejection, and CXCL13 and its specific receptor CXCR5 have a potential role in recruitment of B cells in renal allograft rejection [85].

CCL2, CCL5, CCR1, CCR2, and CCR5 express increased level in acute renal transplant rejection. In particular, CCR1 show high expression prior to rejection and return to baseline levels with antirejection therapy. Therefore CCR1 may have potential use in immunomonitoring in PBMCs and as predictive factors of rejection prior to its clinical manifestation [86]. Another research on CCR1 antagonist BX471 also confirms that CCR1 is a potential therapeutic target. BX471, a competitive antagonist of rabbit CCR1, is able to compete with high affinity with the CCR1 ligands CCL3 and CCL5 in a rabbit kidney transplant rejection model. Animals subcutaneously implanted with slow release pellets of BX471 have increased transplant survival compared with untreated controls or animals implanted with placebo. Furthermore, there is a marked reduction in the urea and creatinine levels in the BX471 treated animals compared with the control and placebo groups. BX471 shows clear efficacy at the single dose tested compared with animals treated with placebo. Pathologic analyses show that BX471 is similar to cyclosporin in its ability to prevent extensive infarction of transplanted kidneys [87]. In addition, the mRNA expressions of CCL2 and CCR2 of all patients with kidney posttransplant are significantly higher than healthy controls. The mRNA expressions of CCL2 and CCR2 in posttransplant patients with hyperlipidemia are much higher than patients with normal lipidemia. After patients with hyperlipidemia are treated with simvastatin, the mRNA expressions of CCL2 and CCR2 are significantly reduced in one and a half months and decrease to the lowest levels in three months. Simvastatin can decrease the expressions of CCL2 and CCR2 in post-kidney transplant patients with hyperlipidemia [88].

Compared to acute renal transplant rejection, chronic rejection, the most important cause of long-term graft failure, is thought to result from both alloantigen-dependent and alloantigen-independent processes which are mediated by cytokines and chemokines. Some chemokine receptors and their ligands could have impact on the development of chronic allograft nephropathy because they are involved in tissue regeneration. The differences in the quantity of expression between the different chemokines and chemokine receptors point to a complex regulation of chemokine expression in renal allografts. Biopsies with chronic allograft nephropathy reveal that the expression of CCL2, CCL5, CCR1, CCR2 and CCR5 are upregulated, and the graft is infiltrated by CCR5 positive mononuclear cells during acute and chronic transplant rejection [89, 90]. During an early reversible allograft rejection episode, CCL5 peaked at 2 weeks; CCL2 increased dramatically to 10 times, presaging intense peak macrophage infiltration at 16 weeks. CCL2 is maximally expressed at 52 weeks, commensurate with a progressive increase in infiltrating macrophages. Chronic rejection of kidney allografts in rats is predominantly a local macrophage-dependent event with intense up-regulation of macrophage products such as CCL2, IL-6, and inducible nitric oxide synthase. The dynamics of CCL5 expression between early and late phases of chronic rejection suggest a key role in mediating the events of the chronic process [49, 91].

The risk of acute rejection in renal transplantation is associated with genetic variation in the chemokine receptors CCR2 and CCR5, and chemokine CCL5. In 163 renal transplant recipients, some studies examine the association of human chemokine receptor genetic variants, CCR5Delta32, CCR5-59029-A/G, CCR2-V64I, CX3CR1-V249I, and CX3CR1-T280M. The risk of acute renal transplant rejection is reduced significantly in recipients who possess the CCR2-V64I allele or who are homozygous for the CCR5-59029A allele. Patients homozygous for CCR5Delta32 show longer survival of renal transplants than in the control group, suggesting a pathophysiological role for CCR5 in transplant loss [90, 92, 93]. However, there are also opposite results that investigate the Turkish population. They show the risk of acute rejection in renal transplantation may be associated with genetic variation in the chemokine receptor genes CCR5-59029 and CCR2V641 in Turkey, and no significant difference in the incidence of rejection among patients possessing or lacking CCR5-Delta32 [94]. In addition to chemokine receptor genes, CCL2 overproduction and CCL5-109TT allele are as well associated with significant deterioration of graft function. The strength of the alloimmune response after renal transplantation is in part genetically determined. Donor-recipient matching of chemokine and chemokine receptor gene polymorphisms has a marginal effect [95]. These gene polymorphisms may be an ideal target for future interventions intended to prevent renal transplant loss.

African American patients demonstrate higher rates of acute allograft rejection and lower kidney graft survival compared with white patients. An investigation examines Duffy blood group status of African American kidney-transplant recipients. Duffy antigen receptor for chemokines (DARC) on red blood cells has been suggested to attenuate the inflammatory effects of delayed graft function by acting as a "chemokine sink". Only the patients who have Duffy positive antigen don't lose their allograft. In contrast, Duffy negative patients demonstrate low allograft survival. Delayed graft function is strongly associated with graft failure for only Duffy negative patients, that is to say, Duffy negative patients have lower allograft survival in the presence of delayed graft function [96].

Chemokines attract leukocytes bearing specific chemokine receptors, and the specific leukocyte chemokine receptor phenotype is associated with types of immune responses, that is, T helper subtype 1 (Th1; CXCR3, CCR5) versus T helper subtype 2 (Th2; CCR3, CCR4, CCR8). Upregulated mRNAs of CCR2 and CCR5 are documented during allograft rejection. The number of CXCR4, CCR5, and CCR2 mRNAs expressing leukocytes and DARC positive vessels increase during rejection episodes. Leukocytes in diffuse interstitial infiltrates are mainly CCR5 positive, but in areas in which leukocytes form nodular aggregates of infiltrating cells, the number of CCR5 positive cells is low. Instead, leukocyte in these nodular aggregates mainly express CXCR4. DARC is expressed on peritubular capillaries, where it is upregulated in areas of interstitial infiltration. Induction of chemokines during renal allograft rejection is accompanied by infiltration of leukocytes bearing the respective chemokine receptors. The upregulation of the CXCR3 ligand CXCL10, as well as CCR5 and its ligands, in the absence of CCR3 and CCR8 is indicative that renal allograft rejection is primarily the result of a Th1-type immune response [97].

Pancreatic Islet Transplantation

Islet transplantation introduces insulin secreting tissue into type 1 diabetes mellitus recipients, relieving patients from exogenous insulin injection. However, insulitis of grafted tissue and allograft rejection prevent long-term insulin independence [98]. Chemokine receptors and their ligands have a pivotal role in the mobilization and activation of specific leukocyte subsets in acute islet allograft rejection. Islet allograft rejection is associated with a steady increase in intragraft expression of the chemokine receptors CXCR3, CCR5, CCR2, CCR1 and their corresponding ligands CXCL9, CXCL10, CCL5, CCL8, CCL9 [99].

In comparison with untreated wild type recipients, anti-CXCL10 treated wild type recipients and CXCR3-/- recipients demonstrated the same degree of chemokine gene expression but less lymphocytic infiltrate. CXCR3 gene deletion or anti-CXCL10 antibody therapy modulates lymphocytic graft infiltration and statistically prolongs graft survival in murine islet allograft recipients. The mean length of allograft survival is markedly increased from 13 days in untreated WT to 20 days for anti-CXCL10 treated WT and CXCR3-/- recipients [100]. On the contrary, untreated WT recipients demonstrate increased graft-site gene expression for CXCL10, CCL4, CCL5 and heavy graft-site cell infiltrates at day 7 posttransplant.

CCR5 is expressed preferentially by CD4+ Th1 cells. The same as CXCR3, CCR5 also plays a crucial role in islet allograft rejection in a streptozotocin-induced diabetic mouse model. BALB/c islet allografts transplanted into CCR5-/- recipients (C57BL/6) survive significantly longer compared with those transplanted into wild-type control mice. Furthermore, twenty percent of islet allografts in CCR5-/- animals without other treatment survive more than 90 days. The possible mechanism is that intragraft mRNA expression of IL-4 and IL-5 is increased while IFN-γ is decreased in CCR5-/- mice [101]. That means a Th2 pattern of T-cell activation in the target tissues versus a Th1 pattern observed in controls. A similar Th2 response pattern is also observed in the periphery (splenocytes responding to donor cells). It can be concluded that CCR5 plays an important role in orchestrating the Th1 immune response which leads to islet allograft rejection [102].

According to above mentioned findings, the effect of a novel, small molecule compound TAK-779 by targeting CCR5 and CXCR3 in acute islet allograft rejection is tested in vivo. Treatment of TAK-779 significantly prolongs allograft survival across the MHC barrier in two distinct transplant models. Furthermore, TAK-779 treatment significantly attenuated the development of chronic vasculopathy, fibrosis and cellular infiltration [103]. The treatment of anti-CCR5 and anti-CXCR3 has an evident therapeutic effect on inhibiting both acute and chronic allograft rejection. Therefore, targeting the CCR5 and CXCR3 may provide a clinically useful strategy to prevent islet allograft rejection in the future.

Another important target is CCR2, which is highly induced and plays a specific role in early islet allograft rejection. In fully MHC mismatched transplant model, islet allograft is transplanted from BALB/c mice into C57BL/6 wild-type and CCR2-/-. The median survival time of islet allograft is prolonged obviously from 12 days for wild type recipients to 24 days for CCR2-/- recipients. However, these changes are only transient in CCR2-/- recipients that ultimately rejected their grafts [99]. In contrast to the islet transplants, CCR2 deficiency offered only marginal prolongation of heart allograft survival. This study highlights the tissue specificity of the chemokine receptor system in vivo in regulating allograft rejection.

Liver Transplantation

Graft rejection after liver transplantation is associated with a lymphocytic infiltrate, the nature of which will be determined by the local activity of chemokines that attract particular subsets of effector cells to the graft. Ischemia-reperfusion injury causes induction of hepatic transcripts for CCL5, CCL2, CCL3, CXCL2, and CXCL10. CCL2, CCL5, and CXCL10 are notable as induced chemokines that are chemotactic to T lymphocytes. The induction of chemokines may contribute to transient lymphopenia and neutrophilia that occur after liver ischemia-reperfusion injury [104]. The chemokine receptors CCR5, CCR6, CXCR3, and CXCR4 are reported to increase on circulating and graft-infiltrating lymphocytes after liver transplantation. Liver-derived T cells responded to the ligands for these receptors in vitro, which suggests that the receptors are functionally active. CXCR3 ligands CXCL9 and CXCL10 are detected on sinusoidal endothelium and CXCL11 is detected on portal and hepatic vascular endothelium, whereas the CXCR4 ligand CXCL12 is restricted to biliary epithelium. CCR5 ligands show on portal endothelium. An in vitro model of T-cell alloactivation demonstrates a similar pattern of expression of functional CXCR3, CXCR4, and CCR5 on T cells. Increased expression of chemokine receptors, especially CCR3 and CCR5, is associated with redistribution of activated Kupffer cells in rejecting grafts. Although ligands for the receptors CXCR3 and CCR5 are important for recruitment, the restriction of CXCL12 to bile ducts suggests that CXCR4 may be involved in the retention of alloactivated lymphocytes at sites of graft damage [105]. CCL20 and CCR6 cells are detected in the portal fields of all acute allograft rejection biopsy specimens. The C4d deposits along the portal capillaries indicate a humoral mediated alloresponse caused by the accumulated B and plasma cells, which are promoted by the expression of B-cell activating chemokine receptor system in acute liver rejection [106].

The production of some chemokine receptors and their ligands varies among individuals and these variations may be determined by genetic polymorphisms, most commonly within the regulatory region of the gene. Ischemic-type biliary lesions are a major complication following orthotopic liver transplantation. Unlike in renal transplants, the non-function CCR5delta32 polymorphism is a significant risk factor for the development of ischemic-type biliary lesions after liver transplantation. The incidence of ischemic-type biliary lesions in patients increased from 12% with WT CCR5 to 31% with CCR5delta32. The rate of 5 year patient survival decreased from 85% with WT CCR5 to 70% with CCR5delta32 [107]. Therefore the CCR5 status should be screened prospectively before liver transplantation.

Another analysis shows that three variants of genotype CCL2-2518, CCL5-28, and CCR5-59029 neither influence the incidence of acute rejection nor affect long-term allograft survival upon liver transplantation [108].

Dendritic cell trafficking is regulated by chemokine receptor CCR7. Donor DC migrates into the recipient spleen after hepatic transplantation. The CCR7 ligand CCL19 is expressed mainly within the splenic white pulp. Immunological unresponsiveness to rat hepatic allografts can be induced by prior donor-specific blood transfusion (DST). Some studies investigate homing receptor phenotype and splenic distribution of donor DC after allografting and DST. In conclusion, differential splenic migration of CCR5lowCCR7low DC expressing Th2-type cytokines is associated with immunological unresponsiveness to rat hepatic allografts [109]. According to comparing CC chemokine receptor expression by mouse liver myeloid lymphoid-related DC and plasmacytoid DC subsets and their responsiveness to CC chemokines, it is found that immature liver DC does not respond to any CC chemokines tested, despite expression of mRNA encoding appropriate receptors for their ligands. CCR7 expression by each liver DC subset is strongly enhanced in response to maturation. The migratory capacity of liver plasmacytoid DC is similar to that of liver myeloid and lymphoid-related DC. These findings suggest that targeting of CCR7 and its ligands may be a potential approach for manipulation of liver DC trafficking to secondary lymphoid tissue after liver transplantation [110].

Bone Marrow Transplantation

In healthy adults, hematopoiesis takes place in the bone marrow, where the majority of hematopoietic progenitor cells (HPC, CD34+ cells) reside. In patients undergoing chemotherapy or radiotherapy, hematopoiesis is seriously disturbed. Reconstitution of bone marrow function can be achieved by bone marrow transplantation or peripheral blood stem cell transplantation. Recently, much attention has been focused on the close association between hematopoiesis and chemokine receptors, because of the possibility of direct consequence for clinical practice in hematopoietic stem cell transplantation. Chemokines induce rapid hematopoietic stem and progenitor cell mobilization and synergize with hematopoietic cytokines in mobilizing stem and progenitor cells. These proteins offer new paradigms for autologous and allogeneic peripheral blood stem cell transplantation [111].

Chemokine receptor CXCR2 which interacts with selective ligand CXCL2 may be the dominant receptor mediating hematopoietic cell mobilization, and polymorphonuclear neutrophils may be the primary CXCR2 expressing target cell for stem and progenitor cell mobilization. A better understanding of the mechanisms responsible for hematopoietic stem cell (HSC) mobilization either with growth factors or chemokines will permit the development of novel, more rapid and efficacious regimens [112].

Graft versus host disease (GVHD) is a major complication of allogeneic hematopoietic stem cell transplantation. It is initiated by infiltrating donor T cells specific against the host antigens [113]. To investigate the role of CXCR3 on donor cells in acute GVHD, some studies investigate an experimental model of bone marrow transplantation (BMT) where acute GVHD is mediated by donor CD8+ T cells against minor histocompatibility antigens. Significantly higher numbers of donor CD8+ CXCR3-/- T cells are found in the spleen on days 7 and 14 after BMT compared to donor wild-type T cells. By contrast, the number of

CD8+ T cells in the small bowel of BMT recipients from CXCR3-/- donors is sevenfold lower than from wild-type donors. Animals that received CXCR3-/- donor T cells demonstrate diminished gastrointestinal tract and liver damage and show improved survival after BMT compared to recipients of wild-type donor cells. The migration of donor CD8+ T cells to GVHD target organs such as the intestine depends on the expression of CXCR3 and contributes significantly to GVHD damage and overall mortality [114]. With regard to idiopathic pneumonia syndrome (IPS), it is a frequently fatal complication after allogeneic stem cell transplantation (allo-SCT) that responds poorly to standard immunosuppressive therapy. CXCR3 is expressed on activated Th1/Tc1 T cell subsets and the expression of its ligands CXCL9 and CXCL10 can be induced in a variety of cell types by IFN-γ alone or in combination with TNF-α. The expression levels of CXCL9 and CXCL10 proteins, which correlate with the infiltration of IFN-γ-secreting CXCR3+ donor T cells into the lung, are significantly enhanced in the bronchoalveolar lavage fluid of allo-SCT recipients compared with syngeneic controls. The neutralization of either CXCL9 or CXCL10 in vivo significantly reduces the severity of IPS compared with control-treated animals, and shows an additive effect when both ligands are blocked simultaneously. Complementary experiments using CXCR3-/- mice as SCT donors also result in a significant decrease in IPS. These data demonstrate that interactions of CXCR3 and its ligands CXCL9 and CXCL10 significantly contribute to donor T cell recruitment to the lung after allo-SCT. Therefore, approaches focusing on the abrogation of these interactions may prove successful in preventing or treating lung injury that occurs in this setting [115].

The success of stem cell transplantation depends on the ability of intravenously infused stem cells to lodge in the bone marrow, a process referred to as homing. Homing is a multistep process, consisting of adhesion of the HPC to endothelial cells of the marrow sinusoids, followed by transendothelial migration directed by chemoattractants, and finally anchoring within the extravascular bone marrow spaces where proliferation and differentiation will occur. One of the most important factors which determine the engraftment potential of stem cells is the role of the CXCR4 and its ligand CXCL12 [116, 117]. Improving approaches for HSC and HPC mobilization is clinically important because increased numbers of these cells are needed for enhanced transplantation. The CXCL12-CXCR4 axis is believed to be involved in retention of HSCs and HPCs in bone marrow. AMD3100, a selective antagonist of the CXCR4, is evaluated in murine, dog and human systems for mobilizing capacity, alone and in combination with granulocyte colony-stimulating factor (G-CSF). AMD3100 mobilizes a population of hematopoietic stem cells with intrinsic characteristics different from those of hematopoietic stem cells mobilized with G-CSF, suggesting fundamental differences in the mechanism of AMD3100 mediated and G-CSF mediated hematopoietic stem cell mobilization [118]. Human CD34+ cells isolated after treatment with G-CSF plus AMD3100 express a phenotype that is characteristic of highly engrafting mouse HSC. Synergy of AMD3100 and G-CSF in mobilization is due to enhanced numbers and perhaps other characteristics of the mobilized cells [119]. Surprisingly, HSC also express mRNA for CCR3 and CCR9, although they failed to migrate to the ligands for these receptors. The sharply restricted chemotactic responsiveness of HSC is unique among leukocytes and may be necessary for the specific homing of circulating HSC to bone marrow, as well as for the maintenance of HSC in hematopoietic microenvironments [120].

Co-expression of CXCR4 on CD34+ progenitor cells may be an important determinant of posttransplant engraftment [121]. The increased migration of cord blood (CB) CD34+ cells may favor homing of these cells to the bone marrow, which might reduce the number of cells required for hematological reconstitution after transplantation. These results shed new light on the potential role of this CXCL12 in the stem cell engraftment process, which involves migration, adhesion, and proliferation. Manipulating the interaction between CXCL12 and CXCR4 may be of clinical relevance for improving cell therapy settings in stem cell transplantation [122, 123]. In addition, other studies suggest that G-CSF induced mobilization of HPC from bone marrow (BM) involves the matrix metalloproteinase 9, without reversing the positive gradient of CXCL12 between BM and peripheral blood (PB). A clear relationship is between the levels of circulating HPC, both at steady state and after mobilization by cyclophosphamide and G-CSF administration, and those of secreted Mmp9 but not of CXCL12. However, a negative correlation is observed between mobilizing capacity and CXCR4 expression on CD34+ cells [124]. The human stem cell compartment is heterogeneous for CXCR4 expressions, which suggest that the relationship between CXCR4 expression and stem cell repopulating function is not obligatory [125].

Human natural killer (NK) and NK T cells play an important role in allogeneic BM transplantation and graft-versus-leukemia (GVL) effect. The retention of NK and NK T cells within the spleen and BM is dependent on Galphai signaling and CXCR4 function. The chemokine receptors CXCR4 and CXCR3 are expressed predominantly on the cell surface of NK T cells. Following activation with IL-2, the levels of CXCR4 on NK and NK T cells decrease significantly. Treatment of cells with IL-2 inhibited their migration in response to CXCL12 and their homing and retention in the BM and spleen of NOD/SCID mice. In contrast to CXCR4, the expression levels of the chemokine receptor CXCR3 and the migration of cells in response to CXCL9 and CXCL10 increased after IL-2 treatment. Moreover, CXCR4 is an autonomous cell essential for long-term lymphoid and myeloid reconstitution in adult bone marrow. Thus, upregulation of CXCR4 expression may be useful for improving engraftment of repopulating stem cells in clinical transplantation [126]. Whereas down-regulation of CXCR4 and up-regulation of CXCR3 may direct the trafficking of cells to the site of inflammation, rather than to hematopoietic organs, and therefore may limit their alloreactive potential [127].

Some experiments show that quantitative monitoring of the gene expression of CXCR3, CCR1, CCR5, and CCR2 may be a valuable molecular method to monitor and diagnose acute GVHD, although they are not specific for acute GVHD [128]. In addition, the leukocyte recruitment during IPS is dependent in part upon interactions between CCR2 and its primary ligand CCL2. Compared with syngeneic controls, pulmonary expression of CCL2 and CCR2 mRNA is significantly increased after allogeneic bone marrow transplantation. Transplantation of CCR2-/- donor cells result in a significant reduction in IPS severity compared with transplantation of wild type donor cells. In addition, neutralization of CCL2 result in significantly decreased lung injury compared with control-treated allogeneic recipients. Collectively, these data demonstrate that CCR2/CCL2 interactions significantly contribute to the development of experimental IPS and suggest that interventions blocking these receptor-ligand interactions may represent novel strategies to prevent or treat this lethal complication after allogeneic bone marrow transplantation [129].

With regard to other members of chemokine and chemokine receptor family, the analysis of gene polymorphisms, which relate to immune function for association with human cytomegalovirus disease in patients after allogeneic stem cell transplantation, show two relevant markers. One is CCR5 and IL-10 genes conferring a higher risk for the development of human cytomegalovirus disease. The other is CCL2 gene associated with human cytomegalovirus reactivation. Testing of high-risk patients for the presence of these single nucleotide polymorphisms might be useful for individualizing antiviral prophylaxis [130].

Skin Transplantation

CXCR3, a receptor for both CXCL10 and CXCL9, is predominantly expressed on memory/activated T cells. It is reported that CXCL10 and CXCL9 play a critical role in the allograft rejection. CXCR3 is a dominant factor directing T cells into mouse skin allograft to induce acute rejection, without interfering with other functions of the T cells [131].

Using double color flow cytometry, some studies analyze the distribution and modulation of CCR5 or CXCR3 on CD3+ spleen T cells from mice. The percentage of CCR5+ cell fractions in freshly isolated spleen CD3+ T cells is less than 8%. During 7 days after skin allograft transplantation, CCR5+ cell fraction in spleen T cells increase gradually and reach to 66%. CXCR3 is also expressed less than 10% in freshly isolated CD3+ spleen T cells. Within 7 days after skin allograft transplantation, CXCR3+ cell fractions in spleen T cells also gradually increase to 98%. Using real-time quantitative RT-PCR assay and Northern blots, it is observed a similar pattern of CCR5 and CXCR3 mRNA expression in allografts at the different time intervals after allotransplantation. Furthermore, to quantitatively characterize the subpopulation of infiltrating cells that are expressing CXCR3, the cells from the allograft are analyzed after skin transplantation. It is observed that CXCR3 is highly expressed on CD4+ and CD8+ T cells from the grafts at 7 days after skin transplantation compared with native skin biopsies, whereas the expression of CXCR3 is not significantly changed on CD19+ B cells and CD14+ monocytes [131].

Chemokines are likely to play a critical role in directing leukocytes to skin allograft sites and in amplifying intragraft inflammation during rejection. Two general patterns of chemokine gene expression in each of the allografts are observed. Intragraft expression of first group of chemokine genes, such as CCL3 and CCL4, is observed at peak levels 3 days posttransplant in allograft models, and expression of levels reach 10 to 17 folds higher than control isografts on day 5 after transplantation [132]. A second group of chemokine genes, including CCL5 and CXCL10, is expressed at low levels at early times after transplantation but at high levels 4 days before rejection of the allografts is complete. Isograft expression of CCL5 and CXCL10 is undetectable at the late time points. The results suggest that these two patterns of chemoattractant cytokine gene expression may be representative of the early inflammatory and the late T cell mediated phases of the allograft rejection process, respectively [133]. Furthermore, the mRNA expression of different CC and CXC chemokines are investigated in the grafts at different time intervals after allotransplantation. After allograft transplantation, the CCL4, CCL5, and CCL11 mRNA expressions are significantly changed in the skin grafts at days 3, 5, and 7. CXCL9 and CXCL10 mRNA expressions are highly up-regulated in the grafts at days 3, 5, and 7. In addition, the abilities of CXCL9 and CXCL10 to induce CD3+ spleen T cell chemotaxis are as well highly increased. The increases start by day 3 after allograft transplantation and persist by day 5 and day 7 after transplantations [131].

Following figure gives a brief summary of all the mentioned chemokines and chemokine receptors, which are involved in transplant rejectin of various organs or tissue (figure 1). With further research, many more chemokine receptors with more functions may be discoverd.

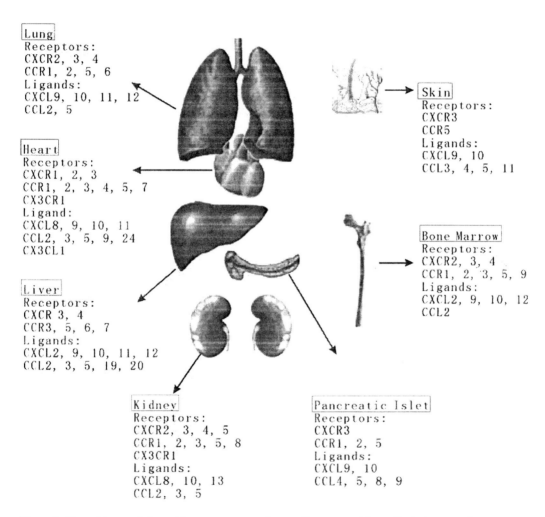

Figure 1. Chemokines and chemokine receptors are abnormally expressed in grafts during transplants rejection.

B. Chemokine Receptors and Transplantation Tolerance

It is well-documented that certain chemokine receptors and their ligands guide homeostatic recirculation of T cells and others promote recruitment of activated T cells to inflammatory sites. However, little is known about the chemokine receptors another function, which they maintain unresponsiveness and transplantation tolerance.

CXCR6 is highly expressed on Vα14+ NKT cells. Blocking the interaction between CXCR6 and CXCL16 result in the failure to maintain graft tolerance and thus induce the acceleration of graft rejection. In a mouse transplant tolerance model, the expression of CXCL16 is up-regulated in the tolerated allograft, and anti-CXCL16 mAb inhibits intragraft accumulation of NKT cells [134]. These results prove the unique role of CXCR6 and CXCL16 molecules in the maintenance of cardiac allograft tolerance mediated by NKT cells.

Foxp3 expression is specifically up-regulated within allograft of mice displaying donor-specific tolerance, which recruitment of Foxp3+ regulatory T cells to an allograft tissue depends on intragraft up-regulating of CCR4 and its ligand CCL22. This particular tolerance induction could not be achieved in CCR4-/- recipients [135].

Immature dendritic cells can induce T-cell hyporesponsiveness, thus interfering with the process of DC maturation maybe provide a novel approach to inducing allograft tolerance. During the process of maturation, DC differentiated from monocytes are exposed to mycophenolic acid (MPA), which is an immunosuppressive agent currently used in transplantation. MPA-DC had a mature phenotype for chemokine receptor expression, exhibiting down-regulation of CCR5 and up-regulation of CCR7. Interestingly, the abilities of the MPA-DC to induce CD4+ T cell proliferation in response to alloantigens are impaired via not only direct but also indirect pathways. The maintenance of endocytosis and the inhibition of syngeneic T cell activation suggest that these cells could have a potential role to avoid chronic rejection. All these characteristics suggest that MPA-DC may be used in cell therapy to induce allograft tolerance [136].

Donor-specific tolerance to heart allografts in the rat can be achieved by donor-specific blood transfusions (DST) before transplantation. This tolerance induction requires the presence of host CD8+ T cells and is characterized by the infiltration of numerous leukocytes. To identify new mediators involved in tolerance induction, gene searching is performed and, shows that CX3CR1 is highly expressed in tolerated allografts. The high CX3CR1 mRNA accumulation in tolerated allografts is related to the active recruitment of monocytes. CX3CR1 transcript accumulation is preceded by an early expression of its ligand CX3CL1 by graft endothelial cells. Interestingly, depletion of recipient CD8+ cells leads to a dramatic decrease in both CX3CR1 and CX3CL1 mRNA levels. Moreover, in vitro, CD8+ T cells from DST primed animals are found to strongly induce CX3CL1 expression in an allogeneic endothelial cell line. These results demonstrate that CX3CR1 and CX3CL1, usually described in inflammatory processes, are expressed in a model of allograft tolerance mediated by host CD8+ T cells [137].

C. Summary

Although almost every known chemokine receptor and its ligand are expressed at some stage during development of allograft rejection, mechanistic studies indicate that the actual key chemokine receptors are rather few (table 2). From the table 2, it can be summarized that CXCR3 and CCR5 are involved in most of the organ/tissue transplant rejection. Antagonists for a number of chemokine receptor have been developed, which promote the possibility of interfering with chemokine function as a therapeutic tool [138]. In addition, it is a viable therapeutic strategy to target chemokine intracellular signaling pathways. One of the key signalling targets downstream of a variety of chemokine receptors identified to date is PI3K-γ (phosphoinositide 3-kinase gamma), a member of the class I PI3K family [1]. Data regarding the chemokine receptor system pathways in ischemia/reperfusion, as well as chronic rejection and tolerance induction following antagonism, provide some new potential entry points for immune monitoring and therapeutic intervention of transplants rejection [92, 139].

**Table 2. The expression of key chemokine receptors
in transplanted organs/tissue [25, 79, 137, 140]**

Organ/tissue	Allograft rejection	Allograft tolerance
Heart	CXCR3, CCR1, CCR2, CCR4, CCR5, CX3CR1	CXCR6, CCR4, CCR7, CX3CR1
Lung	CXCR2, CXCR3, CXCR4, CCR2, CCR5	Unknown
Kidney	CXCR2, CXCR3, CXCR5, CCR1, CCR5	Unknown
Islet	CXCR3, CCR2, CCR5	Unknown
Liver	CXCR3, CXCR4, CCR5	Unknown
Bone marrow	CXCR2, CXCR3, CXCR4, CCR2	Unknown
Skin	CXCR3, CCR5	Unknown

V. Insights into the Mechanism or Pathway of Chemokine Receptor Roles in Allogeneic Transplant Rejection

Certain chemokine receptors expressed on early innate response leukocytes and inflamed graft tissues play essential roles in promoting leukocyte migration into the graft, as well as in facilitating dendritic and T cell trafficking between lymph nodes and transplant in both early and late stage of the allogeneic response. Chemokine system might influence the allograft biology at least three aspects. Firstly, chemokines recruit leukocytes in the process of ischemia-reperfusion injury which is caused by restoration of blood flow in the allograft. Secondly, when activated by their ligands, chemokine receptors might recall the host responses to infection even during immune suppression situation. Thirdly, the inflammatory components of acute and chronic rejection are likely to be controlled by chemokines [15]. Following will discuss the mechanism of roles of several chemokine receptors in allogeneic transplant rejection.

Just as above mentioned, CXCR3 is a dominant factor directing T cells into mouse skin allograft. Then further studies show that peptide nucleic acid (PNA) CXCR3 antisense can significantly prolong skin allograft survival. To explore the mechanism of this observation, the surface chemokine receptor expression on spleen T cells from mice are analyzed after received different treatments by day 7 after skin allograft transplantation. The PNA CXCR3 significantly blocks the expression of CXCR3 in spleen CD3+ T cells, compared to other two control groups treated with normal physiological saline and mismatched PNA. PNA CXCR3 significantly and indirectly reduce CD25 and CD69 but not CD45RB expression in activated/memory subsets of CXCR3-bearing spleen T cells compared with the cells from untreated mice, whereas PNA CCR5, PNA mismatch, and normal physiological saline do not. In addition, the mRNA expression level of CXCR3 in CD3+ spleen T cells is as well dramatically inhibited by their corresponding PNA, compared to two control groups. The same pattern of CXCR3 mRNA expression in allografts is observed from animals receiving different treatments as that seen in the CD3+ spleen T cells [131].

The different treatments have not changed the chemokine expression patterns (CXCL9 and CXCL10) in the allografts from the animals that received different treatments by day 7 after transplantation, despite PNA CXCR3 having an obvious effect of prolonging skin allograft survival. This observation is interpreted that PNA CXCR3 regulate the progression of skin allograft rejection by means of a blockade of CXCR3 expression directing T cells into grafts, but without change in chemokine ligand expression. PNA CXCR3 significantly and specifically inhibit the chemotactic migration of spleen T cells toward CXCL9 and CXCL10, implying that PNA CXCR3 affects the process of skin allograft rejection by means of interfering with the T cell chemotaxis toward CXCL9 and CXCL10, which is the result of blockade of CXCR3 expression in the cells. PNA mismatch does not affect chemotactic migration of CD3+ spleen T cells after allograft transplantations. In conclusion, the mechanism of prolongation of skin allograft survival is that PNA CXCR3 directly blocks the CXCR3 expression in T cells, which is responsible for directing T cells into skin allograft to induce acute rejection, without interfering with other functions of the T cells.

CXCR4 and its ligand CXCL12 have been reported to be key players in the nesting of haematopoietic progenitors within the bone marrow. Therefore, some studies focus on the role of CXCR4 and its downstream signaling cascade. Signalling through the CXCL12 and CXCR4 has been recognized as a key event in the migratory response of HPC. Small GTPases of the Rho/Rac family might be involved in CXCL12 signalling at several different levels. The small GTPase Rho is required for the induction of $Ca(2+)$ transients in HPC, which in turn are necessary for the coordinated migratory response of HPC both in vitro and in vivo. It is reported that two toxins from Clostridium species which inhibit the small GTPase Rho suppress CXCL12-induced generation of intracellular calcium transients in HPC. Chelation of intracellular $Ca(2+)$ with BAPTA or depletion of intracellular $Ca(2+)$ stores with thapsigargin demonstrate that calcium transients are essential for CXCL12-induced chemotactic migration of HPC. Furthermore, transplantation of HPC pretreated with $Ca(2+)$ flux inhibitors into mice reveal a suppression of HPC homing to the bone marrow and increase levels of cells remaining in the bloodstream or circulating to the spleen [141]. Disturbance of CXCR4 signaling, as demonstrated by reduced basal Janus kinase JAK-2 phosphorylation [142], may result in functional impairment of cell mobilization and may participate in leukaemia extramedullary infiltration, thus, providing a rationale for therapeutic intervention. By recruiting quiescent progenitors, by participating in their survival\cycling and by sensitizing them to further cytokine synergistic action, CXCL12 likely contributes to haematopoiesis homeostasis under physiological conditions and in stress situations. The complexity of the CXCR4\CXCL12 interactions in the regulation of haematopoiesis illustrates a dynamic and sequential cross-talk between chemokine and cytokine\growth factor worlds. Because of their pleiotropic effects on haematopoietic progenitor trafficking, survival and proliferation, the CXCR4\CXCL12 couple could be considered as promising molecules for improvement of cell-based therapy protocols in haematopoietic transplantation [143].

GVHD is a major complication of allogeneic hematopoietic stem cell transplantation. Migration of donor-derived T cells into GVHD target organs plays a critical role in the development of GVHD and chemokine receptors and their ligands are important molecules involved in this process. The factors involved CCL2, CCR2 ligand, secreted by sites of neuroinflammation are attractive to neural progenitor cells that will migrate toward damaged areas of the brain [144]. In murine bone marrow transplantation models, the expression of the CCR2 on donor-derived CD8+ T cells is relevant for the control of CD8+ T cell migration and development of GVHD. Recipients of CCR2-/- CD8+ T cells develop less damage of gut and liver than recipients of wild-type CD8+ T cells, which correlate with a reduction in overall GVHD morbidity and mortality. Assessments of donor CD8+ T cell target organ infiltration reveal that CCR2-/- CD8+ T cells have an intrinsic migratory defect to the gut and liver. Other causes for the reduction in GVHD could be excluded, as alloreactive proliferation, activation, IFN-γ production and cytotoxicity of CCR2-/- CD8+ T cells are intact. Interestingly, the graft-versus-tumor (GVT) effect mediated by CCR2-/- CD8+ T cells is preserved, which suggests that interference with T cell migration by blockade of CCR2 signaling can separate GVHD from GVT activity [145].

CD4+CD25+ regulatory T cells (T regs) show function of inhibiting GVHD in murine model. T regs lacking expression of the CCR5 are demonstrated far less effective in preventing lethality from GVHD. Survival of irradiated recipient animals given transplants supplemented with CCR5-/- T regs is significantly decreased, and GVHD scores are enhanced compared with animals receiving wild type T regs. CCR5-/- T regs are functional in suppressing T cell proliferation in vitro and ex vivo. However, although the accumulation of T regs within lymphoid tissues during the first week after transplantation is not dependent on CCR5, the lack of function of CCR5-/- T regs correlate with impaired accumulation of these cells in the liver, lung, spleen, and mesenteric lymph node, more than one week after transplantation. These data definitively demonstrate a requirement for CCR5 in T reg function, and indicate that in addition to their previously defined role in inhibiting effector T cell expansion in lymphoid tissues during GVHD, later recruitment of T regs to both lymphoid tissues and GVHD target organs is important in their ability to prolong survival after allogeneic bone marrow transplantation [146].

The chemokine receptor CCR7 and its ligands regulate migration and colocalization of T cells and mature dendritic cells to and within secondary lymphoid organs. CCR7 is required in efficient priming of allospecific cytotoxic CD8+ T cells. Some experiments demonstrate a role for CCR7 in the initiation of an alloimmune response and in the development of transplant rejection. In a model of acute allogeneic tumor rejection, CCR7-/- mice completely fail to reject subcutaneously injected MHC class I mismatched tumor cells and cytotoxic activity of allospecific T cells is severely compromised. Tumor allografts transplanted from CCR7-/- donors into CCR7-/- recipients show significant prolongation of allograft survival, suggesting a critical function of CCR7 on donor-type passenger leukocytes in the initiation of cytotoxic CD8+ T cell responses. As for CCR7 ligand, overexpression of chemokine CCL19 in tumour cells has been shown to result in accelerated tumour rejection under certain experimental conditions [147]. In a heterotopic heart transplantation model CCR7 deficiency result in significantly prolonged but not indefinite allograft survival. Additional prolongation of graft survival is observed when hearts from CCR7-/- mice are used as donor organs. These results define a key role for CCR7 in allogeneic T cell priming within the context of draining lymph nodes [148].

To sum up, the emigration of leukocytes from the peripheral circulation into an allograft is an essential component of organ transplant rejection. Ischemic damage and surgical trauma start up the stage of leukocyte infiltration and activation, which in turn lead to the recruitment of additional effecter leukocytes to the graft. The migration of dendritic cells from the allograft into secondary lymphoid tissue is also of paramount importance to the rejection process [28]. The biology of chemokine receptors underlies both leukocyte recruitment and important aspects of the adaptive immune response. It is a brief model (figure 2) that indicates the effects of chemokine receptors and their ligands in organ transplant rejection [15]. In addition to their primary role in regulating cell motility, chemokine receptors can also influence cell survival and proliferation.

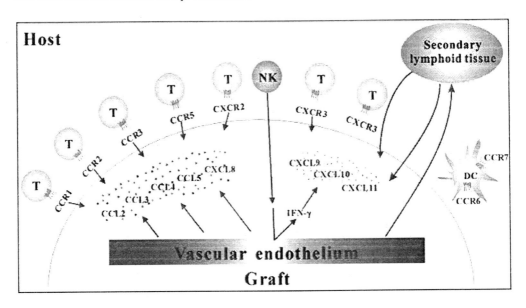

Figure 2. A brief model of the functions of chemokine receptors in organ transplant rejection. Several corresponding ligands are released from the vascular endothelium of allograft in the early stage, and then attract CCR1-, CCR5-, CXCR2-expressing T cells and other types of leukocytes. As a result of MHC mismatch, host NK cells migrate into graft and stimulate the vascular endothelium to produce IFN-γ. Then IFN-γ induces endothelium to synthesize and locally secrete the CXCR3 ligand, CXCL9, CXCL10 and CXCL11, which lead to recruiting CXCR3+ T cells and plasmacytoid dendritic cells. According to these mechanisms, the acute and chronic rejections take place by host cells invading the graft.

In general, signal transduction induced by chemokine receptors leads to the activation of heterotrimeric G proteins and phospholipase C, and the elevation of cytosolic free calcium (calcium influx). Biochemical studies have showed that agonist binding to chemokine receptors can result in activation of phospholipases A2 and C, phosphatidylinositol-3-kinase, Janus kinase (or protein kinase C) signal transducer and activator of transcription proteins, mitogen activated protein, and cytoskeletal remodeling by a G protein-dependent process [149-159]. Following that, these activated proteins and lipid kinases mediate actin cytoskeleton rearrangement, changes in integrin affinity and avidity, leukocyte proliferation, differentiation, and apoptosis [160, 161]. Stimulation of chemokine receptors results in the transient activation of the mitogen-activated protein kinase extracellular signal-regulated kinase (ERK)-2 [162-165]. Activation of ERK-2 is Ras-dependent, and prolonged activation causes its nuclear translocation and activation of transcription [166]. Chemokines also stimulate phosphatidylinositol 3-kinase, leading to the formation of phosphatidyl 3, 4, 5-triphosphate [156, 167] and the activation of protein kinase B [168]. Phosphatidylinositol 3-kinase activity is necessary and sufficient to stimulate protein kinase B. Binding of its pleckstrin homology domain to 3-phosphoinositides and the phosphorylation of two critical residues accomplish activation of protein kinase B by phosphoinositide-dependent kinase [169]. Responsiveness to chemokines is further regulated by desensitization of receptors after chemokine binding. Homologous desensitization occurs in a ligand dependent manner and involves phosphorylation of the receptor by specific G-protein coupled receptor kinases, followed by β-arrestin mediated targeting for endocytosis [170]. Ligand independent desensitization also occurs, when stimulation of a heterologous G-protein coupled receptor leads to phosphorylation of others through second messenger-dependent kinases such as protein kinase C, and subsequent G-protein decoupling [171]. In this manner, cross talk between chemokine receptors has been demonstrated [172, 173].

VI. Chemokine Receptor Associated Therapeutic Issue of Transplant Rejection

A. Analytic Techniques of Chemokine Receptors and Their Ligands Gene Expression During Allograft Rejection

It is crucial for the clinical assessment of many conditions to analyze expression of genes rapidly in small samples of tissue, including allograft transplant rejection. Chemokine receptors have shown to play an essential role in leukocyte recruitment to transplants and in leukocyte localization within graft. Therefore the analysis of chemokine receptor and ligand expression in allograft after transplantation may be a useful early predictor of the onset of rejection.

RT-PCR techniques are the most sensitive for the detection of low abundance mRNA when the amount of tissue sample is limited. In a fully MHC mismatched mouse cardiac allograft model, real-time PCR is compared with competitive-quantitative RT-PCR (CQ-PCR) for the sequential quantification of chemokine transcripts after transplantation. It is found that real-time PCR is more sensitive and reproducible, although CQ-PCR is an accurate and sensitive technique. Real-time PCR analysis, which avoids the potential sample contamination during post-PCR manipulations and offers the advantage that several genes can be analyzed from small graft biopsy samples in a shorter period of time, can distinctly distinguish expression of chemokine and chemokine receptor gene from during rejecting allogeneic grafts and in non-rejecting syngeneic grafts. To illustrate, expression of CXCL5 and CCL2 within graft is found by real-time PCR to be independent of T cell infiltration while expression of CXCL9, CXCL10, CCL1, CCL3, CCL4, CCL5, and XCL1 is clearly T cell dependent and increases significantly after transplantation [174]. To sum up, real-time PCR analysis could distinguish distinctly expression of chemokine and chemokine receptor gene from during rejecting allogeneic grafts and in non-rejecting syngeneic grafts.

Some research develop a genetic system, called degrakine, which specifically and stably inactivates chemokine receptors by redirecting the ability of the HIV-1 protein, Vpu, to degrade CD4 in the endoplasmic reticulum via the host proteasome machinery. To harness Vpu's proteolytic targeting capability to degrade new receptors, a chemokine is fused with the C terminal region of Vpu. The fusion protein, or degrakine, accumulates in the endoplasmic reticulum, trapping and functionally inactivating its target chemokine receptors. It has demonstrated that degrakines based on CXCL12, CCL5 and CCL22 specifically inactivate their respective receptor functions. Thus the degrakine provides an effective genetic tool to dissect receptor functions in a number of biological systems in vitro and in vivo [175].

B. New Therapeutic Strategies Targeting Chemokine Receptor for Transplant Rejection

The chemokines are a large superfamily of chemotactic cytokines that are utilized to direct the trafficking and migration of leukocytes within the immune system. The chemokines mediate their activity through a large family of G-protein-coupled receptors, and thus are highly tractable as therapeutic targets. Exciting advances have been made in the field within the past year, not the least of which is the disclosure of potent antagonists of several chemokine receptors. New biological insights have been gained from the demonstration that the targeting of cells to inflammatory sites is tissue specific, such that different chemokine and chemokine receptor pairs are utilized in recruitment of T-lymphocytes to the skin and to the intestine [176]. The clarification of chemokine receptor effects in allograft transplant will shed a new light on how to prevent allograft transplant rejection, such as blocking or activating particular target chemokine receptors in therapy.

The chemokines CXCL9, CXCL10 and CXCL11 and associated CXCR3 receptor are expressed during the inflammatory process from organ transplantation resulting in the recruitment of lymphocytes leading to tissue damage. Blocking the interaction of the ligands and CXCR3 has potential to provide opportunity for development of agents that would block tissue rejection. Antisense oligodeoxynucleotides represent a unique example of gene specific drugs that can be used to selectively inhibit the expression of target genes. Second and third generation oligodeoxynucleotides have been synthesized that possess improved chemical characteristics regarding stability in biological fluids, cellular uptake, and molecular specificity for the target sequence. Among the various alterations of the standard phosphodiester structure, the PNA backbone is optimal in terms of specificity and affinity for the target and resistance to degradation. PNA is a structural mimic of natural nucleic acids, composed of a pseudo peptide carrying nucleobases. PNA/DNA hybrids are more stable than dsDNA. PNA is resistant to degradation caused by nucleases and proteases, and it has been shown to interfere in a sequence specific manner with several DNA- and RNA-based processes [177-182]. The therapeutic and diagnostic potentials of PNA have been attracting considerable attention with attempts at treatments, such as those for HIV infection and cancers, and of speeding diagnosis, such as for infectious diseases [177-183].

After a number of pioneer experiments in vitro and in vivo, PNA CCR5 and PNA CXCR3 antisenses are designed and selected to treat mice that received skin allograft transplantations. The PNA CXCR3 at a high dosage (10 mg/kg/day) can significantly prolong mouse skin allograft survival compared with physiological saline treatment, whereas the low dosage (0.5 mg/kg/day) failed to prolong mouse skin allograft survival. The high dosage (10 mg/kg/day) of PNA CCR5 can marginally but significantly prolonged mouse skin allograft survival, whereas low dosage (0.5 mg/kg/day) has no such effect. Meanwhile, PNA mismatch and DNA CXCR3 do not have any effects on prolonging mouse skin allograft survival. PNA CXCR3 and PNA CCR5 together seem to be more effective. Without any treatment, skin allografts in recipients are rejected between days 6 and 8 (table 3). Histological analyses also confirm the PNA CXCR3 at a high dosage can significantly prolong mouse skin allograft survival. By day 7 after transplantation, histological analyses of allografts show widespread subcutaneous necrosis and leukocyte infiltration. Most of the infiltrating leukocytes are T cells, identified morphologically. Immunohistologically, CCR5 is moderately expressed, whereas CXCR3 is highly expressed in infiltrating cells (figure 3A). In contrast, there are only a few leukocytes infiltrating subcutaneously and skin structure is almost normal anatomically at day 7 after allograft transplantation from PNA CXCR3 treated animals. Immunohistologically, these cells are expressing a few CCR5 and seldom CXCR3 (figure 3B). The expression of CXCR3 is totally abolished on CD4+ T cells, CD8+ T cells, CD19+ B cells, and CD14+ monocytes from allografts at day 7 after transplantation in PNA CXCR3 treated animals. This phenomenon is not seen in the PNA CCR5-, PNA mismatch- and normal physiological saline-treated animals. PNA CXCR3 significantly and indirectly reduces CD25 and CD69 but not CD45RB expressions in CXCR3-expressing graft-infiltrating CD3+ T cells, whereas PNA CCR5, PNA mismatch, and normal physiological saline do not. The spleen T cells from the animals that received PNA CCR5 and PNA CXCR3 treatments show identical mitogen-induced cell proliferation to that of animals receiving saline treatment, whereas mitogen-induced cell proliferations in animals that received CsA treatment are significantly inhibited implying that CsA does affect the proliferation of T cells in this case. In summary, CXCR3 PNA antisense only inhibits CXCR3 expression on T cells to significantly prolong mouse skin allograft survival but does not interfere with other T cell functions such as proliferation, indicating the therapeutic potential of PNA CXCR3 to prevent acute transplantation rejection [131].

Apart from PNA CXCR3, other studies also show that utilization of neutralizing antibodies to the CXCR3 ligands in murine allograft transplantation models has demonstrated the importance of CXCR3 in orchestrating T cell mediated tissue rejection [176]. Four classes of natural product inhibitors have been described that block the CXCR3 interaction of CXCL10. These include a cyclic thiopeptide, polyketide glycosides, steroidal glycosides and a novel alkyl pyridinium alkaloid that are isolated by bioassay-guided fractionation of the organic extracts derived from actinomycete, fungal, plant and marine sources and discovered using 125I CXCL10/CXCR3 binding assay [184].

Table 3. The survival time of mouse skin allograft in response to different treatments

Treatment	Dosage (mg/kg/day)	Survival time (days)[a]
PNA CCR5	10	11
PNA CXCR3	10	17
PNA CCR5 + PNA CXCR3	10 + 10	20
PNA mismatch	10	7
DNA CXCR3	10	7
Normal physiological saline	—[b]	7
CsA	1	21

[a] The data are mean values ± standard deviation of eight experiments performed. For simplification, the SDs are not shown.

[b] Normal physiological saline is applied in equal volume to PNA treatment.

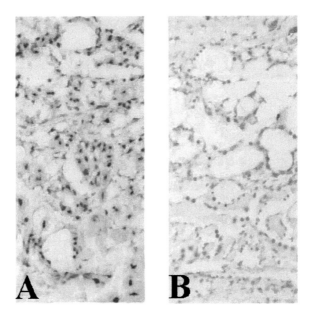

Figure 3. Histological analyses of skin allografts from BALB/c (H-2^d) recipients that received PNA CXCR3 treatment. The donors are C57BL/6 (H-2^b) mice. The recipient mice have been treated without (A) or with PNA CXCR3 (B). Allograft are harvested at day 7 after transplantation and fixed with 10% buffered formalin. Frozen sections are prepared and stained with anti-CXCR3 polyclonal antibody. The positively staining cells in representative areas of the slides are shown in brown color. Magnification: ×200.

CXCL12, the only chemokine binding to CXCR4, contributes to host versus graft rejection in bone marrow transplantation because it is responsible for attracting mature lymphocytes to the bone marrow. Clearly, it is a possible aid in bone marrow transplantation by manipulating CXCL12 activity. CXCL12 binds to CXCR4 primarily via the N terminus, which appears flexible in the recently determined three dimensional structure of CXCL12. Strikingly, short N-terminal CXCL12 peptides have been shown to have significant CXCL12 activity. By using nuclear magnetic resonance, the analyses of conformation of the N terminus of CXCL12 show that the major conformation may be important for recognition in receptor binding, that is to say, there may be a link between structuring of short N-terminal chemokine peptides and their ability to activate their receptor. These studies will act as a starting point for synthesizing non-peptide analogs that act as CXCR4 antagonists [185].

HPCs traffic to and are retained in the marrow through the trophic effects of the chemokine CXCL12 binding to its receptor CXCR4. AMD3100 reversibly inhibits CXCL12/CXCR4 binding, and AMD3100 administration mobilizes CD34+ cells into the circulation. The combination of AMD3100 plus G-CSF can be superior to G-CSF alone in mobilizing HPCs and that AMD3100 plus G-CSF-mobilized cells can engraft as well as G-CSF-mobilized cells. These demonstrate that the combination of A+G is generally safe, effective, and superior to G alone for autologous HPC mobilization [186].

Accelerated coronary arteriosclerosis remains a major problem in the long-term survival of cardiac transplant recipients. However, the pathogenesis of graft vasculopathy is poorly understood, and there is no effective therapy. Transplant arteriosclerosis is characterized by early mononuclear cell attachment on the transplanted vessel followed by development of concentric neointimal hyperplasia. Early and persistent expression of CCL2 in cardiac allografts has been implicated for the pathogenesis of transplant arteriosclerosis. The NH2-terminal deletion mutants of CCL2 gene which can antagonize CCL2 reduce monocytes/macrophages infiltration in cardiac allografts [187]. The CCL2/CCR2 signaling pathway plays a critical role in the pathogenesis of graft vasculopathy. This new anti-CCL2 gene therapy might be useful to treat graft vascular disease [188].

In organ transplantation, successful immunosuppression requires that both rejection and infection episodes be minimized. Unfortunately it is currently impossible to predict individual dose requirement for immunosuppressive drugs, but a number of studies of various immune response genes are now being performed with a view to identifying genotypes associated with rejection and infection [189]. The chemokine receptor CCR5 plays an important role in transplant rejection by affecting the trafficking of effector T cells and monocytes to diseased tissues. Antagonists of CCR5 are believed to be of potential therapeutic value for the allograft rejection. Now some studies have reported on the structure-activity relationship of a new series of highly potent and selective competitive CCR5 antagonists [190]. (5R)-5-hydroxytriptolide (LLDT-8) is a new compound which has potent immunosuppressive activities. LLDT-8 administered orally significantly decreases CCR5 and their ligands CCL3 and CCL4 mRNA expressions in allografts, and induces the survival prolongation of allogeneic cardiac graft. The results outline the great potential of LLDT-8 as a therapeutic tool in transplant rejection [191].

With respect to CCR5 ligands, topical treatment with soluble tumor necrosis factor receptor type I (sTNFR-I) significantly enhance allogeneic corneal allograft survival and inhibit gene expression of CCL4 and CCL5 associated with corneal graft rejection. The postoperative messenger RNA levels of CCL4 and CCL5 in sTNFR-I treated eyes are substantially suppressed compared with vehicle-treated eyes. Vehicle-treated eyes bearing rejected allografts express higher levels of messenger RNA for CCL4 and CCL5 than control eyes bearing accepted allografts [192]. In addition, the NH2-terminal deletion (8ND) mutant of CCL5 gene which can antagonize CCL5 reduce graft infiltration by monocytes/macrophages and CD8+ T cells. In mixed leukocyte reactions in vitro, proliferation of host lymphocytes from regional lymph nodes in response to donor splenocytes is unaffected by 8ND-CCL5 gene transfer. 8ND-CCL5 gene transfer and a short course of low dose CsA synergistically prolong markedly graft survival compared with cyclosporine alone [187]. Another antagonist, the reagent Met-RANTES, is being tested in murine models of renal transplantation. The systemic treatment with the CCL5 based antagonist Met-RANTES can suppress acute damage to transplanted kidneys by blocking effector cell recruitment [193]. It is demonstrated that early application of Met-RANTES can protect renal allografts from long-term deterioration as well. Met-RANTES treatment reduce the infiltration of lymphocytes and macrophages in allografts at 2 weeks after transplantation, accompanied by decreased mRNA expression of CCL5, IL-2, IL-1β, and TNF-α. At posttransplantation week 28, Met-RANTES treatment reduces urinary protein excretion and significantly ameliorates glomerulosclerosis, interstitial fibrosis, tubular atrophy, intimal proliferation of graft arteries and mononuclear cell infiltration. However, creatinine clearance is not influenced by Met-RANTES. Blockade of chemokine receptors by Met-RANTES diminishes early infiltration and activation of mononuclear cells in the grafts, and thus reduces the pace of chronic allograft nephropathy [194]. These findings support the feasibility of an anti-chemokine strategy as a means of reducing allograft rejection without resorting to the use of potentially toxic immunosuppressive drugs.

The CCL21-ΔCT mutant is derived from mouse CCL21 whose 41 amino acids at the C-terminal is truncated while construction. The truncated part includes the site at which CCL21 binds to the surface of high endothelial venule. The rest peptide contains the receptor binding site so that the mutant can effectively bind to CCR7. DCs are widely accepted to be the most potent and versatile antigen-presenting cell in the immune system. The mobilization of DCs from the periphery to the lymph nodes is regulated by the "gatekeeper" chemokine receptor CCR7 [195, 196]. CCL21-ΔCT, as a competitive ligand for CCR7, can effectively inhibit CCR7- bearing DCs migration to wild-type CCL21, and thus block T cell migration in vivo and in vitro. Recent study demonstrates that topical application of CCL21-ΔCT can effectively prolong skin graft survival in murine model [our unpublished data].

By targeting chemokine receptors and their ligands, there are also potential therapeutic strategies else. Some experiments demonstrate plasmid-, retroviral-, or adenoviral-mediated vIL-10 gene transfer can prolong allograft survival. Feline immunodeficiency virus (FIV) can integrate into genomic DNA of nondividing cells, thus FIV-mediated gene transfer can provide long-term gene expression and improved allograft survival. In allogeneic grafts transduced with FIV-IL-10, a number of the chemokine and chemokine receptor genes are suppressed. Therefore, FIV-mediated vIL-10 gene transfer prolongs allograft survival and, in combination with other agents, produces an additive effect [197]. Enhancing dendritic cell tolerogenicity is a potent approach for the promotion of cell or organ allograft survival. Delivery of genes encoding molecules that subvert T-cell responses by various mechanisms, and targeting of dendritic cell migration by selective manipulation of chemokine and chemokine receptor expression, represent additional promising strategies [198].

To sum up, graft rejection is a major barrier to successful outcome of transplantation surgery. Leukocyte trafficking is necessary for the launch of successful immune responses to pathogen or allograft. Chemokines direct the migration of leukocytes through their interaction with chemokine receptors found on cell surfaces of immune cells. Unique receptor expressions of leukocytes, and the specificity of chemokine secretion during various states of immune response, suggest that the extracellular chemokine milieu specifically homes certain leukocyte subsets. Thus, only those leukocytes required for the current immune task are attracted to the inflammatory site. CsA mediated immune suppression individuals undergoing organ transplantation are at increased risk of recurrences of initial cancers, although how immunosuppressive therapy increases early cancer metastasis remains unclear [199]. Chemokine blockade, using antagonists and monoclonal antibodies directed against chemokine receptors, is an emerging and specific immunosuppressive strategy. Importantly, chemokine blockade may potentiate tolerance induction regimens to be used following transplantation surgery, and prevent the need for life-long immunosuppression of transplant recipients. While selection of mentioned above strategies may allow a more individualised therapy, the special immunosuppressive potential of each chemokine receptor has to be weighed against adverse reactions for an individual patient [98, 200].

VIII. Further Investigation of Chemokine Receptors in Allograft Transplant

Allograft rejection is mediated to a significant degree by the influx of monocytes and T cells. The induction of chemokines during allograft rejection is accompanied by the infiltration of leukocytes bearing the respective chemokine receptors [28]. The chemokine receptors expressed by different T cell populations have been linked to Th1/Th2-like effector responses of receptor-expressing cells [41]. Allograft rejection is thought to be primarily the result of a Th1 type immune response. The Th1 effector cells often express CXCR3 and CCR5, while Th2 cells can express CCR3, CCR4, and CCR8 [28]. In particular, recent studies from different independent groups have documented that CXCR3 and corresponding ligands CXCL10 and CXCL9 are most significantly associated with acute allograft rejection in heart [43, 54, 201, 202], lung [203], kidney [60], pancreatic islet [100], liver [105], and skin [131]. CCR5 is also found to be highly expressed on infiltrating mononuclear cells during allograft rejection [77, 60, 204]. Thus, a rather complex picture is now beginning to take shape of how T cells selectively enter different transplanted organs, nest on sites, are further activated, and transmigrate to final destinations to cause physiological and pathophysiological events under continuous interaction with chemokines and cytokines.

Most studies in the transplantation field have so far concentrated on chemokines rather than their receptors and on rather few chemokines. Whether they are in fact playing a biologically significant role and whether their inhibition by any of several strategies would be of actual therapeutic value are largely unknown [2]. Some tools are now becoming available to analyze these roles in a meaningful manner, including commercially available multiprobe RNA protecting assays, anti-chemokine and anti-chemokine-receptor mAbs, and gene-knockout animals. It is a reasonable expectation that the fundamental significance of chemokine receptors and their ligands for therapeutic targeting will become available from experimental systems [43, 44, 201, 205, 206]. However, many data from in vitro experiments demonstrating the presence of multiple ligands for a given chemokine receptor, and often multiple receptors for a given chemokine, have led to concerns of biologic redundancy [2]. The biologic redundancy of chemokine receptors leads us to consider the selection of target chemokine receptor regarding the treatment of allograft rejection. This finding could be a meaningful event along the lines of accumulating knowledge of the roles of chemokines and chemokine receptors in allograft rejection and providing important insight into the physiological and pathophysiological processes under continuous interaction between host and allografts. Demonstrating the chemokine receptors roles in transplantation will contribute to find a novel potential strategy in the exploration and treatment of transplant rejection [131].

Recently developed PNAs, which are synthetic homologs of nucleic acids in which the phosphate-sugar polynucleotide backbone is replaced by a flexible polyamide, allow the formation of a PNA-DNA hydrogen-bonded double helix, which is more stable than the one formed by DNA-DNA interaction [207]. PNAs are resistant to nucleases and proteases [208] and consequently are more stable in cells than oligonucleotides. Though potentially capable of blocking gene expression in a selective and specific manner [209], PNAs have never been shown to be effective anti-gene agents in intact live cells in culture because of their limited ability to reach cell nuclei [210]. But recent study demonstrates that PNA CXCR3 significantly and specifically inhibit CXCR3 mRNA and protein expression in the spleen T cells and skin grafts. Taking a number of previous observations into account [211], these indications of the potential of PNA CXCR3 to prevent acute transplantation rejection will lead to exciting new therapeutic approaches.

Stem cell transplantation, whether autologous or allogeneic, improves the outcome of patients with a number of hematologic malignancies or solid tumors. A relevant proportion of these patients are excluded from this treatment because sufficient numbers of hematopoietic stem cells cannot be obtained by standard cytokine assisted mobilization. Previous studies have investigated the physiology of peripheral blood progenitor cell (PBPC) mobilization and discussed the role of chemokine receptors and their ligands, such as CXCR4 and CXCL12, adhesion molecules, and proteolytic enzymes. Based on this knowledge, several innovative pharmacologic approaches have been proposed to boost the stem cell harvest. Some of them are still subject of pre-clinical development, others, such as CXCR4 antagonist AMD3100, have recently been introduced in clinical trials and already deliver promising results. It appears possible to harvest PBPC successfully in poor mobilizers and to cut down the number of collections required in the remaining PBPC donors [212].

The goal of immunosuppression in allograft transplantation is to blunt the immune response of the patient to the allograft, while maintaining sufficient resistance to avoid opportunistic infections and malignancy. Despite progress in this field, rejection processes, particularly of the chronic form, remain an important cause of morbidity and graft loss. The recent advances in drug development and pharmacology as well as in immunobiology are likely to lead to more potent, effective and selective regimens to improve the therapeutic efficacy and overcome the range of adverse side effects now plaguing the transplant enterprise. The future era of transplantation is likely to focus on chemokine receptor or cytosolic enzyme targets more specifically represented on or in lymphocytes as opposed to other cells or tissues [213].

References

[1]   Johnson, Z; Power, CA; Weiss, C; Rintelen, F; Ji, H; Ruckle, T; Camps, M; Wells, TN; Schwarz, MK; Proudfoot, AE; Rommel, C. Chemokine inhibition--why, when, where, which and how? *Biochem. Soc. Trans*, 2004, 32, 366-77.

[2]   Hancock, WW; Gao, W; Faia, KL; Csizmadia, V. Chemokines and their receptors in allograft rejection. *Curr. Opin. Immunol*, 2000, 12, 511-6.

[3]   Pfeffer, W. Locomotorische richtungsbewegungen durch chemische reize. *Untersuchungen aus dem botanischen institut tübingen*, 1884, 1, 363-482.

[4]   Leber, T. Ueber die enstehung der entzündung und die wirkung der entzündung und die wirkung der entzunddungerregenden schadlichkeiten. *Fortschr. Med*, 1888, 6, 460-4.

[5]   Leber, T. Die enstehung der entzündung. Die wirkung der entzunddungerregenden schadlichkeiten nach vorzugsweise am auge angestellten untersuchungen. *Engelmann Leipzig*, 1891, 1891, 1-535.

[6]   Boyden, S. The chemotactic effect of mixture of antibody and antigen on polymorphonuclear leukocytes. *J. Exp. Med*, 1962, 115, 453-66.

[7]   Falk, W; Goodwin, RK; Leonard, EJ. A 48-well micro chemotaxis assembly for rapid and accurate measurement of leukocyte migration. *J. Immunol. Methods*, 1980, 33, 239-47.

[8]   Oppenheim, JJ; Zachariae, CO; Mukaida, N; Matsushima, K. Properties of the novel proinflammatory supergene "intercrine" cytokine family. *Ann. Rev. Immunol*, 1991, 9, 617-48.

[9]   Cocchi, F; DeVico, AL; Garzino-Demo, A; Arya, SK; Gallo, RC; Lusso, P. Identification of RANTES, MIP-α, and MIP-1β as the major HIV-suppressive factors produced by CD8+ T cells. *Science*, 1995, 270, 1811-5.

[10] Baggiolini, M. Chemokines and leukocyte traffic. *Nature*, 1998, 392, 565-8.

[11] Mackay, CR. Chemokines: immunology's high impact factors. *Nat. Immunol*, 2001, 2, 95-101.

[12] Luther, SA; Cyster, JG. Chemokines as regulators of T cell differentiation. *Nat. Immunol*, 2001, 2, 102-7.

[13] Taub, DD; Oppenheim, JJ. Review of the chemokine meeting the Third International Symposium of Chemotatic Cytokines. *Cytokine*, 1993, 5, 175-79.

[14] Teixeira, MM; Gazzinelli, RT; Silva, JS. Chemokines, inflammation and Trypanosoma cruzi infection. *Trends Parasitol*, 2002, 18, 262-5.

[15] Gerard, C; Rollins, BJ. Chemokines and disease. *Nat. Immunol*, 2001, 108-15.

[16] Rossi, D; Zlotnik, A. The biology of chemokines and their receptors. *Annu. Rev. Immunol*, 2000, 18, 217-42.

[17] Zlotnik, A; Yoshie, O. Chemokines: a new classification system and their role in immunity. *Immunity*, 2000, 12, 121-7.

[18] Muller, A; Homey, B; Soto, H; Ge, N; Catron, D; Buchanan, ME; McClanahan, T; Murphy, E; Yuan, W; Wagner, SN; Barrera, JL; Mohar, A; Verastegui, E; Zlotnik, A. Involvement of chemokine receptors in breast cancer metastasis. *Nature*, 2001, 410, 50-6.

[19] Fischereder, M; Luckow, B; Hocher, B; Wuthrich, RP; Rothenpieler, U; Schneeberger, H; Panzer, U; Stahl, RA; Hauser, IA; Budde, K; Neumayer, H; Kramer, BK; Land, W; Schlondorff, D. CC chemokine receptor 5 and renal-transplant survival. *Lancet*, 2001, 357, 1758-61.

[20] Sallusto, F; Lanzavecchia, A; Mackay, CR. Chemokines and chemokine receptors in T-cell priming and Th1/Th2-mediated responses. *Immunol. Today*, 1998, 19, 568-74.

[21] Jinquan, T; Anting, L; Jacobi HH; Glue, C; Jing, C; Ryder, LP; Madsen, HO; Svejgaard, A; Skov, PS; Malling, HJ; Poulsen, LK. CXCR3 Expression on CD34+ Hemopoietic Progenitors Induced by Granulocyte-Macrophage Colony-Stimulating Factor: II. Signaling Pathways Involved. *J. Immunol*, 2001, 167, 4405-13.

[22] Rollins, BJ. Chemokines. *Blood*, 1997, 90, 909-28.

[23] Rodriguez-Frade, JM; Vila-Coro, AJ; de Ana, AM; Albar, JP; Martinez-A, C; Mellado, M. The chemokine monocyte chemoattractant protein-1 induces functional responses through dimerization of its receptor CCR2. *Proc. Natl. Acad. Sci. USA*, 1999, 96, 3628-33.

[24] Vila-Coro, AJ; Rodriguez-Frade, JM; Martin De Ana, A; Moreno-Ortiz, MC; Martinez-A, C; Mellado, M. The chemokine SDF-1alpha triggers CXCR4 receptor dimerization and activates the JAK/STAT pathway. *FASEB J*, 1999, 13, 1699-710.

[25] Colvin, BL; Thomson, AW. Chemokines, their receptors, and transplant outcome. *Transplantation*, 2002, 74, 149-55.

[26] Murphy, PM; Baggiolini, M; Charo, IF; Hebert, CA; Horuk, R; Matsushima, K; Miller, LH; Oppenheim, JJ; Power, CA. International union of pharmacology. XXII. Nomenclature for chemokine receptors. *Pharmacol. Rev*, 2000, 52, 145-76.

[27] Eis, V; Vielhauer, V; Anders, HJ. Targeting the chemokine network in renal inflammation. *Arch. Immunol. Ther. Exp. (Warsz)*, 2004, 52, 164-72.

[28] Nelson, PJ; Krensky, AM. Chemokines, chemokine receptors, and allograft rejection. *Immunity*, 2001, 14, 377-86.

[29] Le, YY; Zhou, Y; Iribarren, P; Wang, JM. Chemokines and chemokine receptors: their manifold roles in homeostasis and disease. *Cell Mol. Immunol*, 2004, 1, 95-102.

[30] Lisa, M. Schwlebert. Chemokines; Chemokine Receptors; and Disease. *Current Topics in Membranes;* Volume 55. California; USA: Elsevier Academic Press; 2005.

[31] Peter J. Morris. Tissue Transplantation. Clinical Surgery International; Volume 3. Edinburgh London Melbourne and New York: Churchill Livingstone; 1982.

[32] Jensen, MK. Chromosome studies in patients treated with azathioprine and amethopterin. *Acta Med. Scand*, 1967, 182, 445-55.

[33] Koranda, FC; Loeffler, RT; Koranda, DM; Penn, I. Accelerated induction of skin cancers by ultraviolet radiation in hairless mice treated with immunosuppressive agents. *Surg. Forum*, 1975, 26, 145-6.

[34] Russell, ME; Adams, DH; Wyner, LR; Yamashita, Y; Halnon, NJ; Karnovsky, MJ. Early and persistent induction of monocyte chemoattractant protein 1 in rat cardiac allografts. *Proc. Natl. Acad. Sci. USA*, 1993, 90, 6086-90.

[35] Bang, H; Brune, K; Nager, C; Feige, U. Interleukin-8 is a cyclosporin A binding protein. *Experientia*, 1993, 49, 533-8.

[36] DeVries, ME; Ran, L; Kelvin, DJ. On the edge: the physiological and pathophysiological role of chemokines during inflammatory and immunological responses. *Semin. Immunol*, 1999, 11, 95-104.

[37] Clavien, PA; Harvey, PR; Strasberg, SM. Preservation and reperfusion injuries in liver allografts. An overview and synthesis of current studies. *Transplantation*, 1992, 53, 957-78.

[38] Engler, RL; Dahlgren, MD; Peterson, MA; Dobbs, A; Schmid-Schonbein, GW. Accumulation of polymorphonuclear leukocytes during a 3-h experimental myocardial ischemia. *Am. J. Physiol*, 1986, 251, H93-100.

[39] Ivey, CL; Williams, FM; Collins, PD; Jose, PJ; Williams, TJ. Neutrophil chemoattractants generated in two phases during reperfusion of ischemic myocardium in the rabbit. Evidence for a role for C5a and interleukin-8. *J. Clin. Invest*, 1995, 95, 2720-8.

[40] Kukielka, GL; Smith, CW; LaRosa, GJ; Manning, AM; Mendoza, LH; Daly, TJ; Hughes, BJ; Youker, KA; Hawkins, HK; Michael, LH. Interleukin-8 gene induction in the myocardium after ischemia and reperfusion in vivo. *J. Clin. Invest*, 1995, 95, 89-103.

[41] Sallusto, F; Lanzavecchia, A. Understanding dendritic cell and T lymphocyte traffic through the analysis of chemokine receptor expression. *Immunol. Rev*, 2000, 177, 134-40.

[42] Le, MA; Goldman, M; Abramowicz, D. Multiple pathways to allograft rejection. *Transplantation*, 2002, 73, 1373-81.

[43] Hancock, WW; Lu, B; Gao, W; Csizmadia, V; Faia, K; King, JA; Smiley, ST; Ling, M; Gerard, NP; Gerard, C. Requirement of the chemokine receptor CXCR3 for acute allograft rejection. *J. Exp. Med*, 2000, 192, 1515-20.

[44] Gao, W; Topham, PS; King, JA; Smiley, ST; Csizmadia, V; Lu, B; Gerard, CJ; Hancock, WW. Targeting of the chemokine receptor CCR1 suppresses development of acute and chronic cardiac allograft rejection. *J. Clin. Invest*, 2000, 105, 35-44.

[45] Zhang, Z; Kaptanoglu, L; Haddad, W; Ivancic, D; Alnadjim, Z; Hurst, S; Tishler, D; Luster, AD; Barrett, TA; Fryer, J. Donor T cell activation initiates small bowel allograft rejection through an IFN-γ-inducible protein-10-dependent mechanism. *J. Immunol*, 2002, 168, 3205-12.

[46] Hayry, P; Myllarniemi, M; Calderon, RL; Aavik, E; Loubtchenkov, M; Koskinen, P; Lemstrom, K; Raisanen-Sokolowski, A. Immunobiology and pathology of chronic rejection. *Transplant. Proc*, 1997, 29, 77-8.

[47] Tullius, SG; Heemann, U; Hancock, WW; Azuma, H; Tilney, NL. Long-term kidney isografts develop functional and morphologic changes that mimic those of chronic allograft rejection. *Ann. Surg*, 1994, 220, 425-32.

[48] Glassock, RJ; Feldman, D; Reynolds, ES; Dammin, GJ; Merrill, JP. Human renal isografts: a clinical and pathologic analysis. *Medicine (Baltimore)*, 1968, 47, 411-54.

[49] Nadeau, KC; Azuma, H; Tilney, NL. Sequential cytokine dynamics in chronic rejection of rat renal allografts: roles for cytokines RANTES and MCP-1. *Proc. Natl. Acad. Sci. USA*, 1995, 92, 8729-33.

[50] Pattison, JM; Nelson, PJ; Huie, P; Sibley, RK; Krensky, AM. RANTES chemokine expression in transplant-associated accelerated atherosclerosis. *J. Heart Lung Transplant*, 1996, 15, 1194-9.

[51] Russell, ME; Wallace, AF; Hancock, WW; Sayegh, MH; Adams, DH; Sibinga, NE; Wyner, LR; Karnovsky, MJ. Upregulation of cytokines associated with macrophage activation in the Lewis-to-F344 rat transplantation model of chronic cardiac rejection. *Transplantation*, 1995, 59, 572-8.

[52] Stark, VK; Hoch, JR; Warner, TF; Hullett, DA. Monocyte chemotactic protein-1 expression is associated with the development of vein graft intimal hyperplasia. *Arterioscler. Thromb. Vasc. Biol*, 1997, 17, 1614-21.

[53] Nagano, H; Mitchell, RN; Taylor, MK; Hasegawa, S; Tilney, NL; Libby, P. Interferon-gamma deficiency prevents coronary arteriosclerosis but not myocardial rejection in transplanted mouse hearts. *J. Clin. Invest,* 1997, 100, 550-7.

[54] Meyer, M; Hensbergen, PJ; van der Raaij-Helmer, EM; Brandacher, G; Margreiter, R; Heufler, C; Koch, F; Narumi, S; Werner, ER; Colvin, R; Luster, AD; Tensen, CP; Werner-Felmayer, G. Cross reactivity of three T cell attracting murine chemokines stimulating the CXC chemokine receptor CXCR3 and their induction in cultured cells and during allograft rejection. *Eur. J. Immunol*, 2001, 31, 2521-7.

[55] Horiguchi, K; Kitagawa-Sakakida, S; Sawa, Y; Li, ZZ; Fukushima, N; Shirakura, R; Matsuda, H. Selective chemokine and receptor gene expressions in allografts that develop transplant vasculopathy. *J. Heart Lung. Transplant*, 2002, 21, 1090-100.

[56] Melter, M; Exeni, A; Reinders, ME; Fang, JC; McMahon, G; Ganz, P; Hancock, WW; Briscoe, DM. Expression of the chemokine receptor CXCR3 and its ligand IP-10 during human cardiac allograft rejection. *Circulation*, 2001, 104, 2558-64.

[57] Zhao, DX; Hu, Y; Miller, GG; Luster, AD; Mitchell, RN; Libby, P. Differential expression of the IFN-gamma-inducible CXCR3-binding chemokines, IFN-inducible protein 10, monokine induced by IFN, and IFN-inducible T cell alpha chemoattractant in human cardiac allografts: association with cardiac allograft vasculopathy and acute rejection. *J. Immunol*, 2002, 169, 1556-60.

[58] Chen, D; Ding, Y; Zhang, N; Schroppel, B; Fu, S; Zang, W; Zhang, H; Hancock, WW; Bromberg, JS. Viral IL-10 gene transfer inhibits the expression of multiple chemokine and chemokine receptor genes induced by inflammatory or adaptive immune stimuli. *Am. J. Transplant*, 2003, 3, 1538-49.

[59] Horuk, R; Clayberger, C; Krensky, AM; Wang, Z; Grone, HJ; Weber, C; Weber, KS; Nelson, PJ; May, K; Rosser, M; Dunning, L; Liang, M; Buckman, B; Ghannam, A; Ng, HP; Islam, I; Bauman, JG; Wei, GP; Monahan, S; Xu, W; Snider, RM; Morrissey, MM; Hesselgesser, J; Perez, HD. A non-peptide functional antagonist of the CCR1 chemokine receptor is effective in rat heart transplant rejection. *J. Biol. Chem*, 2001, 276, 4199-204.

[60] Fairchild, RL; VanBuskirk, AM; Kondo, T; Wakely, ME; Orosz, CG. Expression of chemokine genes during rejection and long-term acceptance of cardiac allografts. *Transplantation*, 1997, 63, 1807-12.

[61] Huser, N; Tertilt, C; Gerauer, K; Maier, S; Traeger, T; Assfalg, V; Reiter, R; Heidecke, CD; Pfeffer, K. CCR4-deficient mice show prolonged graft survival in a chronic cardiac transplant rejection model. *Eur. J. Immunol*, 2005, 35, 128-38.

[62] Fahmy, NM; Yamani, MH; Starling, RC; Ratliff, NB; Young, JB; McCarthy, PM; Feng, J; Novick, AC; Fairchild, RL. Chemokine and receptor-gene expression during early and late acute rejection episodes in human cardiac allografts. *Transplantation*, 2003, 75, 2044-7.

[63] Luckow, B; Joergensen, J; Chilla, S; Li, JP; Henger, A; Kiss, E; Wieczorek, G; Roth, L; Hartmann, N; Hoffmann, R; Kretzler, M; Nelson, PJ; Perez de Lema, G; Maier, H; Wurst, W; Balling, R; Pfeffer, K; Grone, HJ; Schlondorff, D; Zerwes, HG. Reduced intragraft mRNA expression of matrix metalloproteinases Mmp3; Mmp12; Mmp13 and Adam8; and diminished transplant arteriosclerosis in Ccr5-deficient mice. *Eur. J. Immunol*, 2004, 34, 2568-78.

[64] Fildes, JE; Walker, AH; Howlett, R; Bittar, MN; Hutchinson, IV; Leonard, CT; Yonan, N. Donor CCR5 Delta32 polymorphism and outcome following cardiac transplantation. *Transplant. Proc*, 2005, 37, 2247-9.

[65] Simeoni, E; Vassalli, G; Seydoux, C; Ramsay, D; Noll, G; von, Segesser, LK; Fleury, S. CCR5, RANTES and CX3CR1 polymorphisms: possible genetic links with acute heart rejection. *Transplantation*, 2005, 80, 1309-15.

[66] Athanassopoulos, P; Vaessen, LM; Maat, AP; Zondervan, PE; Balk, AH; Bogers, AJ; Weimar, W. Preferential depletion of blood myeloid dendritic cells during acute cardiac allograft rejection under controlled immunosuppression. *Am. J. Transplant*, 2005, 5, 810-20.

[67] Haskell, CA; Hancock, WW; Salant, DJ; Gao, W; Csizmadia, V; Peters, W; Faia, K; Fituri, O; Rottman, JB; Charo, IF. Targeted deletion of CX3CR1 reveals a role for fractalkine in cardiac allograft rejection. *J. Clin. Invest*, 2001, 108, 679-88.

[68] Chen, D; Ding, Y; Schroppel, B; Zhang, N; Fu, S; Chen, D; Zhang, H; Bromberg, JS. Differential chemokine and chemokine receptor gene induction by ischemia; alloantigen; and gene transfer in cardiac grafts. *Am. J. Transplant*, 2003, 3, 1216-29.

[69] Van Hoffen, E; Van Wichen, D; Stuij, I; De Jonge, N; Klopping, C; Lahpor, J; Van Den Tweel, J; Gmelig-Meyling, F; De Weger, R. In situ expression of cytokines in human heart allografts. *Am. J. Pathol*, 1996, 149, 1991-2003.

[70] Douglas, IS; Nicolls, MR. Chemokine-mediated angiogenesis: an essential link in the evolution of airway fibrosis? *J. Clin. Invest*, 2005, 115, 1133-6.

[71] Belperio, JA; Keane, MP; Burdick, MD; Gomperts, B; Xue, YY; Hong, K; Mestas, J; Ardehali, A; Mehrad, B; Saggar, R; Lynch, JP; Ross, DJ; Strieter, RM. Role of CXCR2/CXCR2 ligands in vascular remodeling during bronchiolitis obliterans syndrome. *J. Clin. Invest*, 2005, 115, 1150-62.

[72] Medoff, BD; Wain, JC; Seung, E; Jackobek, R; Means, TK; Ginns, LC; Farber, JM; Luster, AD. CXCR3 and its ligands in a murine model of obliterative bronchiolitis: regulation and function. *J. Immunol*, 2006, 176, 7087-95.

[73] Belperio, JA; Keane, MP; Burdick, MD; Lynch JP, 3rd; Xue, YY; Li, K; Ross, DJ; Strieter, RM. Critical role for CXCR3 chemokine biology in the pathogenesis of bronchiolitis obliterans syndrome. *J. Immunol*, 2002, 169, 1037-49.

[74] Belperio, JA; Keane, MP; Burdick, MD; Lynch JP, 3rd; Zisman, DA; Xue, YY; Li, K; Ardehali, A; Ross, DJ; Strieter, RM. Role of CXCL9/CXCR3 chemokine biology during pathogenesis of acute lung allograft rejection. *J. Immunol*, 2003, 171, 4844-52.

[75] Gomperts, BN; Belperio, JA; Rao, PN; Randell, SH; Fishbein, MC; Burdick, MD; Strieter, RM. Circulating progenitor epithelial cells traffic via CXCR4/CXCL12 in response to airway injury. *J. Immunol*, 2006, 176, 1916-27.

[76] Belperio, JA; Keane, MP; Burdick, MD; Lynch JP, 3rd; Xue, YY; Berlin, A; Ross, DJ; Kunkel, SL; Charo, IF; Strieter, RM. Critical role for the chemokine MCP-1/CCR2 in the pathogenesis of bronchiolitis obliterans syndrome. *J. Clin. Invest*, 2001, 108, 547-56.

[77] Belperio, JA; Burdick, MD; Keane, MP; Xue, YY; Lynch JP, 3rd; Daugherty, BL; Kunkel, SL; Strieter, RM. The role of the CC chemokine; RANTES; in acute lung allograft rejection. *J. Immunol*, 2000, 165, 461-72.

[78] Ross, DJ; Cole, AM; Yoshioka, D; Park, AK; Belperio, JA; Laks, H; Strieter, RM; Lynch JP, 3rd; Kubak, B; Ardehali, A; Ganz, T. Increased bronchoalveolar lavage human beta-defensin type 2 in bronchiolitis obliterans syndrome after lung transplantation. *Transplantation*, 2004, 78, 1222-4.

[79] Inston, NG; Cockwell, P. The evolving role of chemokines and their receptors in acute allograft rejection. *Nephrol. Dial. Transplant*, 2002, 17, 1374-9.

[80] Cugini, D; Azzollini, N; Gagliardini, E; Cassis, P; Bertini, R; Colotta, F; Noris, M; Remuzzi, G; Benigni, A. Inhibition of the chemokine receptor CXCR2 prevents kidney graft function deterioration due to ischemia/reperfusion. *Kidney Int*, 2005, 67, 1753-61.

[81] Araki, M; Fahmy, N; Zhou, L; Kumon, H; Krishnamurthi, V; Goldfarb, D; Modlin, C; Flechner, S; Novick, AC; Fairchild, RL. Expression of IL-8 during reperfusion of renal allografts is dependent on ischemic time. *Transplantation*, 2006, 81, 783-8.

[82] Budde, K; Waiser, J; Ceska, M; Katalinic, A; Kurzdorfer, M; Neumayer, HH. Interleukin-8 expression in patients after renal transplantation. *Am. J. Kidney Dis*, 1997, 29, 871-80.

[83] Hoffmann, U; Segerer, S; Rummele, P; Kruger, B; Pietrzyk, M; Hofstädter, F; Banas, B; Kramer, BK. Expression of the chemokine receptor CXCR3 in human renal allografts—a prospective study. *Nephrology Dialysis Transplantation*, 2006, 21, 1373-81.

[84] Romagnani, P. From basic science to clinical practice: use of cytokines and chemokines as therapeutic targets in renal diseases. *J. Nephrol*, 2005, 18, 229-33.

[85] Steinmetz, OM; Panzer, U; Kneissler, U; Harendza, S; Lipp, M; Helmchen, U; Stahl, RA. BCA-1/CXCL13 expression is associated with CXCR5-positive B-cell cluster formation in acute renal transplant rejection. *Kidney Int*, 2005, 67, 1616-21.

[86] Dalton, RS; Webber, JN; Pead, P; Gibbs, PJ; Sadek, SA; Howell, WM. Immunomonitoring of renal transplant recipients in the early posttransplant period by sequential analysis of chemokine and chemokine receptor gene expression in peripheral blood mononuclear cells. *Transplant. Proc*, 2005, 37, 747-51.

[87] Horuk, R; Shurey, S; Ng, HP; May, K; Bauman, JG; Islam, I; Ghannam, A; Buckman, B; Wei, GP; Xu, W; Liang, M; Rosser, M; Dunning, L; Hesselgesser, J; Snider, RM;

Morrissey, MM; Perez, HD; Green, C. CCR1-specific non-peptide antagonist: efficacy in a rabbit allograft rejection model. *Immunol. Lett*, 2001, 76, 193-201.

[88] Wang, J; Zou, H; Li, Q; Wang, Y; Xu, Q. The expression of monocyte chemoattractant protein-1 and C-C chemokine receptor 2 in post-kidney transplant patients and the influence of simvastatin treatment. *Clin. Chim. Acta*, 2006, 373, 44-8.

[89] Ruster, M; Sperschneider, H; Funfstuck, R; Stein, G; Grone, HJ. Differential expression of beta-chemokines MCP-1 and RANTES and their receptors CCR1; CCR2; CCR5 in acute rejection and chronic allograft nephropathy of human renal allografts. *Clin. Nephrol,* 2004, 61, 30-9.

[90] Abdi, R; Tran, TB; Sahagun-Ruiz, A; Murphy, PM; Brenner, BM; Milford, EL; McDermott, DH. Chemokine receptor polymorphism and risk of acute rejection in human renal transplantation. *J. Am. Soc. Nephrol*, 2002, 13, 754-8.

[91] Le Berre, L; Herve, C; Buzelin, F; Usal, C; Soulillou, JP; Dantal, J. Renal macrophage activation and Th2 polarization precedes the development of nephrotic syndrome in Buffalo/Mna rats. *Kidney Int*, 2005, 68, 2079-90.

[92] Hancock, WW. Chemokines and transplant immunobiology. *J. Am. Soc. Nephrol*, 2002, 13, 821-4.

[93] Fischereder, M; Luckow, B; Hocher, B; Wuthrich, RP; Rothenpieler, U; Schneeberger, H; Panzer, U; Stahl, RA; Hauser, IA; Budde, K; Neumayer, H; Kramer, BK; Land, W; Schlondorff, D. CC chemokine receptor 5 and renal-transplant survival. *Lancet*, 2001, 357, 1758-61.

[94] Yigit, B; Bozkurt, N; Berber, I; Titiz, I; Isbir, T. Analysis of CC chemokine receptor 5 and 2 polymorphisms and renal transplant survival. *Cell Biochem. Funct*, 2006, Apr 6; (Epub ahead of print).

[95] Lacha, J; Hribova, P; Kotsch, K; Brabcova, I; Bartosova, K; Volk, HD; Vitko, S. Effect of cytokines and chemokines (TGF-beta, TNF-alpha, IL-6, IL-10, MCP-1, RANTES) gene polymorphisms in kidney recipients on posttransplantation outcome: influence of donor-recipient match. *Transplant. Proc*, 2005, 37, 764-6.

[96] Akalin, E; Neylan, JF. The influence of Duffy blood group on renal allograft outcome in African Americans. *Transplantation*, 2003, 75, 1496-500.

[97] Segerer, S; Cui, Y; Eitner, F; Goodpaster, T; Hudkins, KL; Mack, M; Cartron, JP; Colin, Y; Schlondorff, D; Alpers, CE. Expression of chemokines and chemokine receptors during human renal transplant rejection. *Am. J. Kidney Dis*, 2001, 37, 518-31.

[98] Merani, S; Truong, WW; Hancock, W; Anderson, CC; Shapiro, AM. Chemokines and their receptors in islet allograft rejection and as targets for tolerance induction. *Cell Transplant*, 2006, 15, 295-309.

[99] Abdi, R; Means, TK; Ito, T; Smith, RN; Najafian, N; Jurewicz, M; Tchipachvili, V; Charo, I; Auchincloss, HJr; Sayegh, MH; Luster, AD. Differential role of CCR2 in islet and heart allograft rejection: tissue specificity of chemokine/chemokine receptor function in vivo. *J. Immunol*, 2004, 172, 767-75.

[100] Baker, MS; Chen, X; Rotramel, AR; Nelson, JJ; Lu, B; Gerard, C; Kanwar, Y; Kaufman, DB. Genetic deletion of chemokine receptor CXCR3 or antibody blockade of its ligand IP-10 modulates posttransplantation graft-site lymphocytic infiltrates and

prolongs functional graft survival in pancreatic islet allograft recipients. *Surgery*, 2003, 134, 126-33.

[101] Abdi, R; Smith, RN; Makhlouf, L; Najafian, N; Luster, AD; Auchincloss, HJr; Sayegh, MH. The role of CC chemokine receptor 5 (CCR5) in islet allograft rejection. *Diabetes*, 2002, 51, 2489-95.

[102] Sigrist, S; Ebel, N; Langlois, A; Bosco, D; Toso, C; Kleiss, C; Mandes, K; Berney, T; Pinget, M; Belcourt, A; Kessler, L. Role of chemokine signaling pathways in pancreatic islet rejection during allo- and xenotransplantation. *Transplant. Proc*, 2005, 37, 3516-8.

[103] Akashi, S; Sho, M; Kashizuka, H; Hamada, K; Ikeda, N; Kuzumoto, Y; Tsurui, Y; Nomi, T; Mizuno, T; Kanehiro, H; Hisanaga, M; Ko, S; Nakajima, Y. A novel small-molecule compound targeting CCR5 and CXCR3 prevents acute and chronic allograft rejection. *Transplantation*, 2005, 80, 378-84.

[104] Day, YJ; Marshall, MA; Huang, L; McDuffie, MJ; Okusa, MD; Linden, J. Protection from ischemic liver injury by activation of A2A adenosine receptors during reperfusion: inhibition of chemokine induction. *Am. J. Physiol. Gastrointest. Liver. Physiol*, 2004, 286, G285-93.

[105] Goddard, S; Williams, A; Morland, C; Qin, S; Gladue, R; Hubscher, SG; Adams, DH. Differential expression of chemokines and chemokine receptors shapes the inflammatory response in rejecting human liver transplants. *Transplantation*, 2001, 72, 1957-67.

[106] Krukemeyer, MG; Moeller, J; Morawietz, L; Rudolph, B; Neumann, U; Theruvath, T; Neuhaus, P; Krenn, V. Description of B lymphocytes and plasma cells, complement, and chemokines/receptors in acute liver allograft rejection. *Transplantation*, 2004, 78, 65-70.

[107] Moench, C; Uhrig, A; Lohse, AW; Otto, G. CC chemokine receptor 5delta32 polymorphism-a risk factor for ischemic-type biliary lesions following orthotopic liver transplantation. *Liver Transpl*, 2004, 10, 434-9.

[108] Schroppel, B; Fischereder, M; Lin, M; Marder, B; Schiano, T; Kramer, BK; Murphy, B. Analysis of gene polymorphisms in the regulatory region of MCP-1; RANTES; and CCR5 in liver transplant recipients. *J. Clin. Immunol*, 2002, 22, 381-5.

[109] Furuhashi, T; Yamaguchi, Y; Wang, FS; Uchino, S; Okabe, K; Ohshiro, H; Kihara, S; Yamada, S; Mori, K; Ogawa, M. Hepatic CCR7lowCD62LlowCD45RClow allograft dendritic cells migrate to the splenic red pulp in immunologically unresponsive rats. *J. Surg. Res*, 2005, 124, 29-37.

[110] Abe, M; Zahorchak, AF; Colvin, BL; Thomson, AW. Migratory responses of murine hepatic myeloid; lymphoid-related; and plasmacytoid dendritic cells to CC chemokines. *Transplantation*, 2004, 78, 762-5.

[111] Maekawa, T; Ishii, T. Chemokine/receptor dynamics in the regulation of hematopoiesis. *Intern. Med*, 2000, 39, 90-100.

[112] Pelus, LM; Horowitz, D; Cooper, SC; King, AG. Peripheral blood stem cell mobilization. A role for CXC chemokines. *Crit. Rev. Oncol. Hematol*, 2002, 43, 257-75.

[113] Rao, AR; Quinones, MP; Garavito, E; Kalkonde, Y; Jimenez, F; Gibbons, C; Perez, J; Melby, P; Kuziel, W; Reddick, RL; Ahuja, SK; Ahuja, SS. CC chemokine receptor 2 expression in donor cells serves an essential role in graft-versus-host-disease. *J. Immunol*, 2003, 171, 4875-85.

[114] Duffner, U; Lu, B; Hildebrandt, GC; Teshima, T; Williams, DL; Reddy, P; Ordemann, R; Clouthier, SG; Lowler, K; Liu, C; Gerard, C; Cooke, KR; Ferrara, JL. Role of CXCR3-induced donor T-cell migration in acute GVHD. *Exp. Hematol*, 2003, 31, 897-902.

[115] Hildebrandt, GC; Corrion, LA; Olkiewicz, KM; Lu, B; Lowler, K; Duffner, UA; Moore, BB; Kuziel, WA; Liu, C; Cooke, KR. Blockade of CXCR3 receptor: ligand interactions reduces leukocyte recruitment to the lung and the severity of experimental idiopathic pneumonia syndrome. *J. Immunol*, 2004, 173, 2050-9.

[116] Voermans, C; van Hennik, PB; van der Schoot, CE. Homing of human hematopoietic stem and progenitor cells: new insights, new challenges? *J. Hematother. Stem Cell Res*, 2001, 10, 725-38.

[117] Voermans, C; Gerritsen, WR; von dem Borne, AE; van der Schoot, CE. Increased migration of cord blood-derived CD34+ cells; as compared to bone marrow and mobilized peripheral blood CD34+ cells across uncoated or fibronectin-coated filters. *Exp. Hematol,* 1999, 27, 1806-14.

[118] Larochelle, A; Krouse, A; Metzger, M; Orlic, D; Donahue, RE; Fricker, S; Bridger, G; Dunbar, CE; Hematti, P. AMD3100 mobilizes hematopoietic stem cells with long-term repopulating capacity in nonhuman primates. *Blood*, 2006, 107, 3772-8.

[119] Broxmeyer, HE; Orschell, CM; Clapp, DW; Hangoc, G; Cooper, S; Plett, PA; Liles, WC; Li, X; Graham-Evans, B; Campbell, TB; Calandra, G; Bridger, G; Dale, DC; Srour, EF. Rapid mobilization of murine and human hematopoietic stem and progenitor cells with AMD3100; a CXCR4 antagonist. *J. Exp. Med*, 2005, 201, 1307-18.

[120] Wright, DE; Bowman, EP; Wagers, AJ; Butcher, EC; Weissman, IL. Hematopoietic stem cells are uniquely selective in their migratory response to chemokines. *J. Exp. Med*, 2002, 195, 1145-54.

[121] Spencer, A; Jackson, J; Baulch-Brown, C. Enumeration of bone marrow 'homing' haemopoietic stem cells from G-CSF-mobilised normal donors and influence on engraftment following allogeneic transplantation. *Bone Marrow Transplant*, 2001, 28, 1019-22.

[122] Lataillade, JJ; Clay, D; Dupuy, C; Rigal, S; Jasmin, C; Bourin, P; Le Bousse-Kerdiles, MC. Chemokine SDF-1 enhances circulating CD34(+) cell proliferation in synergy with cytokines: possible role in progenitor survival. *Blood*, 2000, 95, 756-68.

[123] Petit, I; Szyper-Kravitz, M; Nagler, A; Lahav, M; Peled, A; Habler, L; Ponomaryov, T; Taichman, RS; Arenzana-Seisdedos, F; Fujii, N; Sandbank, J; Zipori, D; Lapidot, T. G-CSF induces stem cell mobilization by decreasing bone marrow SDF-1 and up-regulating CXCR4. *Nat. Immunol*, 2002, 3, 687-94.

[124] Carion, A; Benboubker, L; Herault, O; Roingeard, F; Degenne, M; Senecal, D; Desbois, I; Colombat, P; Charbord, P; Binet, C; Domenech, J. Stromal-derived factor 1 and matrix metalloproteinase 9 levels in bone marrow and peripheral blood of patients mobilized by granulocyte colony-stimulating factor and chemotherapy. Relationship

with mobilizing capacity of haematopoietic progenitor cells. *Br. J. Haematol,* 2003, 122, 918-26.

[125] Rosu-Myles, M; Gallacher, L; Murdoch, B; Hess, DA; Keeney, M; Kelvin, D; Dale, L; Ferguson, SS; Wu, D; Fellows, F; Bhatia, M. The human hematopoietic stem cell compartment is heterogeneous for CXCR4 expression. *Proc. Natl. Acad. Sci. USA,* 2000, 97, 14626-31.

[126] Nagasawa, T. A chemokine SDF-1/PBSF and its receptor CXC chemokine receptor 4, as mediators of hematopoiesis. *Int. J. Hematol,* 2000, 72, 408-11.

[127] Beider, K; Nagler, A; Wald, O; Franitza, S; Dagan-Berger, M; Wald, H; Giladi, H; Brocke, S; Hanna, J; Mandelboim, O; Darash-Yahana, M; Galun, E; Peled, A. Involvement of CXCR4 and IL-2 in the homing and retention of human NK and NK T cells to the bone marrow and spleen of NOD/SCID mice. *Blood,* 2003, 102, 1951-8.

[128] Jaksch, M; Remberger, M; Mattsson, J. Increased gene expression of chemokine receptors is correlated with acute graft-versus-host disease after allogeneic stem cell transplantation. *Biol. Blood Marrow Transplant,* 2005, 11, 280-7.

[129] Hildebrandt, GC; Duffner, UA; Olkiewicz, KM; Corrion, LA; Willmarth, NE; Williams, DL; Clouthier, SG; Hogaboam, CM; Reddy, PR; Moore, BB; Kuziel, WA; Liu, C; Yanik, G; Cooke, KR. A critical role for CCR2/MCP-1 interactions in the development of idiopathic pneumonia syndrome after allogeneic bone marrow transplantation. *Blood,* 2004, 103, 2417-26.

[130] Loeffler, J; Steffens, M; Arlt, EM; Toliat, MR; Mezger, M; Suk, A; Wienker, TF; Hebart, H; Nurnberg, P; Boeckh, M; Ljungman, P; Trenschel, R; Einsele, H. Polymorphisms in the genes encoding chemokine receptor 5, interleukin-10, and monocyte chemoattractant protein 1 contribute to cytomegalovirus reactivation and disease after allogeneic stem cell transplantation. *J. Clin. Microbiol,* 2006, 44, 1847-50.

[131] Jiankuo, M; Xingbing, W; Baojun, H; Xiongwin, W; Zhuoya, L; Ping, X; Yong, X; Anting, L; Chunsong, H; Feili, G; Jinquan, T. Peptide nucleic acid antisense prolongs skin allograft survival by means of blockade of CXCR3 expression directing T cells into graft. *J. Immunol,* 2003, 170, 1556-65.

[132] Kondo, T; Watarai, Y; Novick, AC; Toma, H; Fairchild, RL. T cell-dependent acceleration of chemoattractant cytokine gene expression during secondary rejection of allogeneic skin grafts. *Transplantation,* 1997, 63, 732-42.

[133] Kondo, T; Novick, AC; Toma, H; Fairchild, RL. Induction of chemokine gene expression during allogeneic skin graft rejection. *Transplantation,* 1996, 61, 1750-7.

[134] Jiang, X; Shimaoka, T; Kojo, S; Harada, M; Watarai, H; Wakao, H; Ohkohchi, N; Yonehara, S; Taniguchi, M; Seino, K. Cutting edge: Critical role of CXCL16/CXCR6 in NKT cell trafficking in allograft tolerance. *J. Immunol,* 2005, 175, 2051-5.

[135] Lee, I; Wang, L; Wells, AD; Dorf, ME; Ozkaynak, E; Hancock, WW. Recruitment of Foxp3+ T regulatory cells mediating allograft tolerance depends on the CCR4 chemokine receptor. *J. Exp. Med,* 2005, 201, 1037-44.

[136] Lagaraine, C; Hoarau, C; Chabot, V; Velge-Roussel, F; Lebranchu, Y. Mycophenolic acid-treated human dendritic cells have a mature migratory phenotype and inhibit allogeneic responses via direct and indirect pathways. *Int. Immunol,* 2005, 17, 351-63.

[137] Louvet, C; Heslan, JM; Merieau, E; Soulillou, JP; Cuturi, MC; Chiffoleau, E. Induction of Fractalkine and CX3CR1 mediated by host CD8+ T cells in allograft tolerance induced by donor specific blood transfusion. *Transplantation*, 2004, 78, 1259-66.

[138] Bendall, L. Chemokines and their receptors in disease. *Histol. Histopathol*, 2005, 20, 907-26.

[139] Hancock, WW; Wang, L; Ye, Q; Han, R; Lee, I. Chemokines and their receptors as markers of allograft rejection and targets for immunosuppression. *Curr. Opin. Immunol*, 2003, 15, 479-86.

[140] Martine, Reynaud-Gaubert; Valerie, Marin; Xavier, Thirion; Catherine, Farnarier; Pascal, Thomas; Monique, Badier; Pierre, Bongrand; Roger, Giudicelli; Pierre, Fuentes. Upregulation of Chemokines in Bronchoalveolar Lavage Fluid as a Predictive Marker of Post-Transplant Airway Obliteration. *J. Heart Lung Transplant*, 2002, 21, 721–730.

[141] Henschler, R; Piiper, A; Bistrian, R; Mobest, D. SDF-1alpha-induced intracellular calcium transient involves Rho GTPase signalling and is required for migration of hematopoietic progenitor cells. *Biochem. Biophys. Res. Commun*, 2003, 311, 1067-71.

[142] Walter, DH; Haendeler, J; Reinhold, J; Rochwalsky, U; Seeger, F; Honold, J; Hoffmann, J; Urbich, C; Lehmann, R; Arenzana-Seisdesdos, F; Aicher, A; Heeschen, C; Fichtlscherer, S; Zeiher, AM; Dimmeler, S. Impaired CXCR4 signaling contributes to the reduced neovascularization capacity of endothelial progenitor cells from patients with coronary artery disease. *Circ. Res*, 2005, 97, 1142-51.

[143] Lataillade, JJ; Domenech, J; Le Bousse-Kerdiles, MC. Stromal cell-derived factor-1 (SDF-1)\CXCR4 couple plays multiple roles on haematopoietic progenitors at the border between the old cytokine and new chemokine worlds: survival; cell cycling and trafficking. *Eur. Cytokine Netw*, 2004, 15, 177-88.

[144] Belmadani, A; Tran, PB; Ren, D; Miller, RJ. Chemokines regulate the migration of neural progenitors to sites of neuroinflammation. *J. Neurosci*, 2006, 26, 3182-91.

[145] Terwey, TH; Kim, TD; Kochman, AA; Hubbard, VM; Lu, S; Zakrzewski, JL; Ramirez-Montagut, T; Eng, JM; Muriglan, SJ; Heller, G; Murphy, GF; Liu, C; Budak-Alpdogan, T; Alpdogan, O; van den Brink, MR. CCR2 is required for CD8-induced graft-versus-host disease. *Blood*, 2005, 106, 3322-30.

[146] Wysocki, CA; Jiang, Q; Panoskaltsis-Mortari, A; Taylor, PA; McKinnon, KP; Su, L; Blazar, BR; Serody, JS. Critical role for CCR5 in the function of donor CD4+CD25+ regulatory T cells during acute graft-versus-host disease. *Blood*, 2005, 106, 3300-7.

[147] Krautwald, S; Ziegler, E; Forster, R; Ohl, L; Amann, K; Kunzendorf, U. Ectopic expression of CCL19 impairs alloimmune response in mice. *Immunology*, 2004, 112, 301-9.

[148] Hopken, UE; Droese, J; Li, JP; Joergensen, J; Breitfeld, D; Zerwes, HG; Lipp, M. The chemokine receptor CCR7 controls lymph node-dependent cytotoxic T cell priming in alloimmune responses. *Eur. J. Immunol*, 2004, 34, 461-70.

[149] Jinquan, T; Deleuran, B; Gesser, B; Maare, H; Larsen, CG; Thestrup-Pedersen, K. Regulation of human T lymphocyte chemotaxis in vitro by T-cell derived cytokines, IL-13, IL-4 and IL-10. *J. Immunol*, 1995, 154, 3742-52.

[150] Jinquan, T; Quan, S; Feili, G; Larsen, CG; Thestrup-Pedersen, K. Eotaxin activates T cells to chemotaxis and adhesion only if induced to express CCR3 by IL-2 together with IL-4. *J. Immunol*, 1999, 162, 4285-92.

[151] Haribabu, B; Zhelev, DV; Pridgen, BC; Richardson, RM; Ali, H; Snyderman, R. Chemoattractant receptors activate distinct pathways for chemotaxis and secretion. Role of G-protein usage. *J. Biol. Chem*, 1999, 274, 37087-92.

[152] Jinquan, T; Quan, S; Jacobi, HH; Madsen, HO; Glue, C; Skov, PS; Malling, HJ; Poulsen, LK. CXC chemokine receptor 4 expression and stromal cell-derived factor-1alpha-induced chemotaxis in CD4+ T lymphocytes are regulated by interleukin-4 and interleukin-10. *Immunology*, 2000, 99, 402-10.

[153] Jinquan, T; Quan, S; Jacobi, HH; Jing, C; Millner, A; Jensen, B; Madsen, HO; Ryder, LP; Svejgaard, A; Malling, HJ; Skov, PS; Poulsen, LK. CXC chemokine receptor 3 expression on CD34+ hematopoietic progenitors from human cord blood induced by granulocyte-macrophage colony-stimulating factor: chemotaxis and adhesion induced by its ligands, interferon γ-inducible protein 10 and monokine induced by interferon γ. *Blood*, 2000, 96, 1230-8.

[154] Jinquan, T; Jing, C; Jacobi, HH; Reimert, CM; Millner, A; Quan, S; Hansen, JB; Dissing, S; Malling, HJ; Skov, PS; Poulsen, LK. CXCR3 expression and activation of eosinophils: role of interferon γ-inducible protein 10 and monokine induced by interferon γ. *J. Immunol*, 2000, 165, 1548-56.

[155] Oppermann, M; Mack, M; Proudfoot, AE; Olbrich, H. Differential effects of CC chemokines on CC chemokine receptor 5 (CCR5) phosphorylation and identification of phosphorylation sites on the CCR5 carboxyl terminus. *J. Biol. Chem*, 1999, 274, 8875-85.

[156] Turner, SJ; Domin, J; Waterfield, MD; Ward, SG; Westwick, J. The CC chemokine monocyte chemotactic peptide-1 activates both the class I p85/p110 phosphatidylinositol 3-kinase and the class II PI3K-C2alpha. *J. Biol. Chem*, 1998, 273, 25987-95.

[157] Wong, M; Fish, EN. RANTES and MIP-1alpha activate stats in T cells. *J. Biol. Chem*, 1998, 273, 309-14.

[158] Zhao, J; Ma, L; Wu, YL; Wang, P; Hu, W; Pei, G. Chemokine receptor CCR5 functionally couples to inhibitory G proteins and undergoes desensitization. *J. Cell Biochem*, 1998, 71, 36-45.

[159] Zimmermann, N; Conkright, JJ; Rothenberg, ME. CC chemokine receptor-3 undergoes prolonged ligand-induced internalization. *J. Biol. Chem*, 1999, 274, 12611-8.

[160] Wysocki, CA; Panoskaltsis-Mortari, A; Blazar, BR; Serody, JS. Leukocyte migration and graft-versus-host disease. *Blood*, 2005, 105, 4191-9.

[161] Mellado, M; Rodriguez-Frade, JM; Manes, S; Martinez, AC. Chemokine signaling and functional responses: the role of receptor dimerization and TK pathway activation. *Annu. Rev. Immunol*, 2001, 19, 397-421.

[162] Jones, SA; Moser, B; Thelen, M. A comparison of post-receptor signal transduction events in Jurkat cells transfected with either IL-8R1 or IL-8R2: chemokine mediated activation of p42/p44 MAP-kinase (ERK-2). *FEBS Lett*, 1995, 364, 211-4.

[163] Knall, C; Young, S; Nick, JA; Buhl, AM; Worthen, GS; Johnson, GL. Interleukin-8 regulation of the Ras/Raf/mitogen-activated protein kinase pathway in human neutrophils. *J. Biol. Chem*, 1996, 271, 2832-8.

[164] Ganju, RK; Dutt, P; Wu, L; Newman, W; Avraham, H; Avraham, S; Groopman, JE. Beta-chemokine receptor CCR5 signals via the novel tyrosine kinase RAFTK. *Blood*, 1998, 91, 791-7.

[165] Kampen, GT; Stafford, S; Adachi, T; Jinquan, T; Quan, S; Grant, JA; Skov, PS; Poulsen, LK; Alam, R. Eotaxin induces degranulation and chemotaxis of eosinophils through the activation of ERK2 and p38 mitogen-activated protein kinases. *Blood*, 2000, 95, 1911-7.

[166] Cowley, S; Paterson, H; Kemp, P; Marshall, CJ. Activation of MAP kinase kinase is necessary and sufficient for PC12 differentiation and for transformation of NIH 3T3 cells. *Cell*, 1994, 77, 841-52.

[167] Thelen, M; Uguccioni, M; Bösiger, J. PI 3-kinase-dependent and independent chemotaxis of human neutrophil leukocytes. *Biochem. Biophys. Res. Commun*, 1995, 17, 1255-62.

[168] Tilton, B; Andjelkovic, M; Didichenko, SA; Hemmings, BA; Thelen, M. G-protein-coupled receptors and Fcγ-receptors mediate activation of Akt protein kinase B in human phagocytes. *J. Biol. Chem*, 1997, 272, 28096-101.

[169] Didichenko, SA; Tilton, B; Hemmings, BA; Ballmer-Hofer, K; Thelen, M. Constitutive activation of protein kinase B and phosphorylation of p47phox by membrane-targeted phosphoinositide 3-kinase. *Curr. Biol*, 1996, 6, 1271-8.

[170] Luttrell, LM; Lefkowitz, RJ. The role of beta-arrestins in the termination and transduction of G-protein-coupled receptor signals. *J. Cell Sci*, 2002, 115, 455-65.

[171] Ali, H; Richardson, RM; Haribabu, B; Snyderman, R. Chemoattractant receptor cross-desensitization. *J. Biol. Chem*, 1999, 274, 6027-30.

[172] Hecht, I; Cahalon, L; Hershkoviz, R; Lahat, A; Franitza, S; Lider, O. Heterologous desensitization of T cell functions by CCR5 and CXCR4 ligands: inhibition of cellular signaling; adhesion and chemotaxis. *Int. Immunol*, 2003, 15, 29-38.

[173] Honczarenko, M; Le, Y; Glodek, AM. CCR5-binding chemokines modulate CXCL12 (SDF-1)–induced responses of progenitor B cells in human bone marrow through heterologous desensitization of the CXCR4 chemokine receptor. *Blood*, 2002, 100, 2321-29.

[174] Carvalho-Gaspar, M; Billing, JS; Spriewald, BM; Wood, KJ. Chemokine gene expression during allograft rejection: comparison of two quantitative PCR techniques. *J. Immunol. Methods*, 2005, 301, 41-52.

[175] Coffield, VM; Jiang, Q; Su, L. A genetic approach to inactivating chemokine receptors using a modified viral protein. *Nat. Biotechnol*, 2003, 21, 1321-7.

[176] Cascieri, MA; Springer, MS. The chemokine/chemokine-receptor family: potential and progress for therapeutic intervention. *Curr. Opin. Chem. Biol*, 2000, 4, 420-7.

[177] Koppelhus, U; Zachar, V; Nielsen, PE; Liu, X; Eugen-Olsen, J; Ebbesen, P. Efficient in vitro inhibition of HIV-1 gag reverse transcription by peptide nucleic acid (PNA) at minimal ratios of PNA/RNA. *Nucleic Acids Res*, 1997, 25, 2167-73.

[178] Gambacorti-Passerini, C; Mologni, L; Bertazzoli, C; le Coutre, P; Marchesi, E; Grignani, F; Nielsen, PE. In vitro transcription and translation inhibition by anti-promyelocytic leukemia (PML)/retinoic acid receptor-α and anti-PML peptide nucleic acid. *Blood*, 1996, 88, 1411-7.

[179] Mologni, L; Marchesi, E; Nielsen, PE; Gambacorti-Passerini, C. Inhibition of promyelocytic leukemia (PML)/retinoic acid receptor-α and PML expression in acute promyelocytic leukemia cells by anti-PML peptide nucleic acid. *Cancer Res*, 2001, 61, 5468-73.

[180] Boffa, LC; Scarfi, S; Mariani, MR; Damonte, G.; Allfrey, VG; Benatti, U; Morris, PL. Dihydrotestosterone as a selective cellular/nuclear localization vector for anti-gene peptide nucleic acid in prostatic carcinoma cells. *Cancer Res*, 2000, 60, 2258-62.

[181] Stock, RP; Olvera, A; Sanchez, R; Saralegui, A; Scarfi, S; Sanchez-Lopez, R; Ramos, MA; Boffa, LC; Benatti, U; Alagon, A. Inhibition of gene expression in Entamoeba histolytica with antisense peptide nucleic acid oligomers. *Nat. Biotechnol*, 2001, 19, 231-4.

[182] Cutrona, G; Carpaneto, EM; Ulivi, M; Roncella, S; Landt, O; Ferrarini, M; Boffa, LC. Effects in live cells of a c-myc anti-gene PNA linked to a nuclear localization signal. *Nat. Biotechnol*, 2000, 18, 300-3.

[183] Nielsen, PE. Peptide nucleic acid: a versatile tool in genetic diagnostics and molecular biology. *Curr. Opin. Biotechnol*, 2001, 12, 16-20.

[184] Ondeykal, JG; Herath, KB; Jayasuriya, H; Polishook, JD; Bills, GF; Dombrowski, AW; Mojena, M; Koch, G; DiSalvo, J; DeMartino, J; Guan, Z; Nanakorn, W; Morenberg, CM; Balick, MJ; Stevenson, DW; Slattery, M; Borris, RP; Singh, SB. Discovery of structurally diverse natural product antagonists of chemokine receptor CXCR3. *Mol. Divers*, 2005, 9, 123-9.

[185] Elisseeva, EL; Slupsky, CM; Crump, MP; Clark-Lewis, I; Sykes, BD. NMR studies of active N-terminal peptides of stromal cell-derived factor-1. Structural basis for receptor binding. *J. Biol. Chem*, 2000, 275, 26799-805.

[186] Flomenberg, N; Devine, SM; Dipersio, JF; Liesveld, JL; McCarty, JM; Rowley, SD; Vesole, DH; Badel, K; Calandra, G. The use of AMD3100 plus G-CSF for autologous hematopoietic progenitor cell mobilization is superior to G-CSF alone. *Blood*, 2005, 106, 1867-74.

[187] Fleury, S; Li, J; Simeoni, E; Fiorini, E; von Segesser, LK; Kappenberger, L; Vassalli, G. Gene transfer of RANTES and MCP-1 chemokine antagonists prolongs cardiac allograft survival. *Gene Ther*, 2006, 13, 1104-9.

[188] Saiura, A; Sata, M; Hiasa, K; Kitamoto, S; Washida, M; Egashira, K; Nagai, R; Makuuchi, M. Antimonocyte chemoattractant protein-1 gene therapy attenuates graft vasculopathy. *Arterioscler. Thromb. Vasc. Biol*, 2004, 24, 1886-90.

[189] Daly, AK; Day, CP; Donaldson, PT. Polymorphisms in immunoregulatory genes: towards individualized immunosuppressive therapy? *Am. J. Pharmacogenomics*, 2002, 2, 13-23.

[190] Thoma, G; Nuninger, F; Schaefer, M; Akyel, KG; Albert, R; Beerli, C; Bruns, C; Francotte, E; Luyten, M; MacKenzie, D; Oberer, L; Streiff, MB; Wagner, T; Walter, H;

Weckbecker, G; Zerwes, HG. Orally bioavailable competitive CCR5 antagonists. *J. Med. Chem*, 2004, 47, 1939-55.

[191] Tang, W; Zhou, R; Yang, Y; Li, YC; Yang, YF; Zuo, JP. Suppression of (5R)-5-hydroxytriptolide (LLDT-8) on allograft rejection in full MHC-mismatched mouse cardiac transplantation. *Transplantation*, 2006, 81, 927-33.

[192] Qian, Y; Dekaris, I; Yamagami, S; Dana, MR. Topical soluble tumor necrosis factor receptor type I suppresses ocular chemokine gene expression and rejection of allogeneic corneal transplants. *Arch. Ophthalmol*, 2000, 118, 1666-71.

[193] Notohamiprodjo, M; Djafarzadeh, R; Mojaat, A; von Luttichau, I; Grone, HJ; Nelson, PJ. Generation of GPI-linked CCL5 based chemokine receptor antagonists for the suppression of acute vascular damage during allograft transplantation. *Protein Eng. Des. Sel*, 2006, 19, 27-35.

[194] Song, E; Zou, H; Yao, Y; Proudfoot, A; Antus, B; Liu, S; Jens, L; Heemann, U. Early application of Met-RANTES ameliorates chronic allograft nephropathy. *Kidney Int*, 2002, 61, 676-85.

[195] Randolph, GJ; Angeli, V; Swartz, MA. Dendritic-cell trafficking to lymph nodes through lymphatic vessels. *Nat. Rev. Immunol*, 2005, 5, 617-28.

[196] Weninger, W; von Andrian, UH. Chemokine regulation of naive T cell traffic in health and disease. *Semin. Immunol*, 2003, 15, 257-70.

[197] Fu, S; Chen, D; Mao, X; Zhang, N; Ding, Y; Bromberg, JS. Feline immunodeficiency virus-mediated viral interleukin-10 gene transfer prolongs non-vascularized cardiac allograft survival. *Am. J. Transplant*, 2003, 3, 552-61.

[198] Coates, PT; Colvin, BL; Kaneko, K; Taner, T; Thomson, AW. Pharmacologic, biologic, and genetic engineering approaches to potentiation of donor-derived dendritic cell tolerogenicity. *Transplantation*, 2003, 75, 32S-36S.

[199] Ohsawa, I; Murakami, T; Uemoto, S; Kobayashi, E. In vivo luminescent imaging of cyclosporin A-mediated cancer progression in rats. *Transplantation*, 2006, 81, 1558-67.

[200] Fischereder, M; Kretzler, M. New immunosuppressive strategies in renal transplant recipients. *J. Nephrol*, 2004, 17, 9-18.

[201] Hancock, WW; Gao, W; Csizmadia, V; Faia, KL; Shemmeri, N; Luster, AD. Donor-derived IP-10 initiates development of acute allograft rejection. *J. Exp. Med*, 2001, 193, 975-80.

[202] Miura, M; Morita, K; Kobayashi, H; Hamilton, TA; Burdick, MD; Strieter, RM; Fairchild, RL. Monokine induced by IFN-γ is a dominant factor directing T cells into murine cardiac allografts during acute rejection. *J. Immunol*, 2001, 167, 3494-504.

[203] Agostini, C; Calabrese, F; Rea, F; Facco, M; Tosoni, A; Loy, M; Binotto, G; Valente, M; Trentin, L; Semenzato, G. CXCR3 and its ligand CXCL10 are expressed by inflammatory cells infiltrating lung allografts and mediate chemotaxis of T cells at sites of rejection. *Am J Pathol*, 2001, 158, 1703-11.

[204] Strieter, RM; Belperio, JA. Chemokine receptor polymorphism in transplantation immunology: no longer just important in AIDS. *Lancet*, 2001, 357, 1725-6.

[205] Koga, S; Auerbach, MB; Engeman, TM; Novick, AC; Toma, H; Fairchild, RL. T cell infiltration into class II MHC-disparate allografts and acute rejection is dependent on the IFN-induced chemokine Mig. *J. Immunol*, 1999, 163, 4878-85.

[206] Watarai, Y; Koga, S; Paolone, DR; Engeman, TM; Tannenbaum, C; Hamilton, TA; Fairchild, RL. Intraallograft chemokine RNA and protein during rejection of MHC-matched/multiple minor histocompatibility-disparate skin grafts. *J. Immunol*, 2000, 164, 6027-33.

[207] Egholm, M; Buchardt, O; Christensen, L; Behrens, C; Freier, SM; Driver, DA; Berg, RH; Kim, SK; Norden, B; Nielsen, PE. PNA hybridizes to complementary oligonucleotides obeying the Watson-Crick hydrogen-bonding rules. *Nature*, 1993, 365, 566-8.

[208] Demidov, VV; Potaman, VN; Frank-Kamenetskii, MD; Egholm, M; Buchard, O; Sonnichsen, SH; Nielsen, PE. Stability of peptide nucleic acids in human serum and cellular extracts. *Biochem. Pharmacol*, 1994, 48, 1310-3.

[209] Hanvey, JC; Peffer, NJ; Bisi, JE; Thomson, SA; Cadilla, R; Josey, JA; Ricca, DJ; Hassman, CF; Bonham, MA; Au, KG. Antisense and antigene properties of peptide nucleic acids. *Science*, 1992, 258, 1481-5.

[210] Gray, DG; Basu, S; Wickstrom, E. Transformed and immortalized cellular uptake of oligodeoxynucleoside phosphorothioates, 3'-alkylamino oligodeoxynucleotides, 2'-O-methyl oligoribonucleotides, oligodeoxynucleosides methylphosphonates, and peptides nucleic acids. *Biochem. Pharmacol*, 1997, 53, 1465-76.

[211] Pooga, M; Soomets, U; Hallbrink, M; Valkna, A; Saar, K; Rezaei, K; Kahl, U; Hao, JX; Xu, XJ; Wiesenfeld-Hallin Z, Hokfelt T, Bartfai T, Langel U. Cell penetrating PNA constructs regulate galanin receptor levels and modify pain transmission in vivo. *Nat. Biotechnol*, 1998, 16, 857-61.

[212] Fruehauf, S; Seeger, T; Topaly, J. Innovative strategies for PBPC mobilization. *Cytotherapy*, 2005, 7, 438-46.

[213] Kilic, M; Kahan, BD. New trends in immunosuppression. *Drugs Today. (Barc)*, 2000, 36, 395-410.

In: Transplantation Immunology Research Trends
Editor: Oliver N. Ulricker, pp. 87-110

ISBN: 978-1-60021-578-0
© 2007 Nova Science Publishers, Inc.

Chapter III

Immune Tolerance in Transplantation

Phillip Ruiz, Jennifer Barker and Andreas Tzakis
University of Miami School of Medicine, FL USA

Abstract

The advent and successful evolution of human solid organ transplantation over the past 50 years has been a remarkable achievement that has provided thousands of patients with certain types of end stage organ disease an improved life with notably reduced morbidity and mortality. In order to achieve this success there has been the need for significant immunosuppression of the host to prevent recipient alloimmune responses from rejecting the genetically disparate donor organ. Unfortunately, the application of immunosuppression comes at a price and carries with it the potential for numerous life threatening and debilitating side effects. Since donor allograft tolerance has been extensively characterized and accomplished in animal models, transplant physicians have always attempted to achieve immunological tolerance in human transplant recipients in order to attain a state of specific nonreactivity to the donor transplant with little or no immunosuppression but without sacrificing graft function. To date, the realization of true immunological tolerance in human transplantation remains elusive; however, there have been many examples where a state of "operational" tolerance has been achieved. This chapter will describe these clinical occurrences and based upon animal models, an overview of some postulated mechanisms in immune tolerance.

I. Introduction: Definition of Immunological Tolerance

In order to maintain proper homeostasis in the face of exogenous microorganisms and endogenously generated pathological processes with novel antigenic epitopes, a host must have a properly functioning adaptive immune system capable of selectively mounting immune responses to non-self molecules while remaining unresponsive to molecules produced by the host. This state of selective and non-injurious immunity that ignores host structures in a healthy individual is designated as *immune tolerance*. It is the amalgamation of a variety of complex changes that occur among and between different cell lineages of the immune system. As with many aspects of the immune system, there are often overlapping and recapitulating effects of the various components of the immune system so that depending on the particular deficiency there may not be a notable change in the overall immune response or tolerance status. Malleability and induction of alternative cellular pathways may compensate for one or more given defects. However, a more central or critical flaw in the immune networks supporting the maintenance of immune tolerance, such as the steps involved in blocking autoreactive cells from maturation, can result in the generation of systemic autoimmunity or dysfunctional response to neoantigens. While immune tolerance occurs normally in the healthy immunocompetent host, there are also several experimental animal models that have demonstrated how an *alteration* of the immune pathways can make the host artificially tolerant to foreign antigens. The most notable example of beneficial *actively acquired* immune tolerance and the core topic of this chapter is an attempt to induce tolerance in the host response to allogeneic or xenogeneic organ transplants while maintaining normal immunity to other pathogens. This highly desirable state of *transplantation tolerance*, is as of yet, not easily attainable in humans and remains the "holy grail" of transplant physicians.

The modern-day notion of inducing tolerance to foreign grafts was originally conceived in 1945 with the observation by Owen [1] that Freemartin cattle sharing the same placenta exhibited hematopoietic chimerism and accepted allogeneic skin grafts from their twins later in life without the need for immunosuppression. This observation was the basis of ground breaking experiments by Billingham, Brent, and Medawar who attempted in 1953 [2] to *induce* tolerance artificially in experimental animals. These investigators inoculated tissues from allogeneic adult donors into fetal mice which led to hematopoietic chimerism; in adulthood, the inoculated mice showed specific acceptance (i.e., tolerance) to donor strain graft challenge (unrelated third party grafts were rejected) and this provided the first direct experimental evidence that artificial tolerance was attainable. Since then, the field of transplantation immunology has emerged with particular focus upon and investigation of the mechanisms of tolerance and whether tolerance can be induced in the transplanted host. Indeed, our understanding of tolerance has grown tremendously and has been the basis of clinical and preclinical studies developed in an attempt to induce true transplantation tolerance. True transplantation tolerance is measured by long-term graft acceptance due to a specific lack of immune response to the graft and without immunosuppression. While this Holy Grail of transplantation tolerance yet remains to be attained, many studies (some discussed later in this chapter) show promise that this goal is in the not too distant future and ultimately attainable.

The mechanisms operative in normal immune tolerance have direct relevance to the artificial acquisition of allogeneic graft tolerance. Essentially, for the latter to occur there has to be a variety of different interactions between introduced allogeneic cells and subpopulations of host immune cells. These interactions are not restricted to neonatal exposure and can be reproduced under the appropriate conditions in adult experimental animals. In order to understand these interactions it is important to get an overview of the means by which tolerance normally occurs in the host and to which cell populations.

II. Mechanisms of Central and Peripheral Immune Tolerance

A. The Central Compartment

The immune system is organized into two major subdivisions, the innate (nonspecific) immune system and the adaptive (specific) immune system [3, 4]. The innate immune system serves as a primary and major guard against invading organisms while the adaptive immune system affords specific secondary protection and can instill memory responses to the host that defend upon re-exposure to the offending pathogen or antigen.. Cellular and humoral components are present in both of the arms of the immune system and there can be significant interaction between the two systems. Insofar as graft recognition and rejection, there is a role for the innate immune system in recognizing and promoting immunity to alloantigens [5], however, the principal system operative in the response to transplants is the adaptive immune system [6]. In contrast to the nonspecific, constitutive nature of the innate immune system, the adaptive component is antigen specific and exhibits immunological memory. These two latter features make the adaptive immune system a formidable hurdle that must be crossed in transplantation since allografts represent an introduction of foreign tissue. The adaptive system is exemplified by the actions of T cells and B cells in the immune response, essentially responsible for the specificity of cellular and humoral arms of the immune response, respectively. Antigen specificity by T cells and B cells is mediated through heterodimeric antigen receptors expressed on their surfaces. During the development of these cell lineages and the culmination of a series of molecular events, these receptors [T cell receptor (TCR) and B cell receptor (BCR)] [7, 8] are each instilled with a remarkable degree of intrinsic specificity for a particular ligand. The result is that there is a remarkable amount of diversity *between* these molecules and thus, the host upon encounter can identify a vast number of antigen epitopes.

The *generation* of T and B cells in the mammalian host results from central, regulated processes that provide the individual with latent immune cell populations that are capable of recognizing and responding to external antigens but that tend to ignore homologous or self molecules. Therefore, this *central* development of lymphoid cells is the period during which B and T cells are selected in a fashion that eliminates self-reacting cells but promotes those that recognize external antigens; a process characterized as *central tolerance*. T cells develop from hematopoietic stem cells that travel to the thymus. This development in the thymus requires interactions with stromal cells such as thymic epithelial cells (TECs), mesenchymal fibroblasts and bone marrow (BM)-derived dendritic cells (DCs). Signals are provided to these immature thymocytes (no expression of CD4 and CD8, i.e., double negative [DN] cells) to differentiate within distinct thymic anatomic sites [9]. As these cells move through the thymic cortex CD44 and subsequently CD25 are expressed. The two lineages of T cells—α/β and γ/δ separate at this stage, congruent with rearrangement of the T cell receptor (TCR). For α/β T cells there is the CD3, TCRβ, pre-TCRα chain (pTα) complex and for γ/δ T cells, there is the γ/δ/CD3 complex. CD4 and CD8 coreceptors are next expressed (double-positive [DP] thymocytes) and there is rearrangement of the TCR α locus. The specificity of the antigen receptor will then determine whether the cell survives through the process of positive and negative selection, the latter an important component of central tolerance. *Negative selection* is the mechanism by which T cells with unwanted reactivity to self-components are removed in the thymus. The DP thymocytes with high affinities or avidities to self-antigen result in the elimination of the cell (*clonal deletion*) [10]. Thymic *positive selection* of T cells is initiated by interaction of low affinity α/β TCR with self-MHC molecules, and involves rescue from programmed cell death (PCD), as well as induction of differentiation and maturation of certain precursors [11]. Thus, the process of whether a DP thymocyte is positively or negatively selected is determined by the overall avidity of the TCR with self-peptides presented by APC or epithelial cells in the thymus. There are many different molecules participating in these two processes and different pathways, however the ultimate result is that this provides a T-cell population that will respond to foreign antigenic peptides presented by self-major histocompatibility complex molecules. Ultimately, a small fraction of cells (less than 5%) will downregulate either CD4 or CD8, becoming either CD4 single positive (SP) or CD8 SP thereafter leaving the thymus as mature T cells.

Can *clonal deletion* of immune cells directed to given alloantigens be artificially accomplished in the host such that developing alloimmune T cells will no longer be in the repertoire and therefore no reaction to a transplant will take place? Essentially, the answer is yes with clonal deletion of allospecific T cells being one of several methods of achieving tolerance to donor alloantigens *in vivo*. The earliest observation that clonal deletion could be accomplished were the experiments performed in the 1950s by Billingham et al., [2] who first suggested that transplantation tolerance could be a result of neonatal exposure to donor cells. Indeed, there are other clinical examples where fetal and neonatal exposure to noninherited maternal HLA antigens may facilitate a level of lower reactivity in renal transplant recipients [12]. This phenomenon is now understood to be mediated by interactions between allogeneic antigen-presenting cells and responding T cells. These interactions are not limited to neonatal exposure and can be reproduced under the appropriate conditions in adult animals. The intrathymic presence of allogeneic cells or peptides under the appropriate conditions can result in a central deletion of these recipient alloreactive cells. In this regard, the induction of antigen-specific tolerance *within* the thymus has been accomplished but the techniques and results are complicated [13]. For some protein antigens, the use of a viral vector facilitates intrathymic injection and central tolerance induction with negative selection of effector T-cells and positive selection of regulatory T-cells [14]. In addition to the central compartment, chimeric donor strain cells can participate peripherally to clonally delete recipient effector cells [15]. Based on these observations, there have been many experimental systems [16-18] and clinical trials where there is an attempt to induce transplantation tolerance by infusing donor hematopoietic cells. Indeed, blood transfusions or donor bone marrow given before (or near) transplantation have sometimes resulted in enhanced graft survival and reduced responsiveness to donor-specific antigens [19]. Unfortunately, these results have been inconsistent [20] but they have laid foundation to the thought that central and peripheral clonal deletion of alloreactive clones is possible and represents one of the mechanisms by which the central T cell compartment can participate in transplantation tolerance acquisition.

The central compartment development of functional peripheral *B cells* is a regulated process that initiates with hematopoietic stem cells in the fetal liver before birth and afterward in the bone marrow. As with T cell development, there is a crucial role for TdT and recombinase (RAG-1 and RAG-2) synthesis in the maturation of B lymphoid progenitors [21]. Following D-J joining on the H chain chromosome is the development of early pro-B cells and after joining of a V segment to the D-J$_H$ is accomplished is the late pro-B cell stage. Subsequently, Pro-B cells become pre-B cells when they express membrane μ chains; another series of events develops surrogate light chains and the pre-B receptor [22]. There is a cytoplasmic signaling cascade (with μ chain expression) following antigen binding (the dividing large pre-B cell). Subsequently, non-dividing small pre-B cells productively synthesize light chain, which then (no longer dividing) undergo V-J joining on one L chain chromosome (immature B cell). If this latter cell type binds self-antigen in the bone marrow it will die. B cells not binding self antigen leave the marrow and become mature naive (resting) B cells with membrane IgD and IgM (mature naive B cells).

Concurrent with this process of B cell development is an appropriate regulation of self-reactive B cells. It is well known that as with T cells, there are notable proportions of antibodies (and the B cells that produce them) that bear reactivity to self amongst their vast repertoire of specificities. The levels of regulation of B cell differentiation from immature B cell to plasma cell in the central bone marrow compartment primarily involve an elimination of the immature autoreactive B cells that bear high avidity self reactive receptors following their interaction with self antigen. Following their encounter with antigen, these immature highly autoreactive B cells internalize the antigen and proceed to undergo antigen receptor light chain editing (i.e., BCR replacement) and developmental arrest that ultimately results in one of several fates [23]. The cell can now express a receptor that is no longer autoreactive whereupon the B cell undergoes apoptosis via alteration (essentially downregulation) of the Bcl-2 pathway and dies 1 or 2 days later. The other more frequently occurring alternative is that BCR editing results in a B cell with reduced or no autoreactivity; this cell now emigrates from the bone marrow and enters the secondary lymphoid circulation with the typical lifespan of a mature B cell [24].

B. The Peripheral Compartment

Mature T cells and B cells bearing their specific antigen receptors on their surface constitute an armada of cells that potentially can recognize and inactive a preponderance of the offending pathogens that a mammalian host potentially can face. The encounter and subsequent immune response to foreign antigen involves an intricate interplay of different cell populations, particularly antigen presenting cells (APCs) with the B and T cells. Possibly as the result of "danger" signals from tissue [25] containing pathogens, "professional", specialized APCs such as dendritic cells and different types of macrophages bind, process and present antigen via their major histocompatibility complex (MHC) molecules on their cell surface to T cells and B cells [26]. The T cells utilize their T cell receptor to recognize processed peptides of the foreign antigen; the latter presented by the APCs via their MHC molecules. Likewise, each B cell with its unique membrane-bound immunoglobulin B cell receptor protein can bind to one particular antigen. Once the T cell and B cell encounters and binds its cognate antigen by their antigen receptor, there are a multifarious series of biochemical events [27, 28] that ensue within these cells, and which are promoted and regulated by external cell populations (e.g., signals from helper T cells) and secreted cytokines. This activation process in T cells and B cells following antigen binding allows these cells to further differentiate into one of several potential cell types. In the case of the B cell it can become either a memory cell or plasma cell by hypermutation of the variable region of its immunoglobulin gene in an intermediate differentiation step (the germinal center reaction) or in direct fashion. In the case of the T cell, there are varying paths of activation depending on the cell subtype although the two-signal model is generally the best understood. There is an interaction between the TCR and specific MHC/antigen complexes on APCs and this represents signal 1 into the T cell. Signal 2 is a binding between costimulatory molecules such as CD28 on the T cell and B7 molecules on the APC [29]. In reality, there are various co-stimulatory and adhesive interactions between APCs and T cells that help to drive proliferative, proinflammatory cytokine and cytotoxic effector functions of T cells [30, 31]. Finally, there has been proposed a "signal 3", likely a soluble factor such as IL-12 [32] that is required for immune effector cell function. Importantly, without costimulation a T cell will become functionally inert or anergic.

Within the population of newly released mature single positive T cells from the thymus into the peripheral circulation are subpopulations of autoreactive cells that escaped central clonal deletion. An analogous deficiency in the selection of B cells leads to the presence of some cells in the periphery with autoreactive potential. The activity of these autoreactive T and B cell populations must be regulated to avoid autoimmune reactions and is the basis of *peripheral tolerance* mechanisms.

Self-reactive T cells that have escaped into the peripheral circulation can be further controlled by other tolerance mechanisms, some that have significant importance in transplantation tolerance. The first research suggesting that self-tolerance is established by way of T-cell mediated *control* of self-reactive T cells was conducted more than 30 years ago. In 1969, Nishizuka and Sakakura demonstrated that neonatal thymectomy of mice led to the destruction of the ovaries, which later was found to be caused by an autoimmune process [33]. Then, in 1973, Penhale et al. showed that thymectomy of adult rats followed by exposure to sublethal X-irradiation resulted in the development of autoimmune thyroiditis [34]. With inoculation of CD4+ T cells, disease was prevented. Thus, both groups thought that depletion of *suppressor T cells* may lead to autoimmune disorders. Additional studies have been performed suggesting that CD4+ T cells have autoimmune-inhibitory activity, including a study of rodents that developed type 1 diabetes mellitus. When inoculated with CD4+ T cells, diabetes was prevented. Likewise, Kilshaw, Brent and Pinto in 1975 recognized the role of suppressor cells in transplantation tolerance [35]. Suppressor T cells have since been renamed as *regulatory T cells* (Treg). Regulatory T cells (Treg) are critical players in the maintenance of peripheral tolerance and homeostasis of the immune system. Regulatory T cells are involved in the control of autoimmune diseases, transplantation tolerance, and anti-tumor immunity. Essentially, this diverse and pliable T-cell subpopulation serves to restrain T-cell activation and expansion.

Comparable to other T cells, regulatory T cells develop in the thymus. The large majority of Treg cells are (MHC) class II restricted CD4-expressing ($CD4^+$) cells (as are T helper cells) and express high levels of the interleukin-2 receptor alpha chain (CD25), similar to activated T cells. Unlike conventional CD4+ T cells, CD4+ regulatory T cells require high-affinity peptide-MHC class II interactions with agonist peptides that otherwise induce negative selection. However, Treg cells are further defined by expression of the forkhead family *transcription factor FOXP3* (forkhead box p3) (Foxp3 is not expressed on activated T cells). FOXP3 expression is required for regulatory T cell development and controls a genetic program specifying this cell fate [36]. In addition to the Foxp3-expressing CD4$^+$CD25$^+$ cells, there is also a minor population of MHC class I restricted CD8$^+$ Foxp3-expressing regulatory T cells [37]. As defined by CD4 and CD25 expression, Treg cells comprise about 1-2% of CD4$^+$ helper T cells in humans.

CD4$^+$CD25$^+$ Foxp3+ regulatory T cells have also been referred to as "naturally-occurring" regulatory T cells to distinguish them from "suppressor" T cell populations that can be induced *in vitro* or *in vivo*. In fact, the "naturally-occurring" CD4$^+$CD25$^+$ regulatory T cell population is a subset of the total Foxp3-expressing regulatory T cell population. The regulatory T cell field is further complicated by reports of additional "suppressor" T cell populations, including Tr1, CD8$^+$CD28$^-$, NKT cells and Qa-1 restricted T cells [37, 38]. At this point, the contribution of these populations to self-tolerance and immune homeostasis is less well defined.

Currently, it appears that CD4+CD25+ regulatory T cells play a prominent role in transplantation tolerance [39]; in addition, CD8+, CD8+CD28-, T-cell receptor+CD4-CD8-, dendritic cells and natural killer T (NKT) cells have *also* been acknowledged to have the potential to downregulate immune responses [40, 41]. One of the issues with so many potential regulatory cell populations potentially operative during transplantation is our current inability to reliably identify these cells. Recently activated T cells, also known as effector T cells, express CD25 at lower levels and for a limited period of time, whereas CD4+ T cells with the greatest regulatory properties express CD25 at high levels continuously. A concern in using CD25 expression as a marker for regulatory T cells is that there have been several reports claiming regulatory activity in CD4+CD25- T cell populations following transplantation [37]. Therefore, other markers are necessary to further identify regulatory T cells after transplantation. This finding is particularly important for generating effective therapies targeted at achieving tolerance. Markers that are currently being investigated include CD45RB, cytotoxic T-lymphocyte antigen 4 (CTLA4; CD152), glucocorticoid-induced tumor necrosis factor receptor family-related gene (GITR; TNFRSF18), CD122, CD103, and FOXP3 [42, 43]. To date, no gene has fulfilled the criteria of exclusivity and stability.

It is has been known for several years that some T cells are incapable of becoming fully activated and moreover, they enter a state of hyporesponsiveness if rechallenged with the original antigen. This phenomenon known as *T cell anergy* [44] is a means of peripheral tolerance of autoreactive T cells and may also play a role in transplantation tolerance. There are several ways by which T cell anergy can be achieved [44]. The first manner is when there is *only* signal 1 (T cell receptor binds antigen and initiates intracellular biochemical cascade) in the *absence* of signal 2 (costimulation, e.g., the receptor CD28 on T cells binding to B7.1 [CD80] and B7.2 [CD86]). This scenario is present when resting APCs interact with T cells – deficient signal 2 results in T cell anergy [45]. This process requires induction of the transcription factor NF-AT [46] and protein synthesis [47]. Anergy may also result if altered peptide ligands are used to stimulate the T cells [48] even if there is sufficient signal 2 present. The exact mechanisms that place a T cell into the anergic state are unknown but one model proposes that in addition to T cell activation biochemical steps, there are also internal negative factors in the cells that shut down activation [44]. The role of anergic T cells is unclear but it may be a mechanism allowing T cells to respond to classical antigens preventing organ-specific responses that do not provide adequate signal 2. At this point, there are no anergy-promoting immunosuppressive agents – in fact, cyclosporine prevents T cell activation *and* the generation of anergy [47] since it binds to calcineurin and prevents NF-AT from working, the latter needed for the anergic state.

There have been other mechanisms of tolerance induction in T cells that have been described and that will be briefly mentioned here. *Clonal deletion* of T cells, as described above in the central compartment, can also occur in the peripheral circulation. Upon interaction with certain donor cell populations (e.g., certain dendritic cells) there can be an elimination of recipient alloreactive cells. This may be one of the mechanisms by which infused donor hematopoietic cells at the time of solid organ transplant promote the tolerance in experimental animal models. *Clonal ignorance* is felt to be a relatively rare mechanism of tolerance that involves the keeping the recipient's immune system "ignorant" of the presence of donor cells, and thus, an immune response is not mounted. For instance, encapsulating islet cells before being transplanted might allow the immune system to remain unresponsive [49, 50]. *Clonal exhaustion* can occur after episodes of repetitive stimulation of recipient T cells by alloantigen – this can lead to either deletion or inactivation of the immune effector T cells [15, 51]. This occurrence has been described following liver transplantation, where there are a significant number of donor antigen presenting cells that migrate from the liver to the surrounding lymphoid tissues [52]. Finally, many cytokines and other soluble factors are individually immunosuppressive to T cell function (e.g., IL-10) [53]. Any perturbation of their secretion and increase in their levels can markedly alter the surrounding milieu and dampen T cell function.

Some of the B cells that escape central bone marrow deletion and elimination do so because they possess low avidity autoreactive antigen receptors. These cells become *anergic*, a state similar to that with anergic T cells in which the cell undergoes innate biochemical alterations that prevents it from undergoing activation following antigen binding, thereby arresting further differentiation [54]. Alternatively, these anergic B cells in the peripheral circulation may require higher levels of the specific antigen in order to cross the threshold into the activated state [55]. At this point, the block in the activation pathway that occurs in B cell anergy is not well understood although it appears that NF-κB and toll-like receptor signaling via the BCR pathway are inhibited. Anergic B cells express reduced levels of B-cell activating factor (BAFF) receptor [56] ultimately making these cells less able to bind and utilize this crucial cytokine that is needed for B cell survival. Anergic B cells can potentially be reversed from this state of tolerance if the self antigen that induced anergy is no longer present (cessation of anergy signaling) or if the anergic B cell now encounters high avidity antigen in the presence of T cell help. Either of these latter situations may occur in graft transplantation. For example, a loss of donor chimeric cells may result in *reactivation* of anergic B cells since the tolerizing molecule is no longer sending the necessary signal to the B cell. In addition, exogenous antigens (e.g., infectious agents) may be encountered during graft rejection such that two immune responses are simultaneously occurring; in this way, the

T cell involved in the response to the infection may provide the necessary help to break the anergic state of the B cell. This scenario could result in B cells that make anti-pathogen antibodies and recruitment of clones that now make anti-graft antibodies. Finally, during an active immune response in graft rejection, there may be a plethora of growth factors (e.g., BAFF) that can overcome the anergic B cell state.

Costimulation, as with T cells, is an important adjunct that can provide augmentation or inhibition of B cell activation following BCR signaling. There are several B cell molecules capable of behaving as inhibitory receptors [57] including CD22, CD23, and FcγRIIB1. The CD40:CD40 ligand (the latter on T cells) interaction is a potent stimulatory boost to B cell activation, followed by a release of cytokines that promote B cell activation and development. One way in which B cells directed to alloantigens may be prevented from becoming activated is by a reduction or elimination of the T cell help (i.e., T cell tolerance to the same antigens). If CD4+ T cell tolerance to a particular alloantigen is overcome (by a variety of different means, including cross-reaction with other foreign peptides) then the alloreactive B cells against those same antigens can become activated.

Finally, if alloreactive B cells and alloantibodies (as seen with panel reactive antibodies [PRA]) are present in a transplanted patient this does not necessarily mean that injury will occur to the allograft. This phenomenon cannot be simply explained by the effects of immunosuppressive reagents and brings up the possibility that the *allograft itself* is capable of protecting itself to some degree from immune effector injury. For example, there could be concealing or downregulation of crucial alloantigen dominant epitopes seen by antibodies and effector T cells and inherent individual organ capacity to control inflammation. Future therapeutic agents may be able to promote these inherent immunosuppressive effects within the grafted organ. In this regard, *immune privilege* is a term used to describe specific organs that upon their transplantation into a host can *induce* tolerance or organs that upon receiving foreign tissue will *accept* the material due to the lack of an immune response to this antigenically disparate material [58]. The classical organ that can show both forms of immune privilege is the liver [59]. For example, livers that are orthotopically transplanted in several species are readily accepted in the absence of immunosuppression and despite MHC differences with the recipient [60]. In addition, livers can have foreign cells (e.g., pancreatic islets) injected under their capsule and there will not be any significant immune response; some infections in the liver are not exposed to any effective immune response. The anterior chamber of the eye is another example of a site where tissue is not recognized as foreign and has no effective immune response [61]; other sites with immune privilege include some areas of the central nervous system and the testis [62].

III. Tolerance in Human Solid Organ Transplantation

The modern day success story of clinical solid organ transplantation, now over 50 years old [63], is certainly one of the landmark achievements of medicine over the last century. The success of clinical transplantation has inexorably been allied with superior immunosuppression, improved surgical techniques and medical management, and a better understanding of donor and recipient characteristics that promote graft acceptance. In spite of an overall improvement in graft acceptance and patient survival in all forms of organ transplantation, there continue to be significant obstacles. Acute rejection and infections continue to beleaguer the post transplant course [64] of many patients and chronic rejection has been a consistent and unacceptably high hindrance to long term graft survival [65]. Moreover, the nonspecific nature of immunosuppression therapy induces a ubiquitous dampening of the immune response in the recipient that brings with it an array of potential side effects that can cause significant morbidity to the patient including, a higher risk of infections and malignancies [66, 67], increased risk of primary disease recurrence in the allograft, and direct toxic side effects of the immunosuppressive drugs [68]. Thus, there has been an increased focus in recent years from over- immunosuppression and towards achieving clinical immune tolerance. This would essentially allow the immune system to recognize the transplanted organ as if it were the native organ without the need for immunosuppressive agents. As compared to animal models however, achieving tolerance in humans has posed a greater challenge with only rare patients fitting the criteria for "true" immunological tolerance, the latter representing graft acceptance concomitant with a specific absence of immune reactivity to the transplant and therefore no immunosuppressive therapy. In spite of this, the use of new and different approaches and our recognition of underlying immune mechanisms have allowed us to consider that achieving tolerance in the transplant setting is a more realistic goal.

As opposed to "true" immunological tolerance, there have been multiple anecdotal cases of patients, particularly liver transplant recipients, who have been able to cease or be weaned of all immunosuppressive therapy with maintenance of long term graft function [69]. Episodes of acute rejection could still occur (implying an intact immune response to the allograft), but these episodes resolved spontaneously [70]. Patients who do well following cessation of immunosuppressive therapy typically have at least two years of post liver-transplantation follow-up, a low incidence of acute rejection prior to stopping therapy, and non-autoimmune primary liver disease [71]. These patients have been characterized as having *operational tolerance*, a clinical situation defined as stable graft function without clinical features of chronic rejection and in the absence of any immunosuppressive drugs, usually for more than one year [72]. In general it appears that well-selected patients who have been stable post-transplant make more suitable candidates for attempting to achieve operational tolerance. The limited clinical trials have involved a weaning from their immunosuppressive drug regimens with in some cases up to 20% of selected liver transplant recipients capable of full drug removal [73].

Another notion that been forwarded is that of partial or *prope tolerance* [74], a situation where patients sustain stable graft function with minimal immunosuppression. The approach for attaining prope tolerance is to have a powerful induction immunosuppressive regimen, followed by minimal immunosuppression. For example, transplantation can be performed soon after 1 to 2 doses of alemtuzumab (Campath 1H), a humanized anti-CD52 antibody and lytic agent for both T and B lymphocytes that produces a marked lymphopenia, are administered. The recipients are then treated with a low dose calcineurin inhibitor, without the need for additional immunosuppressive agents. This approach has had some success and provides an opportunity for the transplanted patient to receive lower drug doses; however, this is not true immunological tolerance. The underlying basis of prope tolerance is unknown but may be a selective expansion of T regulatory cells over T effector cells as lymphocyte populations are regenerated [75].

Although achieving operational tolerance or prope tolerance has met with some success in occasional liver transplant recipients, attaining tolerance in other solid organ transplant recipients has proven more difficult. In addition to weaning (operational) and induction/monotherapy (prope) approaches, there are other strategies that have been attempted to achieve tolerance in transplant patients. One approach of noteworthy interest is supplementation with infused donor cells to enhance donor hematopoietic chimerism. As described in the previous sections, this method has been very successful in inducing true immune tolerance in animal models for many years. In humans, creating hematopoietic chimerism has been attempted in multiple ways, including bone marrow ablative (eliminating the recipient's bone marrow) and nonablative techniques, as well donor blood transfusions [76]. These cell infusions enhance the donor ("passenger") leucocytes that leave solid organs and populate the host [77]. These supplemental approaches to induce chimerism have met with mixed success and have not shown the striking results seen in animal models. Moreover, ablating and replacement with donor bone marrow is often not practical, frequently requiring powerful drugs and/or irradiation, both of which come with their own toxicities.

Clinical tolerance induction has also been attempted with strategies aimed to disrupt the normal *cooperation* of T cells in order to prevent rejection. Most of these techniques have utilized antibodies that either depletes host peripheral T cells or that temporarily block cell surface receptors. Rodent models have demonstrated that administering CD4 antibody combined with CD8 antibodies is quite successful at achieving a tolerant state [78]. Unfortunately, the high doses of antibodies required to achieve tolerance also have side-effects. CD40L antibodies, as well as antibodies against CD3 are currently being investigated and appear to have less severe side-effects [79]. With all of these approaches to tolerance induction, there is as of yet, no consistent set of reliable immunologic assays that can assess the likelihood of rejection or tolerance [80]. This latter issue is of paramount importance since the post transplant period needs to be carefully assessed with specific immunological assays rather than simple observation of long-term graft survival. These assays, yet to be determined, will hopefully be able to predict whether certain therapeutic regimens are leading to a successful attainment of tolerance, and the need for immunosuppressive therapy.

A. Kidney Transplantation

The overall progress in immunosuppressive therapy and optimizing recipient matching has improved short-term survival of renal allografts (as well as other allografts) by decreasing the frequency of acute rejections. Yet, the long-term survival of renal grafts has not notably improved with many transplanted kidneys having long-term failure as a result of chronic rejection [81]. Certainly, there have always been occasional patients that have had longstanding grafts with normal function and on minimal or no immunosuppression but this is a rare situation. The characteristics of these unusual patients who are seemingly tolerant (operational) of their kidney allografts are often not very different from other organ recipients. In 1992, Starzl et al, found that a group of long-term stable transplant patients (some 30 years post transplant) had multilineage chimeric cells of the donor in many lymphoid and non-lymphoid organs [82]. These and other studies implicated that the presence of donor chimeric cells was necessary for clinical tolerance to occur, although many since then have countered that acute rejection can occur in a host who has a high level of chimerism [83]. Nevertheless, many investigators maintain that the *presence* of chimeric cells is a prerequisite if some of the tolerance-inducing mechanisms (e.g., clonal deletion of immune effector cells) are to take place. A variety of tolerance-inducing strategies in renal transplant recipients have been attempted to enhance chimerism [84] and all have met with marginal or no consistent success [85]. There have been several trials that have been able to induce prope (or partial) tolerance in kidney transplant patients. For example, Cortesini, et al, showed that renal transplant patients could be maintained on minimal immunosuppression following irradiation and low doses of immunosuppression [86]. Roussey-Kesler, et al. [72] reported 10 cases of kidney transplant recipients who maintained operational tolerance for a period of 5 to 15 years. All but one recipient in the study received a kidney from a deceased mismatched donor, and most of the patients stopped taking immunosuppression over a long time period (typically non-compliance). Six patients out of eight transfused patients had low titers of anti-HLA antibodies (low PRA levels). Two of the patients' renal function declined after 9 to 13 years of stopping immunosuppressive agents and unfortunately five out of ten patients were clinically diagnosed with acute rejection during the follow-up. This latter point emphasizes that these patients *did* have a competent immune response to the donor and were therefore not truly tolerant. Some graft pathology of these patients included a moderate and focal infiltrate with an arteriolar intimal hyperplasia, suggestive of early chronic nephropathy, another with a focal interstitial infiltrate, and was described as normal. There have been other cases of operationally tolerant kidney transplants that have been described. Fudaba and colleagues [87] validated the use of nonmyeloablative bone marrow and kidney transplantation to treat patients with multiple myeloma and renal failure. HLA-Identical siblings were transplanted after undergoing nonmyeloablative conditioning, including cyclophosphamide (CP), peritransplant antithymocyte globulin and thymic irradiation. Cyclosporine (CyA) was given for approximately 2 months posttransplant, followed by donor leukocyte infusions. Interestingly, they concluded that long-term acceptance of renal allografts in this particular group of patients did not seem dependent on the persistence of hematopoietic chimerism.

The ability to have a simplified immunosuppressive regimen consisting of only one agent is highly advantageous to kidney transplant patients (Prope tolerance). Shapiro, et al, [88] described 150 renal transplant recipients who were pretreated with Thymoglobulin hours before transplantation, along with bolus doses of prednisone. Following transplantation, they were administered minimal immunosuppression consisting of tacrolimus monotherapy plus steroid pulses if rejection episodes occurred. Patients who had tolerated this treatment well were then weaned from their tacrolimus monotherapy at or after 4 months post-transplantation. Spaced weaning was initiated in 113 of 150 recipients. 23% of the weaned patients experienced acute rejection; however some of the patients were able to be weaned after the episodes of acute rejection subsided. One-year graft survival was 92% with 94 of the 150 patients subsequently taking tacrolimus in a spaced fashion. Only 7% needed long term treatment with agents other than tacrolimus. Calne [89] studied thirty one patients with cadaveric renal transplants that were treated with Campath antibody on day 0 and 1 day post-transplantation. At 48 hours following transplantation, cyclosporine monotherapy was given with no additional immunosuppressants. The patients were then followed up for approximately 24 months. 30/31 patients were living, and 29 had functioning grafts and remained on low dose monotherapy with cyclosporine. Five patients developed rejection, which was treated with steroid pulses. One patient developed a recurrence of the original disease.

B. Liver Transplantation

As mentioned before, the liver is an immunoprivileged organ that has a lower susceptibility to rejection than other transplanted organs. Clinically, this is often reflected by successful transplants in the face of a positive cross-match, minimal importance of HLA matching, reduced incidence of hyperacute rejection, occasional spontaneous recovery following severe rejection, reduced incidence of chronic rejection, and the ability to sometimes reverse chronic rejection. Immunosuppression withdrawal or conversion to monotherapy is possible in certain liver transplant patients (see table 1). Often, these are patients who are non-compliant with their medications or ones with post transplant lymphoproliferative disorder (PTLD) that have had reduced levels of immunosuppressive drugs. There have been several experiences trying to induce tolerance in liver transplant patients. Some studies have attempted to induce tolerance shortly after transplantation, while in others a tolerance protocol is implemented many years following transplantation. This is a significant difference, considering that the longer an organ has been transplanted into a recipient, the more likely the organ will be tolerated. Mazariegos, et al at Pittsburgh [90] electively withheld immunosuppression in 95 recipients; of these 18 patients were able to be off all immunosuppressants and 37 patients were on spaced immunosuppression. Twenty eight patients experienced acute rejection and 12 were withdrawn from the protocol. The mean delay between the initiation of weaning and the biopsy-proven rejection was 13.2 months. All 18 patients off of immunosuppressive agents had a significantly improved health-related quality of life. Devlin, et al (King's College) discontinued immunosuppressive therapy in18 long-term, clinically stable liver transplant patients [91]. They found five (27%) of the patients who could stay off immunosuppressive therapy. The remaining 13 patients had elevated liver function tests and immunosuppression was started again. Four out of the 13 patients with elevated liver function tests had acute rejection on liver biopsy. The predictors of successful cessation of immunosuppression were lower incidence of early post liver transplantation rejection, good HLA matching, nonautoimmune and nonviral primary liver disease. The presence of donor microchimerism was not found to be a predictor of successful immunosuppressive cessation.

Table 1. Clinical trials in organ transplantation attempting tolerance induction

Author	Patient no.	Type of Tolerance	Time between transplant and weaning (years)	Complete IS cessation	Acute/chronic rejection	Maintenance IS	Bone marrow	Follow-up time
Mazariegos(90)	95	Complete IS weaning	mean: 8.4	19%	26/0%	CsA, Aza, Tac	No	median:35.5 months, range: 10-58 months
Devlin (91)	18	Complete IS weaning	median: 7	16.70%	28/5.6%	CsA, Aza	No	>3 years
Takatsuki (92)	26	Complete IS weaning	>2	23.80%	12/0%	Tac	No	median: 21.9 months, range: 3-69 months
Pons (109)	9	Complete IS weaning	median: 5.2	23.80%	22/0%	CsA	No	range: 17-24 months
Eason (93)	18	Complete IS weaning	>0.5	5.60%	61/0%	Tac	No	1 year
Tryphonopoulos (94)	104	Complete IS weaning	mean: 4	19%	67/1.9%	Tac, CsA	45 patients received BM tspl.	median:25.9, range 11-36
Tisone (110)	34		mean: 5.25	23.40%	76.4/0%	CsA	No	mean: 45.5, range: 15-44
Takatsuki (95)	63	Complete IS weaning	>2	38.10%	25.50%	Tac	No	>69 months
De Ruvo (100)	22	Prope tolerance; Thymoglobulin, followed by low dose tacrolimus	4 months	N/A	37.00%	Tac	No	1 year
Roussey-Kesler (72)	10	Complete IS weaning	7.8 +/- 4.3	80%	50% (acute)	Aza and CS, CsA	No	Median: 9.4 +/- 5.7 years
Shapiro (88)	150	Prope tolerance with Thymoglobulin, followed by Tac monotherapy	>4 months	0%/ 63% partially weaned	23% (acute)	Tac	No	6-21 months
Calne (89)	31	Prope tolerance; Campath 1H, followed by cyclosporine	Immediately following transplant	0%/94% remained on monotherapy	16%	Cya	No	2 years

Table 1. (Continued).

Author	Patient no.	Type of Tolerance	Time between transplant and weaning (years)	Complete IS cessation	Acute/chronic rejection	Maintenance IS	Bone marrow	Follow-up time
Fudaba (87)	6	Complete IS weaning via nonmyeloablative conditioning, followed by Cyclosporine A and donor leukocyte infusions	Immediately following transplant	50%	17%	CyA	Nonmyeloablative BM transplant	1.3 to >7 years
Tzakis (104)	16	Prope tolerance: no steroids, tacrolimus at 1/2 normal dose	Immediately following transplant	N/A: 12/16 with functioning grafts	7 mild acute, 2 severe rejection, 3 moderate	Tac at approx. 1/2 dose normally given	No	Avg: 9 months

Abbreviations: CyA = Cyclosporine; Tac = tacrolimus; IS = immunosuppression; BM = bone marrow; Aza = Azathioprine.

The Kyoto study [92] examined 26 pediatric living related liver transplant patients, having one HLA haplotype identity, in which immunosuppression was electively weaned. Six of the 26 patients (23%) were successfully weaned. 15.4% of the patients experienced an episode of acute rejection that resolved with either steroids or with Tacrolimus. In this study, neither the degree of HLA matching nor the early episodes of rejection were found to be indicative of success in weaning immunosuppressive therapy. They suggest that down regulation of intra-graft TH1 cytokines and increased numbers of peripheral blood regulatory CD4+CD25+ T cells are associated with an operationally tolerant state. As compared to long-term patients, Eason et al. [93] attempted to completely wean 18 patients (selected from a larger cohort of 280 patients) who were at least 6 months status-post liver transplantation and who had not experienced an episode of acute rejection. Only 1 patient (5.5%) was able to be completely weaned at one year. Tryphonopoulos, et al (Miami) had 20 out of 104 liver transplant patients who were able to be successfully weaned, regardless of whether or not they had received donor bone marrow infusions [94]. There were no significant differences in donor cell chimerism levels between those patients that were successfully weaned and those who developed graft rejection. The tolerant group had a lower incidence of renal dysfunction, malignancies and infections. Finally, Takatsuki et al. [95] studied 63 patients who were weaned from immunosuppressants. Twenty-four patients (38.1%) achieved a complete weaning with a median drug-free period of 23.5 months (range, 3-69 months).

A negative prognostic factor in the survival of transplant patients with Hepatitis C infection is an increased strength of immunosuppressants [96]. HCV RNA levels are related to the degree of immunosuppression, the higher the viral load, and the higher the degree of chronic hepatitis in the liver graft [97, 98]. Therefore, the level of induction of immunosuppression in an attempt to induce Prope tolerance (with monotherapy) has to be carefully considered. For example, a Pittsburgh study using Campath induction and tacrolimus monotherapy showed that liver transplant patients with hepatitis C had an increase in viral hepatitis in the Campath group (HCV) [99]. De Ruvo et al. [100] described a weaning protocol for HCV patients who received liver transplants due to HCV cirrhosis. Twenty-two patients received Thymoglobulin preoperatively and were given tacrolimus as maintenance therapy. Twelve of 22 patients treated with Thymoglobulin went through the planned weaning schedule; however, none of the patients were totally weaned off of immunosuppression. The recurrence rates of HCV infection in their study were not much different than those seen in patients treated with conventional therapy. There was a lower viral load in the patients in patients who were treated with tacrolimus and steroids. The authors ultimately concluded that although a longer follow up period is needed, Thymoglobulin given preoperatively in addition to tacrolimus monotherapy may be an effective therapy regimen in HCV-infected liver transplant recipients. These studies illustrate that tolerance induction in HCV liver transplant patients may be a difficult proposition at the current time.

C. Bowel Transplantation

Due to the large intrinsic lymphoid mass and immunogenic nature of the bowel, tolerance in intestinal transplantation has long been considered to be a difficult task to achieve. Bowel allografts are very susceptible to acute rejection, and these patients also experience a high risk of infection and PTLD [101]. An intertwining of sepsis, endotoxinemia, and rejection after intestinal transplantation is among reasons why the bowel is so highly immunogenic. Moreover, inflammation associated with intestinal transplantation may create a milieu that enables enterocytes to function as APCs. HLA mismatching is thought to play a role, based on studies in dogs that were less susceptible to rejection when MHC matching occurred [102], however, clinically this is not apparent.

Several clinical studies have been met with partial success in attempting to achieve tolerance in intestinal transplantation. In general, intestinal transplantation is now treated with smaller doses of immunosuppression than just several years ago and a goal of low dose monotherapy (i.e., Prope tolerance) is being actively pursued. A Pittsburgh study described progressively tapered tacrolimus monotherapy (following induction) with no observable compromise in graft function [103]. The University of Miami conducted a study of 21 adult patients receiving either intestinal or multivisceral transplants. They found that Campath induction therapy could be followed by Tacrolimus monotherapy, without the need for steroids and without causing frequent infections [104]. The liver is an immunoprivileged organ that may have a protective effect on other organs transplanted from the same donor as demonstrated in several experimental models [105, 106]. At this point, this has not translated into definitive success in humans. The mechanisms underlying this suppressive liver effect are likely multifactorial and may include soluble HLA molecule blocking factors, generation of Treg cells, induction of anergy and Th2 immune deviation. Multivisceral transplantation (with or without the liver) presents a massive donor antigenic challenge to the host with the potential to lead to exhaustion of the recipient's immune system [107]. This raises the possibility that transplant physicians may be able to take advantage and manipulate the large donor antigen challenge to decrease the anti-graft immune response. However, at this point, multivisceral transplantation still requires a vigorous regimen of immunosuppression to maintain graft function.

IV. Summary

There are many future challenges and budding opportunities in the field of clinical tolerance for autoimmunity, cancer and transplantation. In this regard, the National Institute on Allergy and Infectious Diseases (NIAID) convened an Expert Panel on Immune Tolerance that in 1997 ultimately established the Immune Tolerance Network (ITN) [108]. The goal of the ITN is to develop a collaborative approach to the clinical application of immune tolerance that encompasses a wide range of disease processes, including kidney and islet cell transplantation, autoimmune disease, and allergy and asthma. In addition, there are many other potential strategies for inducing immune tolerance that are at the experimental level and that may eventually be clinically applied in a safe and effective manner. The goal with tolerance in transplantation will be to achieve a specific lack of immune responsiveness to the graft, without immunosuppressive drugs and while maintaining other necessary immune functions. By combining our improved understanding of responses to the human allograft with the exciting possibility of new molecular targets and patient-tailored therapy we may finally be able to give credence to the notion that the upcoming years will let us attain the "Holy Grail" of transplantation tolerance.

References

[1]   Owen RD. Immunogenic consequences of vascular anastomoses between bovine twins. *Science.* 102: 400-404, 1945.

[2]   Billingham RE, Brent L, Medawar PB. Actively acquired tolerance of foreign cells. *Nature.* 172:603-606, 1953.

[3]   Cohn M. The common sense of the self-nonself discrimination. *Springer Sem. Immunopath.* 27(1):3-17, 2005.

[4]   Beutler B. Innate immunity: an overview. *Mol. Immunol.* 40(12):845-59, 2004.

[5]   Andrade CF, Waddell TK, Keshavjee S, Liu M. Innate immunity and organ transplantation: the potential role of toll-like receptors. *Am. J. Transplant.* 5(5):969-975, 2005.

[6]   Gould SJ, Hildreth JE, Booth AM. The evolution of alloimmunity and the genesis of adaptive immunity. *Quar. Rev. Biol.* 79(4):359-382, 2004.

[7]   Garcia KC, Adams EJ. How the T cell receptor sees antigen--a structural view. *Cell.* 122(3):333-336, 2005.

[8]   Pleiman CM, D'Ambrosio D, Cambier JC. The B-cell antigen receptor complex: structure and signal transduction. *Immunol. Today.* 15(9):393-399, 1994.

[9]   He X, Kappes DJ. CD4/CD8 lineage commitment: light at the end of the tunnel? *Curr. Opin. Immunol.* 18(2):135-142, 2006.

[10]   Siggs OM, Makaroff LE, Liston A. The why and how of thymocyte negative selection. *Curr. Opin. Immunol.* 18(2):175-183, 2006.

[11]   Aliahmad P, Kaye J. Commitment issues: linking positive selection signals and lineage diversification in the thymus. *Immunol. Rev.* 209:253-273, 2006.

[12]   Burlingham WJ, Grailer AP, Heisey DM, et al. Effect of tolerance to noninherited maternal HLA antigens on the survival of renal transplants from sibling donors. *N. Engl. J. Med.* 339:1657-1664, 1998.

[13]   Attavar P, Budhai L, Kim BH, et al. Mechanisms of intrathymic tolerance induction to isolated rat hepatocyte allografts. *Hepatology.* 26(5):1287-1295, 1997.

[14]   Marodon G, Fisson S, Levacher B, et al. Induction of antigen-specific tolerance by intrathymic injection of lentiviral vectors. *Blood.* 2006; 108: 2972 – 2978.

[15]   Starzl TE. Chimerism and tolerance in transplantation. *PNAS* (USA) 101 Suppl. 2:14607-14614, 2004.

[16]   Wekerle T, Sayegh MH, Chandraker A, et al. Role of peripheral clonal deletion in tolerance induction with bone marrow transplantation and costimulatory blockade. *Transplant. Proc.* 31(1-2):680, 1999.

[17] Ruiz P, Coffman TM, Howell DN, et al. Evidence that pretransplant donor blood transfusion prevents rat renal allograft dysfunction but not the in situ cellular alloimmune or morphologic manifestations of rejection. *Transplantation.* 45(1):1-7, 1988.

[18] Thomas JM, Neville DM, Contreras JL, et al. Preclinical studies of allograft tolerance in rhesus monkeys: a novel anti-CD3-immunotoxin given peritransplant with donor bone marrow induces operational tolerance to kidney allografts. *Transplantation.* 64(1):124-35, 1997.

[19] Marti HP, Henschkowski J, Laux G, et al. Effect of donor-specific transfusions on the outcome of renal allografts in the cyclosporine era. *Transplant. Internat.* 19(1):19-26, 2006.

[20] Hollander AA, de Waal LP, van Bockel HJ, et al. No tolerance induction with cryopreserved bone marrow cells after allogeneic kidney transplantation and antilymphocyte globulin in rhesus monkeys. *Transplant. Internat.* 10(3):249-50, 1997.

[21] Hagman J, Lukin K. Transcription factors drive B cell development. *Curr. Opin. Immunol.* 18(2):127-34, 2006.

[22] Louzoun Y, Fredman T, Luning Prak E, et al. Analysis of B cell receptor production and rearrangement. Part I. Light chain rearrangement. *Semin. Immunol.* 14:169-170, 2002.

[23] Nemazee D, Weigert M. Revising B cell receptors. *J. Exp. Med.* 191:1813-1817, 2000.

[24] Zhang M, Srivastava G, Lu L. The pre-B cell receptor and its function during B cell development. *Cell* Mol. Immunol. 1(2):89-94, 2004.

[25] Meylan E, Tschopp J, Karin M. Intracellular pattern recognition receptors in the host response. *Nature.* 442(7098):39-44, 2006.

[26] Hugues S, Boissonnas A, Amigorena S, Fetler L. The dynamics of dendritic cell-T cell interactions in priming and tolerance. *Curr. Opin. Immunol.* 18(4):491-495, 2006.

[27] Dorner T, Lipsky PE. Signalling pathways in B cells: implications for autoimmunity. *Curr. Top Microbiol. Immunol.* 305:213-240, 2006.

[28] Ashwell JD. The many paths to p38 mitogen-activated protein kinase activation in the immune system. *Nature Rev. Immunol.* 6(7):532-540, 2006.

[29] Greenwald RJ, et al. The B7 family revisited. *Annu. Rev. Immunol.* 23:515-548, 2005.

[30] Okazaki T, Iwai Y, Honjo T. New regulatory co-receptors: inducible co-stimulator and PD-1. *Curr. Opin. Immunol.* 14(6):779-782, 2002.

[31] Ortaldo JR, Young HA. IL-18 as critical co-stimulatory molecules in modulating the immune response of ITAM bearing lymphocytes. *Sem. Immunol.* 18(3):193-196, 2006.

[32] Brombacher F, Kastelein RA, Alber G. Novel IL-12 family members shed light on the orchestration of Th1 responses. *Trends Immunol.* 24(4):207-212, 2003.

[33] Nishizuka Y, Sakakura T. Thymus and reproduction: sex-linked dysgenesis of the gonad after neonatal thymectomy in mice. *Science.* 166(906):753-755, 1969.

[34] Penhale WJ, Farmer A, McKenna RP, Irvine WJ. Spontaneous thyroiditis in thymectomized and irradiated Wistar rats. *Clin. Exper. Immunol.* 15(2):225-236, 1973.

[35] Kilshaw PJ, Brent L, Pinto M. Suppressor T cells in mice made unresponsive to skin allografts. *Nature.* 255(5508):489-491, 1975.

[36] Sakaguchi, S: Naturally arising Foxp3-expressing CD25+CD4+ regulatory T cells in immunological tolerance to self and non-self. *Nat. Immunol.* 6:345-352, 2005.

[37] Jiang H, Chess L. Regulation of immune responses by T cells. *N. Engl. J. Med.* 354:1166-1176, 2006.

[38] Lohr J, Knoechel B, Abbas AK. Regulatory T cells in the periphery. *Immunol. Rev.* 212:149-162, 2006.

[39] Aluvihare VR, Betz AG. The role of regulatory T cells in alloantigen tolerance. *Immunol. Rev.* 212:330-43, 2006.

[40] McCurry KR, Colvin BL, Zahorchak AF, Thompson AW. Regulatory dendritic cell therapy in organ transplantation. *Transplant. Int.* 19:525-538, 2006.

[41] Kim HJ, Hwang SJ, Kim BK, et al. NKT cells play critical roles in the induction of oral tolerance by inducing regulatory T cells producing IL-10 and transforming growth factor beta, and by clonally deleting antigen-specific T cells. *Immunology.* 118(1):101-11, 2006.

[42] Marazuela M, Garcia-Lopez MA, Figueroa-Vega N, et al. Regulatory T cells in human autoimmune thyroid disease. *J. Clin. Endocrinol. Metab.* 91(9):3639-46, 2006.

[43] Uss E, Rowshani AT, Hooibrink B, et al. CD103 is a marker for alloantigen-induced regulatory CD8+ T cells. *J. Immunol.* 177(5):2775-83, 2006.

[44] Schwartz RH. Models of T cell anergy: is there a common molecular mechanism? *J. Exp. Med.* 184(1):1-8, 1996.

[45] Jenkins MK, Johnson JG. Molecules involved in T-cell costimulation. *Curr. Opin. Immunol.* 5:361-367, 2003.

[46] Macian F, Garcia-Cozar F, Im SH, Horton HR, et al. Transcriptional mechanisms underlying lymphocyte tolerance. *Cell.* 109:719-731, 2002.

[47] Jenkins MK, Chen CA, Jung G, Mueller DL, Schwartz RH. Inhibition of antigen-specific proliferation of type 1 murine T cell clones after stimulation with immobilized anti-CD3 monoclonal antibody. *J. Immunol.* 144(1):16-22, 1990.

[48] Sloan-Lancaster J, Evavold BD, Allen PM. Induction of T-cell anergy by altered T-cell receptor ligand on live antigen-presenting cells. *Nature.* 363:156-159, 1993.

[49] Wood K, Sakaguchi S. Regulatory T cells in transplantation tolerance. *Nature.* 3:199-209, 2003.

[50] Coulombe M. Gill RG. T lymphocyte indifference to extrathymic islet allografts. *J. Immunol.* 156(5):1998-2003, 1996.

[51] Welsh RM, McNally JM. Immune deficiency, immune silencing, and clonal exhaustion of T cell responses during viral infections. *Curr. Opin. Microbiol.* 2(4):382-387, 1999.

[52] Bishop G, Sun J, Sheil A, McCaughan G. High dose/activation-associated tolerance. *Transplantation.* 64: 1377-1382, 1997.

[53] Battaglia M, Gianfrani C, Gregori S, Roncarolo MG. IL-10-producing T regulatory type 1 cells and oral tolerance. *Ann. NY Acad. Sci.* 1029:142-153, 2004.

[54] Gauld SB, Merrell KT, Cambier JC. Silencing of autoreactive B cells by anergy: a fresh perspective. *Curr. Opin. Immunol.* 18(3):292-297, 2006.

[55] Melchers F, Rolink AR. B cell tolerance--how to make it and how to break it. *Curr. Top Microbiol. Immunol.* 305:1-23, 2006.

[56] Ait-Azzouzene D, Gavin AL, Skog P, Duong B. Nemazee D. Effect of cell:cell competition and BAFF expression on peripheral B cell tolerance and B-1 cell survival in transgenic mice expressing a low level of Ig kappa-reactive macroself antigen. *Eur. J. Immunol.* 36(4):985-996, 2006.

[57] Pritchard NR, Smith KG. B cell inhibitory receptors and autoimmunity. *Immunology.* 108(3):263-273, 2003.

[58] Streilein JW. Ocular immune privilege: therapeutic opportunities from an experiment of nature. *Nature Rev. Immunol.* 3(11):879-889, 2003.

[59] Crispe I, Giannandrea M, Klein I, et al. Cellular and molecular mechanisms of liver tolerance. *Immunol. Rev.* 213:101-118, 2006.

[60] Ruiz P, Harland R, Yamaguchi Y, Bollinger RR, Sanfilippo F. In situ and systemic cellular immunity associated with orthotopic rat liver allograft acceptance or rejection. *Transplant. Proc.* 21(1 Pt 1):416-420, 1989.

[61] Niederkorn JY. See no evil, hear no evil, do no evil: the lessons of immune privilege. *Nature Immunol.* 7(4):354-359, 2006.

[62] Schuppe HC, Meinhardt A. Immune privilege and inflammation of the testis. *Chem. Immunol. Allerg.* 88:1-14, 2005.

[63] Murray JE: The 50th anniversary of the first successful human organ transplant. *Rev. Invest. Clin.* 57(2): 118-119, 2005.

[64] Callaghan CJ. Bradley JA. Current status of renal transplantation. *Meth. Mol. Biol.* 333:1-28, 2006.

[65] Nankivell BJ, Chapman JR. Chronic allograft nephropathy: current concepts and future directions. *Transplantation.* 81(5):643-654, 2006.

[66] Hariharan S. BK virus nephritis after renal transplantation. *Kid. Int.* 69(4):655-662, 2006.

[67] Kauffman HM, Cherikh WS, McBride MA, Cheng Y, Hanto DW. Post-transplant de novo malignancies in renal transplant recipients: the past and present. *Transplant. Int.* 19(8):607-620, 2006.

[68] Wilkinson A, Pham PT. Kidney dysfunction in the recipients of liver transplants. *Liver Transplant.* 11(11 Suppl 2):S47-51, 2005.

[69] Calne R. Current status of clinical transplantation tolerance. *Curr. Opin. Org. Transplant.* 11:385-388, 2006.

[70] Calne R, Sells RA, Pena JR, Davis DR, Millard PR, Herbertson BM, *et al.*, Induction of immunological tolerance by porcine liver allografts. *Nature.* 223: 472–476, 1969.

[71] Sanchez-Fueyo A. Immunological tolerance and liver transplantation. *Gastroenterol. Hepatol.* 28(4):250-256, 2005.

[72] Roussey-Kesler G, Giral M, Moreau A, et al. Clinical operational tolerance after kidney transplantation. *Am. J. Transplant.* 6: 736-746, 2006.

[73] Lerut J, and Sanchez-Fueyo A. An appraisal of tolerance in liver transplantation. *Am. J. Transplant.* 6: 1774-1780, 2006.

[74] Calne R. "Prope" tolerance: induction, lymphocyte depletion with minimal maintenance.[comment]. *Transplantation.* 80(1):6-7, 2005.

[75] Suciu-Foca N, Manavalan JS, Cortesini R. Generation and function of antigen-specific suppressor and regulatory T cells. *Transplant. Immunol.* 11:235-244, 2003.

[76] Opelz G. The role of HLA matching and blood transfusions in the cyclosporine era. Collaborative Transplant Study. *Transplant. Proc.* 21(1 Pt 1):609-612, 1989.

[77] Morris PJ. Recognition of an allograft. *Nephrologie.* 7(3 Suppl):19-22, 1986.

[78] Wise M, Zelenika D, Bemelman F, Latinne D, Bazin H, Cobbold S, Waldmann H. CD4 T cells can reject major histocompatibility complex class I-incompatible skin grafts. *Eur. J. Immunol.* 29(1):156-167, 1999.

[79] Waldmann H. Transplantation tolerance—where do we stand? *Nature Med.* 5 (11): 1245-1248, 1999.

[80] Newell KA, Larsen CP. Toward transplantation tolerance: a large step on a long road. *Am. J. Transplant.* 6: 1989-1990, 2006.

[81] Nankivell BJ, Chapman JR. Chronic allograft nephropathy: current concepts and future directions. *Transplantation.* 81(5):643-654, 2006.

[82] Starzl TE, Demetris AJ, Murase N, Ildstad S, Ricordi C, Trucco M. Cell-migration, chimerism, and graft acceptance. *Lancet.* 339 (8809): 1579-1582, 1992.

[83] Lechler RI, Garden OA, Turka LA. The complementary roles of deletion and regulation in transplantation tolerance. *Nature Rev. Immunol.* 3(2):147-58, 2003.

[84] Guenther DA, Madsen JC. Advances in strategies for inducing central tolerance in organ allograft recipients. *Ped. Transplant.* 9(3):277-281, 2005.

[85] Garcia-Morales R, Esquenazi V, Zucker K, et al. An assessment of the effects of cadaver donor bone marrow on kidney allograft recipient blood cell chimerism by a novel technique combining PCR and flow cytometry. *Transplantation.* 62(8):1149-1160, 1996.

[86] Cortesini R, Renna-Molajoni E, Cinti P, Pretagostini R, Ho E, Rossi P, Suciu-Foca Cortesini N. Tailoring of immunosuppression in renal and liver allograft recipients displaying donor specific T-suppressor cells. *Hum. Immunol.* 63(11):1010-1018, 2002.

[87] Fudaba Y, Spitzer TR, Shaffer J, Kawai T, Fehr TI, Delmonico F, Preffer F, Tolkoff-Rubin N, Dey B, Saidman SL, Kraus A, Bonnefoix T, McAfee S, Kattleman K, Colvin RB, Sachs DH, Cosimi AB, Sykes M. Myeloma responses and tolerance following combined kidney and non-myeloablative marrow transplantation: in vivo and in vitro analyses. *Am. J. Transplant.* 6: 2121-2133, 2006.

[88] Shapiro R, Jordan M, Basu A, Scantlebury V, Potdar S, Tan H, Gray E, Randhawa P, Murase N, Zeevi A, Demetris A, Woodward J, Marcos A, Fung J, Starzl T. Kidney transplantation under a tolerogenic regimen of recipient pretreatment and low-dose postoperative immunosuppression with subsequent weaning. *Ann. Surg.* 238(4): 520–525, 2003.

[89] Calne R. Prope Tolerance: A step in the search for tolerance in the clinic. *World J. Surg.* 24(7): 793-796, 2000.

[90] Mazariegos GV, Reyes J, Marino IR et al. Weaning of immunosuppression in liver transplant recipients. *Transplantation.* 63:243-249. 1997.

[91] Devlin J, Doherty D, Thomson L, et al. Defining the outcome of immunosuppression withdrawal after liver transplantation. *Hepatology.* 27: 926-933, 1998.

[92] Takatsuki M, Uemoto S, Inomata Y et al. Analysis of alloreactivity and intragraft cytokine profiles in living donor transplant recipients with graft acceptance. *Transpl. Immunol.* 8: 279-286, 2001.

[93] Eason JD, Cohen AJ, Nair S, Alcantera T, Loss GE. Tolerance: is it worth the risk? *Transplantation.* 79(9):1157-1159, 2005.

[94] Tryphonopoulos P, Tzakis AG, Weppler D et al. The role of donor bone marrow infusions in withdrawal of immunosuppression in adult liver allotransplantation. *Am. J. Transplant.* 5: 608-613, 2005.

[95] Takatsuki M, Uemoto S, Inomata Y, Egawa H, Kiuchi T, Fujita S, Hayashi M, Kanematsu T, Tanaka K. Weaning of immunosuppression in living donor liver transplant recipients. *Transplantation.* 72(3):449-454, 2001.

[96] Berenguer M. Host and donor risk factor before and after liver transplantation that impact HCV recurrence. *Liver Transpl.* 9(11):S44-S47, 2003.

[97] Gane EJ, Naoumov NV, Qian KP, et al. A longitudinal analysis of hepatitis C virus replication following liver transplantation. *Gastroenterology.* 110: 167-177, 1996.

[98] Everson G. Impact of immunosuppressive therapy on recurrence of hepatitis C. *Liver Transpl.* 8(10): S19-S27, 2002.

[99] Marcos A, Eghtesad B, Fung JJ, et al. Use of alemtuzumab and tacrolimus monotherapy for cadaveric liver transplantation: with particular reference to hepatitis C virus. *Transplantation.* 78: 966-971, 2004.

[100] De Ruvo N, Cucchetti A, Lauro A, Masetti M, et al. Preliminary results of immunosuppression with thymoglobulin pretreatment and hepatitis C virus recurrence in liver transplantation. *Transplant. Proc.* 37: 2607-2608, 2005.

[101] Pirenne J, Kawai M. Tolerogenic protocols for intestinal transplantation. *Transplant. Immunology.* 13: 131-137, 2004.

[102] Meijssen MA, Heineman E, deBruin RW, Wolvekamp MC, Marquet RL, Molenaar JC. Long-term survival of DLA-matched segmental small-bowel allografts in dogs. *Transplantation.* 56(5):1062-1066, 1993.

[103] Starzl TE, Murase N, Abu-Elmagd K, et al. Tolerogenic immunosuppression for organ transplantation. *Lancet.* 361:1502-1510, 2003.

[104] Tzakis AG, Kato T, Nishida S, et al. Alemtuzumab (Campath 1H) combined with tacrolimus in intestinal and multivisceral transplantation. *Transplantation.* 75: 1512-1517, 2003.

[105] Calne RY, Sells RA, Pena JR, et al. Induction of immunological tolerance by porcine liver allografts. *Nature.* 223: 472-476, 1969.

[106] Kamada N, Wight DGD. Antigen-specific immunosuppression induced by liver transplantation in the rat. *Transplantation.* 38:217-221, 1984.

[107] Meyer D, Baumgardt S, Loeffeler S, et al. Apoptosis of T lymphocytes in liver and/or small bowel allografts during tolerance induction. *Transplantation.* 66(11)1530-1536, 1998.

[108] Bluestone J, Matthews J, Krensky A. The Immune Tolerance Network: The "Holy Grail" Comes to the Clinic. *J. Am. Soc. Nephrol.* 11: 2141-2146, 2000.

[109] Pons J, Yelamos J, Ramirez P et al. Endothelial cell chimerism does not influence allograft tolerance in liver transplantation patients after withdrawal of immunosuppression. *Transplantation.* 75:1045-1047, 2003.

[110] Tisone G, Orlando G, Palmieri G, et al. Complete weaning off immunosuppression in HCV liver transplant recipients is feasible and favourably impacts on the progression of disease recurrence. *J. Hepatol.* 44: 702-709, 2006.

In: Transplantation Immunology Research Trends   ISBN: 978-1-60021-578-0
Editor: Oliver N. Ulricker, pp. 111-145   © 2007 Nova Science Publishers, Inc.

Chapter IV

Measurement of Intracellular Cytokines to Improve Therapeutic Monitoring of Immunosuppressive Drugs Following Lung Transplantation

Greg Hodge[1,2], Sandra Hodge[1], Paul Reynolds[1] and Mark Holmes[1]
[1] Department of Thoracic Medicine, Royal Adelaide Hospital, Adelaide;
[2] Haematology Department, Women's and Children's Hospital,
North Adelaide, South Australia;

Abstract

Lung transplantation has become established therapy in the treatment of selected patients with end stage lung diseases. However, five year survival after lung transplantation is little better than 50%, largely due to chronic graft failure. The basis of this failure is poorly understood but chronic rejection is probably a major factor. At the cellular level, graft rejection is associated with an increase in graft T-cell infiltration, alveolar macrophages, and pro-inflammatory cytokine expression. Although most effective transplantation immunosuppressive strategies are based on interruption of IL-2 signaling by calcineurin inhibitors, Cyclosporin A (CsA) and Tacrolimus (Tac), intensification of immuno-supressive therapies has not lead to any improvement in chronic graft failure. In addition, treatment with these drugs is associated with serious adverse side effects including specific organ toxicities, susceptibility to infections and an increased risk of developing a range of malignancies. Pharmacokinetic properties of both drugs show high inter- and intra-individual variability which may mean some patients do not require the high levels of drugs (that cause adverse side effects) for effective therapeutics. With the availability of novel flow cytometric techniques, recent research has focused on the measurement of inflammatory cytokines at the cellular level as a strategy to assess the physiological response to treatment. Importantly, cytokine levels in both peripheral blood and in the airways have been investigated, which has highlighted important differences in responses seen locally versus systemically. These techniques may complement or ultimately replace current standard approaches which rely on the measurement of plasma drug levels and monitoring by invasive biopsy. The application of these techniques has the potential to improve current immunosuppression protocols, optimise individual therapy and possibly provide new therapeutic options to improve the morbidity of lung transplant patients.

Introduction

Lung transplantation has become established therapy in the treatment of selected patients with end stage lung disease due to a variety of causes. However, five year survival after lung transplantation in many series is little better than 50%, clearly a dissapointing statistic given the huge expenses involved in lung transplatation and post-transplant care, and the critical shortage of donor organs. The principle reason for graft failure is believed to be chronic rejection, a problem which is seen much more frequently in transplanted lungs than in other solid organ transplants. Clinically, chronic graft failure is manifested by progressive airways obstruction (fall in forced expiratory volume in one second, FEV1) and worsening shortness of breath. The clinical syndrome is referred to as "bronchiolitis obliterans syndrome" (BOS). In many cases, there is a defined pathological correlate, "obliterative bronchiolitis" (OB), although this pattern is not seen in all subjects with the clinical syndrome. Histologically, OB is characterised by fibro-proliferative obstruction and obliteration of small airways [1].

Although the precise pathogenesis of chronic graft failure is unclear, there are certain recognised associations. The strongest risk factor is acute rejection; with early and repeated episodes of acute rejection significantly increasing the risk of subsequent OB. This association clearly suggests that imuune mechanisms may in part underly OB and have thus lead to the hypothesis that the disorder is a form of chronic rejection. However, no clear association with, for example, HLA mismatching has been proven. Further, many patients with acute rejection do not develop OB, and some patients with OB have never experienced clinically detected acute rejection. Several non-immune associations also exist, including variable associations with pulmonary infection. In some studies the closest association seems to be with CMV infection, and there is also evidence that CMV prophylaxis reduces subsequent OB. However, this association remains controversial. Other factors that have been proposed are pulmonary ischemia, gastro-oesophageal reflux disease (and micro-aspiration) and several less well-supported associations including donor asthma and when primary pulmonary hypertension is the recipient disease. In summary, OB appears to represent a final common pathway of response to a variety of noxious insults. This heterogeneity of associations has thus made it difficult to determine a single treatment strategy that will benefit all patients.

Allograft Rejection

Allograft rejection is mediated primarily by T cells and antigen presenting cells, with B cells playing a role via antibody production. Acute cellular rejection involves recipient T cell recognition of HLA molecules expressed on donor-derived, antigen presenting cells (direct allorecognition) or presentation of donor derived peptides by recipient antigen-presenting cells to recipient T cells (indirect allorecognition). Once the alloantigens are recognised as foreign, the activation and production of cytokines by T lymphocytes, monocytes and other immune cells lead to the amplification of the alloimmune response.

At the cellular level, acute graft rejection is associated with a marked increase in graft T-cell infiltration, alveolar macrophages, and pro-inflammatory cytokine expression including IL-2, IFN-γ and TNF-α [2].

OB is also associated with a moderate increase in graft airway T-cell infiltration, alveolar macrophages, and pro-inflammatory cytokine expression [3, 4]. An additional feature is airway fibrosis, which may be due to the presence of pro-fibrotic chemokines/cytokines such as MCP-1, IL-4 and TGFβ [4]. Pharmacological immunosuppression is required to prevent the allo-immune response to the transplanted lungs. Immunosuppression has improved graft survival but leaves patients susceptible to infectious complications, of which pulmonary infections are the leading cause of morbidity and mortality. Although immunosuppressants used to prevent and treat rejection involve several classes of drugs, many target the production of pro-inflammatory cytokine by T cells, monocytes and other immune cells.

Immunosuppressants

Corticosteroids

Glucocorticoids were the first immunosuppressants used in transplantation. Although glucocorticoids are potent, they are the least selective agents and affect multiple cell lines, including T and B cells, monocytes, macrophages and neutrophils. In lymphocytes and monocytes, glucocorticoids exert negative regulatory effects on cytokine gene expression by directly inhibiting two transcription factors: activator protein-1 and nuclear factor-κB [5].

Calcineurin Inhibitors: Cyclosporin A (CsA) and Tacrolimus (Tac)

The calcineurin inhibitors CsA and Tac have greatly decreased the incidence of allograft rejection. As they are more T-cell selective, their use has helped preserve other cell lines and has reduced the overall incidence of infection by facilitating the lowering of corticosteroid doses [6]. These immunosuppressants inhibit T-cell activation by binding to intracellular immunophilins. Both CsA and Tac inhibit production of IL-1β, IL-2, IL-6, IL-8, IFNγ and TNFα. Tac preferentially suppresses T-helper-type-1 (Th1) cells over Th2 cells [5].

Both agents have been shown to upregulate TGFβ, which although having several immunosuppressive properties on pro-inflammatory cytokines, promotes matrix formation and may contribute to allograft fibrosis. This effect may play a role in chronic rejection. Thus by inhibiting T-cell activation, proliferation and cytokine production, the calcineurin inhibitors are potent immunosuppressants.

Antimetabolites: Azathioprine (AZA) and Mycophenolate Mofetil (MMF)

AZA and MMF are antimetabolites that inhibit the production of purine which is required for T and B-cell activation and proliferation. AZA also acts by inhibiting CD28 costimulation [7] while MMF inhibits glycostlation of leucocyte adhesion molecules, thereby decreasing recruitment of lymphocytes and monocytes to areas of inflammation and reduces cytokine production through inhibition of clonal expansion [7, 8].

Other agents such as sirolomis and everolomis inhibit mRNA responsible for cell cycle progression thus blocking IL-2 postreceptor signalling and preventing T-cell proliferation [7].

Anti-Lymphocyte Antibodies

Polyclonal anti-lymphocyte antibodies have a long history of use for induction of immuno-suppression and in the treatment of acute rejection, targeting different cell lines such as lymphocytes, thymocytes or specific cell lines. For example, OKT3 or Muromonab-CD3 is a murine monoclonal anti-lymphocyte antibody directed against the epsilon unit of the T-cell receptor. Binding causes T-cell opsinisation and removal by mononuclear phagocytes [7].

Anti-Cytokine Receptor Antibodies

Anti-cytokine receptor monclonal antibodies directed against the α-chains of the CD25 molecule, a key unit of the IL-2 receptor, have also been used successfully in the transplant setting due to the central role of IL-2 in regulating T-cell activation, differentiation and apoptosis.

Standard immunosuppression therapy usually comprises combinations of either cyclosporin A (CsA) or tacrolimus (Tac) with prednisolone and azathioprine. Trough plasma drug levels of either CsA or Tac are kept within recommended therapeutic ranges (range for CsA (80-250 µg/L) and Tac (5-20 µg/L)). Therapeutic drug plasma concentrations however are broad and may vary according to the clinical situation and the choice of immunosuppressive agents being given. Recent data supports the use of therapeutic monitoring of CsA by measurment of the blood concentration two hours after administration of the dose with data showing better prediction of clinical effects [9]. Nevertherless, therapeutic drug monitoring has certain limitations with blood concentrations not necessarily reflecting the concentration of drug at the site of action. In addition, the combined therapeutic effect of all drugs used should be assessed for each patient. An alternative approach has recently been suggested [10].

Measurement of Inflammatory Cytokines in Transplant Patients

There are three potential sites from which cells or fluid can can be assessed for cytokine analysis in transplant patients; blood, the lung airways and within the allograft itself. For routine diagnostic purposes, assays based on peripheral blood would be advantageous.

Previous methodology to measure cytokine levels in transplant patients include ELISA quantification from serum and peripheral blood mononuclear cell culture [11, 12] and RTPCR of cytokine mRNA levels [13]. Measurement of soluble cytokines by ELISA or more recently by cytometric bead arrays have proven useful for diagnosis in several disease states [14, 15]. However, cytokines bind to proteoglycan components of the cell surface or extramedullary matrix [16] and have a very limited availability within the blood, effectively limiting the prognostic value of assay of soluble cytokines. Standard techniques such as ELISA give no indication of cytokine-producing cell types and is time consuming and expensive if several cytokines are quantified. Cell purification techniques lead to loss of specific cell subsets [17] and increased apoptosis of cells [18]. While RTPCR is a sensitive technique, results depend on purification of cells from heterogeneous cell populations and are subject to technical error.

The production of cytokines by individual immune cell types can be assessed using a range of techniques. These assays require cell activation prior to analysis. In the case of T cells this is accomplished by polyclonal stimulation with mitogens active on the cell surface or within the cell or by antigenic stimulation. In the case of alloreactive cells, when the frequency of the responding cells is relatively high, activation by alloantigen presentation can provide a useful technique to assess the potential to mount an antigraft immune response using ELISPOT [19] or limiting dilution analysis [20]. Following polyclonal stimulation, multiparameter flow cytometry offers a powerful tool to analyse multiple pro- and anti-inflammatory intracellular cytokines in thousands of cells by individual cell types.

Measurement of T-cell intracellular cytokines has been used to investigate differences in several clinical situations such as between cord and adult blood in the context of graft versus host disease [21] and effects of other therapeutics [22]. This approach has also been used in preliminary studies in lung transplant patients.

Effect of Immunosuppression Protocols on Intracellular Cytokines in Blood T Cells

It is currently unknown if levels of immunosuppressive drugs correlate with pro-inflammatory cytokine expression in peripheral blood T cells. Lymphocytes are known to traffic from the blood stream to the lung and later rejoin the peripheral circulation [23] suggesting that measurement of blood T cell cytokines may be reflective of graft infiltrating T-cell cytokine profiles.

To investigate the immunomodulatory effects of currently used immunosuppressive regimes, whole blood from a group of 9 stable, non-infected lung transplant patients (9 patients, 13 episodes) and 15 control volunteers was stimulated *in vitro* and intracellular T cell cytokine production determined using multiparameter flow cytometry [10]. This is the first report of intracellular pro- and anti-inflammatory cytokines in peripheral blood T cells from lung transplant patients and provides important new information regarding the immunosuppressive effect of current drug protocols in these patients. We found evidence that current immunosuppression protocols have a significant immunosuppressive effect on pro-inflammatory cytokine production by peripheral blood CD4+ T cells consistent with therapeutic intention. However, there was a limited effect on peripheral blood CD8+ T-cells, particularly IFNγ inflammatory cytokine production in lung transplant patients (figure 1).

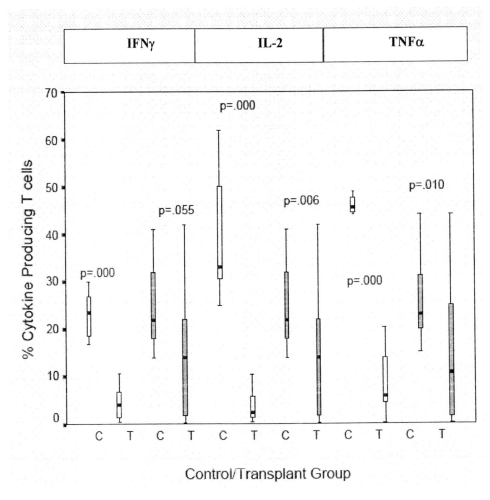

Figure 1. Box plot graphs showing the production of pro-inflammatory cytokines by CD4+ (clear bars) and CD8+ T-cells (grey bars) from lung transplant (T) and control (C) subjects following *in vitro* stimulation (mean ± SD and range). The percentage of CD4+ and CD8+ T-cells producing IL-2 and TNFα was significantly reduced from lung transplant patients compared to control. The percentage of CD4+ T-cells producing IFNγ was also significantly reduced from lung transplant patients but not the percentage of CD8+ T cells producing IFNγ. Note the marked inhibition of inflammatory T-cell cytokines in CD4+ cells compared with CD8+ cells in transplant patients compared to control group.

All transplant patients in this study had plasma levels of CsA or Tac within their therapeutic ranges suggesting that analysis of cytokine production may provide a more accurate assessment of immunosuppression than drug levels.

In contrast to these results [10] a recent report failed to show any differences between inflammatory T-cell cytokines in stable renal transplant patients and controls [24]. However, this study did not distinguish between CD8+ and CD8- T-cell cytokine production while our results showed that immunosuppression protocols are adequate for CD8- (CD4+) but not CD8+ T-cell inflammatory cytokines, particularly IFNγ. We also showed that current immunosuppression agents increased anti-inflammatory cytokine production of IL-4 and TGFβ by T cells from lung transplant patients compared to controls (table 1).

Table 1. The percentage of T cell subsets producing anti-inflammatory cytokines, IL-4 and TGFβ from 9 lung transplant patients (T) compared with 15 control subjects (C) (mean ± SD). There was a significant increase in IL-4 by both T-cell subsets and TGFβ by CD8+ T-cell subsets by tranplant patients compared with control subjects (bold)

	IL-4		TGFβ	
	CD4	CD8	CD4	CD8
C	0.4±0.3	0.0±0.0	5.3±3.2	3.0±2.6
T	1.0±0.8	1.4±0.0	4.9±3.1	4.6±2.4
P	**.019**	**.010**	.890	**.017**

IL-4 negatively regulates Th1 cytokines IFNγ and IL-2 [25] that have been reportedly increased during acute rejection episodes [13]. TGFβ has also been shown to inhibit IL-2 and IFNγ production by T cells [26]. Thus, these findings of increased IL-4 and TGFβ production by T-cells in lung transplant patients may partially explain the significantly reduced levels of IFNγ and IL-2 in peripheral blood T cells. The increased sensitivity of CD4+ T cells to TGFβ in reducing Th1 responses compared to CD8+ T cells [27] may help explain the observation of increased inhibition of these cytokines in CD4+ cells compared to CD8+ T cells.

The previous reports that IL-2 and IFNγ are inhibited in the presence of methylprednisolone [22, 28] are similar to the reported effects of CsA and Tac [29]. However, although Tac and CsA have been shown to inhibit T-cell IL-4 production in vitro [29], low levels of corticosteroids have previously been shown to be stimulatory for T-cell IL-4 production [30] and may be acting similarly in transplant patients. Nevertheless the net combined effect of CsA or Tac, methylprednisolone and AZA may probably accounts for the significant reduction in these pro-inflammatory T-cell cytokines in transplant patients.

We also found increased absolute numbers of CD8+ T cells in transplant patients which is consistent with a previous report [31]. TGFβ has been shown to be co-stimulatory for CD8+ T cells but not CD4+ T cells [32]. IL-4 enhances the proliferation of precursors of cytotoxic lymphocytes and their differentiation into active cytotoxic CD8+ T cells [33]. In CsA or Tac treated mice, T-cell proliferation was shown to be suppressed in CD4+ but not CD8+ subsets [34]. These findings of increased TGFβ by CD8+T cells and increased IL-4 production by both CD4+ and CD8+ T-cell subsets may therefore be causative factors in the significant increase in cytotoxic T cells in these patients. The relative increase in absolute numbers of CD8+ T cells and excellent correlation between the percentage of CD8+ T cells and the amount of IFNγ being produced by these cytotoxic cells suggests that current immunosuppressive protocols are ineffective at reducing this inflammatory cytokine.

In contrast to acute rejection, chronic graft failure is associated with increased fibrosis in the lung. Both IL-4 [35] and TGFβ [36] have been shown to promote fibroblast proliferation in the lung. Therefore, although TGFβ and IL4 are anti-inflammatory cytokines, their increased production by cytotoxic lymphocytes that migrate to the lung may contribute to increased fibrosis in chronic graft rejection.

Current immunosuppression protocols are not without significant toxic side effects [37]. In an attempt to minimise these side effects a number of low toxicity protocols have been developed [38]. One could hypothesise that if a transplant patient was showing signs of drug toxicity and levels of intracellular T-cell inflammatory cytokines were markedly reduced compared to control (eg., Patient B in figure 2), the dose of drug could be reduced and therapeutic effects monitored or tailored to suit the individual patient. Alternately, if intracellular T-cell inflammatory cytokines were not reduced (eg., CD8 T cells in Patient A, figure 2), other immunosuppressive drugs should be considered.

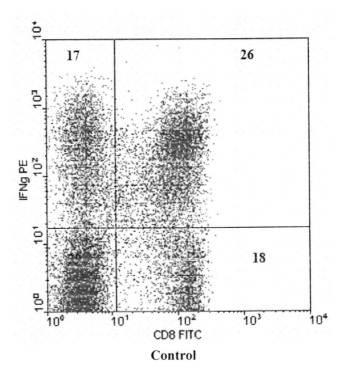

Figure 2 continued

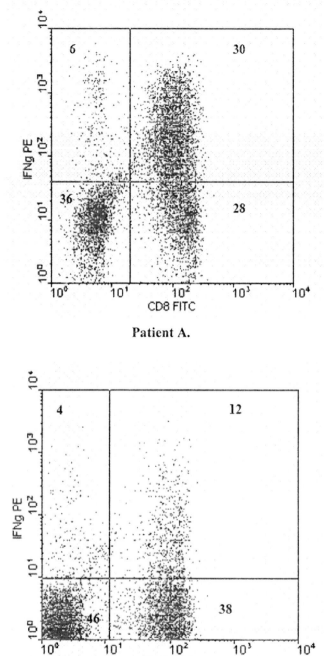

Patient A.

Patient B.

Figure 2. Representative dot plots showing the effect of immunosuppression therapy on IFNγ production by CD8+ and CD8- (CD4+) T cells from 2 lung transplant patients and control. T cells were identified by CD3 PC5 versus side scatter characteristics. Patient A shows immunosuppression of IFNγ in CD8- (CD4+) T cells but not CD8+ T cells. Patient B shows immunosuppression of IFNγ in both T-cell subsets. Note the reduced percentage of CD4 T cells and increased CD8 T cells in transplant patients compared to control.

The conclusions drawn from this study were that current immunosuppression protocols have limited effect on peripheral blood IFNγ production by CD8+ T-cells but do upregulate T-cell anti-inflammatory cytokines, TGFβ and IL4. Drugs that effectively reduce IFNγ production by CD8+ T cells may improve current protocols for reducing graft rejection in these patients. Intracellular cytokine analysis using flow cytometry may be a more appropriate indicator of immunosuppression of all therapeutic drugs used than measurement of plasma CsA or Tac levels in these patients. This technique may prove useful in optimising therapy for individual patients.

Effect of Immunosuppression Protocols on Blood Monocyte Intracellular Cytokine and Chemokine Production

Alveolar macrophages are a major source of inflammatory cytokines/chemokines involved in the pathogenesis of lung transplant rejection and are derived from blood monocytes that migrate to the lung. Chemokines are inflammatory mediators that specifically stimulate the directional migration of T cells and monocytes and play an important role in immune cell recruitment into sites of antigenic challenge [39] such as in lung transplant. Chemokines such as IL-8 and MCP-1 have been reportedly increased in BAL of transplant patients undergoing rejection [40]. MCP-1 induces monocyte migration and differentiation to macrophages and plays a pivotal role in BOS [41]. MCP-3 has also been shown to be chemotactic for T cells and monocytes [39] and may also play a role in the pathogenesis of transplant rejection. Thus we investigated monocyte production of cytokine/chemokine mediators in peripheral blood of lung transplant patients [42]. We studied intracellular cytokine/chemokine production by peripheral blood monocytes following stimulation with LPS from a group of 9 stable lung transplant patients and 15 control volunteers using multiparameter flow cytometry. There was a significant increase in the percentage of monocytes producing chemokines MCP-1, MCP-3 and IL-8 and anti-inflammatory cytokine IL-10, but no change in the percentage of monocytes producing IL-6, TNFα, IL-1α, IL-12, MIP-1α, MIP-1β and TGFβ (table 2). Representative histograms showing the increase in the percentage of monocytes producing chemokines MCP-1, MCP-3 from a transplant patient is shown in figure 3.

We found that current immunosuppression protocols have limited effect on peripheral blood monocyte inflammatory cytokine production and are inadequate at suppressing monocyte chemokine production in lung transplant patients. This was the first report of increased MCP-3 in lung transplant patients. MCP-3 has been shown to be a mediator in the activation of extracellular matrix gene expression in addition to promoting leucocyte trafficking in systemic sclerosis [43]. Monocytes migrating to the lung may be acting similarly in lung transplant patients. Interestingly, it has been shown that the effects of MCP-3 can be diminished by neutralising antibody to TGFβ [43]. As TGFβ has been reported to play a major role in OB, the possible role of TGFβ – MCP-3 mediated effects clearly warrants further study.

Table 2. Monocyte cytokine/chemokine production in 9 lung transplant and 15 control subjects (% positive cells) following LPS stimulation. The percentage of monocytes producing IL-8, IL-10 and MCP-1 and MCP-3 was significantly increased in lung transplant patients (bold) but levels of IL-6, TNFα, IL-1α, IL-12, MIP-1α, MIP-1β and TGFβ were unchanged

		IL-8	IL-6	TNFα	IL-10	IL-1α	IL-12	MCP-1	MCP-3	MIP1α	MIP1β	TGFβ
Controls	Mean	82.4	72.9	82.7	4.3	79.5	24.7	11.4	5.5	13.6	71.6	6.2
	SD	7.6	20.2	7.2	1.5	13.1	9.3	5.7	3.1	11.4	15.9	3.1
Patients	Mean	92.3	65.1	82.1	8.8	73.9	20.1	28.8	18.9	13.9	72.2	5.5
	SD	6.6	21.8	8.2	3.7	16.6	12.3	16.9	16.3	9.1	23.1	2.6
	P =	.039	.731	.612	.042	.714	.542	.006	.010	.875	.788	.468

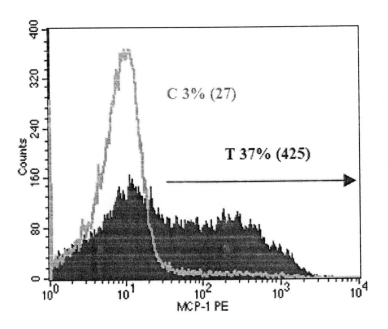

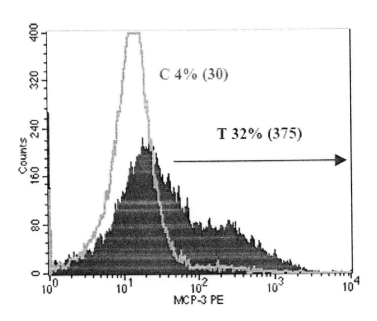

Figure 3. Representative histograms showing intracellular staining of MCP-1 and MCP-3 in peripheral blood monocytes from a transplant patient (T) and control subject (C) following LPS stimulation. The percentage of monocytes producing MCP-1 and MCP-3 was significantly increased in the lung transplant patient compared to control (marker set on negative control-not shown). The amount of MCP-1 and MCP-3 (as indicated by MFI) was also significantly increased in the lung transplant patient compared to control.

MCP-1 levels have been reported to be increased in lung allograft rejection, especially in OB [41]. Alveolar macrophages were identified as the major source of MCP-1. Blood monocytes migrating to the lung are the probable source of these high MCP-1 producers, indicating that these cells are producing MCP-1 before entering the lung. Interestingly MCP-3 has been shown to be a functional ligand for MCP-1 receptor [44]. The increased levels of monocyte MCP-3 identified in transplant patients may enhance the chemoattractant effects of MCP-1, leading to further increases in lymphocyte and monocyte recruitment in the lung. In the mouse model, treatment with neutralising antibody to MCP-1 reduced mononuclear phagocyte recruitment to the lung and led to an attenuation of OB [41]. These findings suggest that treatments aimed at reducing MCP-3 may also be of benefit at reducing monocyte recruitment in lung transplant patients.

IL-10 is a regulatory Th2 cytokine that has been shown to prevent acute rejection and OB in the animal models [45]. IL-10 and IL-4 negatively regulate Th1 cytokines IFNγ and IL-2 [25], two cytokines that are increased during acute rejection episodes [2]. MCP-1 has also been shown to upregulate IL-4 [46] and enhance Th2 polarisation [47]. Monocyte production of IL10 and MCP-1 was increased in the present study. We have previously reported increased T-cell production of IL-4 in lung transplant patients [10]. Taken together, these findings may explain the previous findings of significantly reduced levels of IFNγ and IL-2 in peripheral blood T cells of lung transplant patients. Increased production of IL-10 may be partially caused by treatment with immunosuppressive drugs as it has previously been shown that monocyte IL-10 production is upregulated in the presence of methylprednisolone [22, 28]. IL-12, a Th1 cytokine that has been shown to be downregulated in the presence of methylprednisolone [28], was unchanged in monocytes from transplant patients compared with control. IL-12 synthesis has been shown to be unaltered in the presence of CsA [48] and downregulated by tacrolimus but only when combined with rhG-CSF treatment [49]. As IL-12 is a potent inducer of cell-mediated immunity and IFNγ in T cells [25], drugs that help reduce this important regulatory cytokine may be of benefit for transplant patients. Upregulation of MCP-1 and IL-8 in BAL has recently been shown to be a predictive marker of post-transplant airway obliteration [40] which is consistent with these findings. Treatment with dexamethasone [22] and pulse methylprednisolone [50] has been shown to be associated with a substantial decrease in monocyte MCP-1 synthesis and may be of benefit in the treatment of lung transplant patients.

As described for T cells, detection of intracellular cytokines in blood monocytes may help to provide a more accurate assessment of immunosuppression than systemic therapeutic drug levels as all patients had drug plasma trough levels within their therapeutic range. The technique is relatively rapid, easy to perform and provides a detailed analysis of cytokine/chemokine levels in specific leucocyte subtypes in individual patients. The relatively large standard deviation for chemokines MCP-1 and MCP-3 in the transplant patients indicate these patients are a heterogeneous group. It would thus be of interest to serially monitor intracellular cytokines/chemokines from transplant patients with a view to detect shifts in cytokine/chemokine profiles that are indicative of transplant rejection status. These studies may reveal that patients with elevated MCP-1 and MCP-3 progress to transplant rejection earlier than patients with "normal" levels. Our studies show that current immunosuppression protocols have limited effect on peripheral blood monocyte inflammatory cytokine production and are inadequate at suppressing monocyte chemokine production. Drugs that modulate these cytokines/chemokines may improve current protocols for reducing graft rejection in these patients.

Increased Intracellular Pro- and Anti-Inflammatory Cytokines in Bronchoalveolar Lavage T Cells of Stable Lung Transplant Patients

Analysis of cells and cytokines in bronchoalveolar lavage (BAL) has previously been used as an indicator of transplant rejection in humans [52, 53] and the canine model [54]. While changes in CD4/CD8 in BAL have been associated with acute and chronic rejection [52, 53], surface phenotyping gives little information regarding cytokine production by cells. It has previously been shown that analysis of inflammatory cytokines in BAL and blood using ELISA may not be as reliable as analysis of intracellular cytokines using flow cytometry [55].

To overcome these problems and to investigate the immunomodulatory effects of currently used immunosuppressive regimens on BAL T-cell cytokine production, whole blood and BAL from 9 stable lung transplant patients and 10 control volunteers were stimulated *in vitro* and cytokine production by CD8+ and CD8- (CD4+) T-cell subsets determined using multiparameter flow cytometry [56]. We showed that there was no difference in T-cell pro-inflammatory cytokines between blood and BAL compartments in stable lung transplant patients (table 3). In contrast, the control group showed significantly less pro-inflammatory T-cell cytokine production in BAL compared with blood (table 4). Although there was no difference in T-cell pro-inflammatory cytokine production between blood and BAL compartments in lung transplant patients there was a significant increase in Th1 cytokines by T cells in the BAL compared to the control group (figure 4).

It has previously been shown that there was a good correlation between the percentage of CD8+ T cells in blood of stable lung transplant patients and IFNγ production by these cells [10]. In contrast, the present study showed that there is a poor correlation between the percentage of CD8+ T cells in BAL and IFNγ production suggesting that previous methods to quantify cytotoxic cells in BAL by immunophenotyping [53, 57] do not give accurate results of functional characteristics of these cytotoxic CD8+ T cells. Interestingly, there was a significant increase in the anti-inflammatory cytokine, IL-4 in the BAL compared to blood of both the transplant and control group. Representative dot plots showing IL-4 and IFNγ production by BAL CD8+ and CD8- (CD4+) T cells from 2 lung transplant patients and controls are shown in figure 5.

Table 3. The percentage of T-cells producing intracellular cytokines in blood and BAL of the 9 stable lung transplant patients (mean ± SD). There was a significant increase in the percentage of T cells producing IL-4 and TGFβ in BAL compared to blood (bold)

	CD3		IFNγ		IL-2		IL-4		TGFβ		TNFα	
	CD4	CD8	CD4	CD8	CD4	CD8	CD4	CD8	CD4	CD8	CD4	CD8
Blood	55±18	44±18	7±5	17±15	6±5	5±4	1±1	1±1	4.9±2	5±2.5	12±7	14±12
BAL	44±16	55±16	6±5	13±8	4±3	5±4	5±2	9±6	2±2	2.3±1	9±7	14±11
P	.251	.251	.965	.965	.289	.935	.001	.000	.001	.018	.479	.989

Table 4. The percentage of T-cells producing intracellular cytokines in blood and BAL of the Control group(mean ± SD). There was a significant decrease in the percentage of CD4+ and CD8+ T cells producing IFNγ, IL-2, TGFβ and TNFα and a significant increase in the percentage of CD4+ and CD8+ T cells producing IL-4 in BAL compared to blood (bold)

	CD3		IFNγ		IL-2		IL-4		TGFβ		TNFα	
	CD4	CD8	CD4	CD8	CD4	CD8	CD4	CD8	CD4	CD8	CD4	CD8
Blood	62±7	37±8	19±5	21±8	36±16	8±4	0.4±.3	.5±.3	5±3	3±2	43±11	24±11
BAL	70±15	29±15	2±2	1±.8	1±1	.5±.4	6±6	3±2.6	1±1	.8±.7	8±5	6±6
P	.141	.141	.000	.000	.000	.010	.003	.024	.008	.006	.000	.000

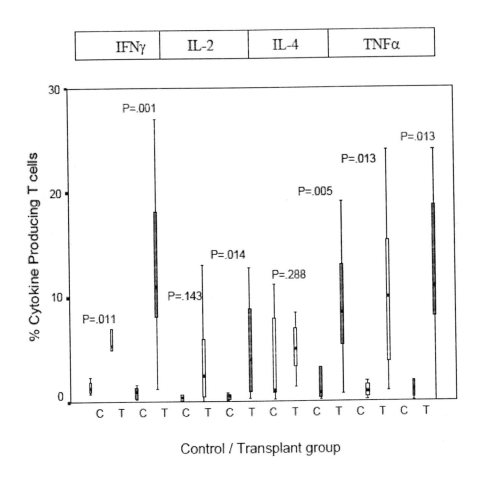

Figure 4. Box plot graphs showing the production of cytokines by BAL CD4+ and CD8+ T-cells from 9 lung transplant (T) and 10 control (C) subjects following *in vitro* stimulation (mean ± 2SD and range). The percentage of CD8+ T-cells producing IFNγ, IL-2 and IL-4 and the percentage of CD4+ cells producing IFNγ and TNFα was significantly increased in lung transplant patients. The percentage of CD4+ T-cells producing IL2 and IL4 was unchanged in lung transplant patients compared to control.

IL-4 is a Th2 cytokine that provides a negative feedback on Th1 cytokine production [25], thus its reduced expression by CD8+ T cells suggests that this regulatory mechanism may be ineffective in stable transplant patients. The Th2 response may be systemic, as the same authors have recently shown increased levels of IL-10, another Th2 cytokine, by monocytes from stable lung transplant patients [42]. The anti-inflammatory cytokine, TGFβ, was also increased in CD8+ T cells in BAL of transplant patients compared with control. TGFβ has previously been shown to inhibit T-cell production of IFNγ and IL-2 [26] suggesting that the function of this regulatory mechanism is also altered in stable transplant patients. The increased sensitivity of CD4+ T cells to TGFβ in reducing Th1 responses compared to CD8+ T cells [27] may help explain the observation of increased inhibition of these cytokines in CD4+ cells compared to CD8+ T cells.

Controls

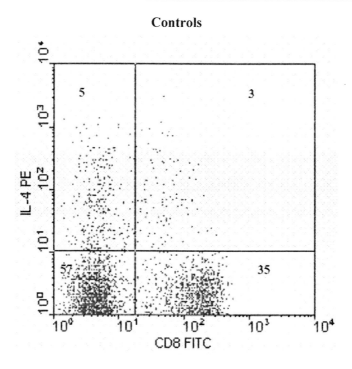

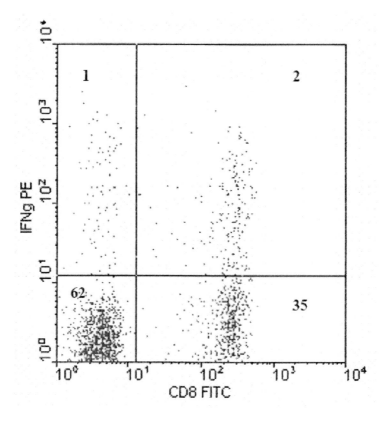

Figure 5 continued

Transplant

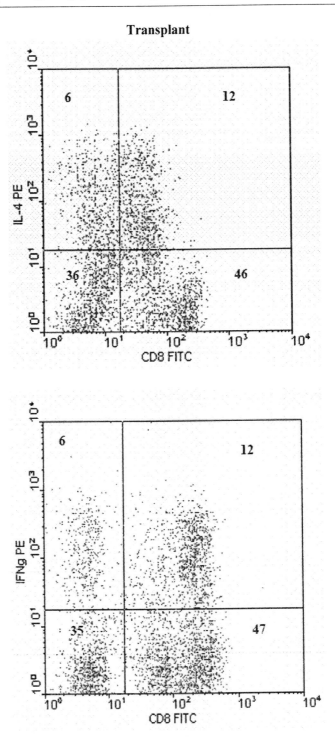

Figure 5. Representative dot plots showing IL-4 and IFNγ production by BAL CD8+ and CD8- (CD4+) T cells from 2 lung transplant patients and controls. T cells were identified by CD3 PC5 versus side scatter characteristics. Transplant patients showed an increase in IL-4 in CD8 dim but not CD8- (CD4+) T cells. Transplant patients showed an increase in IFNγ in both CD4+ and CD8 bright T cells. Note the reduced percentage of CD4+ T cells and increased CD8+ T cells in transplant patients compared to control.

TGFβ has been shown to be co-stimulatory for CD8+ T cells but not CD4+ T cells [32]. IL-4 enhances the proliferation of precursors of cytotoxic lymphocytes and their differentiation into active cytotoxic CD8+ T cells [33]. In CsA or Tac treated mice, T-cell proliferation was shown to be suppressed in CD4+ but not CD8+ subsets [58]. Increased TGFβ and IL-4 by CD8+T cells in BAL and IL-4 and TGFβ by CD4+ and CD8+T cells respectively in blood, may therefore be causative factors in the significant increase in cytotoxic T cells in both blood and BAL in these patients. Chronic graft rejection is associated with increased fibrosis in the lung. Both IL-4 [35] and TGFβ [4] have been shown to promote fibroblast proliferation in the lung. Therefore, although TGFβ and IL4 are anti-inflammatory cytokines, their increased production by cytotoxic lymphocytes in the lung may contribute to increased fibrosis (as observed in chronic graft rejection).

Although this study shows that measurement of blood T-cell cytokine production in lung transplant recipients is reflective of BAL T-cell cytokine production, comparison of T-cell cytokine balance between the two compartments may give a more acurate indication of rejection episodes. All transplant patients in this study had plasma levels of CsA or Tac within their therapeutic range, again suggesting that analysis of cytokine production may provide a more accurate assessment of immunosuppression than drug levels and show that these patients are inadequately immunosuppressed. This study confirms previous findings that current immunosuppression protocols have a limited effect on peripheral blood CD8+ T-cell pro-inflammatory cytokine production in stable lung transplant patients [10]. A longitudinal surveillance of BAL cell phenotypes in individuals has been suggested to identify a preclinical state of rejection [40]. Monitoring intracellular T-cell cytokine profiles may be more appropriate indicator of patient immunosuppression and transplant status than cell phenotypes and we are currently undertaking such a study to investigate this. One could hypothesise that an increase in longitudinal IL-4 and TGFβ may be predictive of chronic rejection whereas an increase in IFNγ, IL-2 and TNFα may be predictive of acute rejection episodes [2-4]. Transplant patients were a very heterogeneous group and exhibited a broad range of inflammatory cytokines compared with controls (figure 1). Aerosolised CsA treatment has been used successfully and safely in reducing inflammatory cytokines in refractory acute rejection [59]. This therapy may be of benefit in treating lung transplant patients identified with high percentages of inflammatory cytokine producing T cells whilst minimising systemic side effects of immunosuppressive agents.

In conclusion, this study demonstrates that it is possible to monitor intracellular T-cell cytokine production in BAL. The study showed decreased T-cell pro- and anti-inflammatory cytokine production in BAL compared with blood in control subjects but not in stable lung transplant patients. Current immunosuppression protocols have limited effect on pro-inflammatory cytokine production by T cells in BAL, especially CD8+ T-cells, but do upregulate T-cell anti-inflammatory cytokines IL-4 and TGFβ. Drugs that effectively reduce T-cell pro-inflammatory cytokines in BAL may improve current protocols for prolonging graft survival in these patients.

Table 5. The percentage of T-cells producing intracellular cytokines in blood and BB of 13 lung transplant patients (mean ± SD). There was a significant decrease in the percentage of CD4+ and a significant increase in the percentage of CD8+ T cells in BB (bold). There was a significant increase in the percentage of CD8+ T cells producing IFNγ, IL-4 and TNFα, a significant decrease in the percentage of CD4+ T cells producing IL-2 and CD4+ and CD8+ T cells producing TGFβ in BB compared to blood

	CD3		IFNγ		IL-2		IL-4		TGFβ		TNFα	
	CD4	CD8	CD4	CD8	CD4	CD8	CD4	CD8	CD4	CD8	CD4	CD8
Blood	53±11	47±11	13±7	26±15	18±13	4±4	1±.8	.9±.4	3.2±2	3±1.7	18±14	16±12
BB	37±11	63±11	17±7	40±13	8±4	3±1.6	1.2±.6	2.3±.8	2±.9	1.7±1	18±7	30±11
P	.002	.002	.085	.026	.042	.300	.179	.043	.039	.028	.738	.002

Table 6. The percentage of T-cells producing intracellular cytokines in BAL and BB of the 13 lung transplant patients (mean ± SD). There was a significant decrease in the percentage of CD4+ and a significant increase in the percentage of CD8+ T cells in BB (bold). There was a significant increase in the percentage of CD4 and CD8+ T cells producing IFNγ and CD8 T cells producing TNFα, and a significant decrease in the percentage of CD4+ and CD8+ T cells producing IL-4 and TGFβ in BB compared to BAL

	CD3		IFNγ		IL-2		IL-4		TGFβ		TNFα	
	CD4	CD8	CD4	CD8	CD4	CD8	CD4	CD8	CD4	CD8	CD4	CD8
BAL	50±11	50±11	10±9	17±15	5±5	3±3	5±4	5±4	4.6±2	5±2.1	19±10	12±11
BB	37±11	63±11	17±7	40±13	8±4	3±1.6	1.2±1	2.3±2	2±.9	1.7±1	18±7	30±11
P	.006	.006	.029	.001	.100	.210	.002	.025	.035	.028	.657	.002

Table 7. The percentage of T-cells producing intracellular cytokines in blood and BB of 10 control volunteers (mean ± SD). There was a significant decrease in the percentage of CD4+ and a significant increase in the percentage of CD8+ T cells in BB (bold). There was a significant increase in the percentage of CD8+ T cells producing IFNγ and TNFα, a significant decrease in the percentage of CD4+ and CD8+ T cells producing IL-2 in BB compared to blood.

	CD3		IFNγ		IL-2		IL-4		TGFβ		TNFα	
	CD4	CD8	CD4	CD8	CD4	CD8	CD4	CD8	CD4	CD8	CD4	CD8
Blood	69±4.4	31±6.9	18±7.8	20±5	40±17	6±4	.8±4	.5±.3	4±2	3±2	43±12	20±6
BB	36±19	64±19	15±6	45±17	10±8	3±2	.5±.3	.9±.7	3±1	1±.3	20±6	37±17
P	.003	.003	.065	.019	.001	.038	.560	.189	.185	.064	.017	.025

Table 8. The percentage of T-cells producing intracellular cytokines in BAL and BB of 10 control volunteers (mean ± SD). There was a significant decrease in the percentage of CD4+ and a significant increase in the percentage of CD8+ T cells in BB (bold). There was a significant increase in the percentage of CD4+ and CD8+ T cells producing IFNγ and IL-2 and CD8+ T cells producing TNFα in BB. There was a significant decrease in the percentage of CD4+ and CD8+ T cells producing IL-4 in BB compared to BAL.

	CD3		IFNγ		IL-2		IL-4		TGFβ		TNFα	
	CD4	CD8	CD4	CD8	CD4	CD8	CD4	CD8	CD4	CD8	CD4	CD8
BAL	71±11	29±11	4±2.7	6±5	3±.8	.8±.7	8.5±2.4	.8±.7	2±2	5±2	14±8	.5±.5
BB	36±19	64±19	15±6	45±17	10±8	3±2	.5±.3	3±.2	3±1	.9±.7	20±6	7.5±6
P	.002	.003	.041	.000	.028	.000	.001	.042	.198	.002	.530	.000

Compartmentalisation of Intracellular Pro-Inflammatory Cytokines in Bronchial Intra-Epithelial T Cells of Stable Lung Transplant Patients

Analysis of inflammatory cytokine profiles of intra-epithelial T cells in bronchial brushing (BB) may provide additional information to assess immune graft status in lung transplant patients. To investigate the immunomodulatory effects of currently used immunosuppressive regimens on bronchial intra-epithelial T-cell cytokine production, whole blood, BAL and BB from 13 stable lung transplant patients and 10 control volunteers were stimulated *in vitro* and cytokine production by T-cell subsets quantified [60].

This is the first report of the use of flow cytometry to measure intracellular pro- and anti-inflammatory cytokines in BB-derived intra-epithelial T cells. Although there was a decrease in T-cell pro-inflammatory cytokine production in blood of transplant patients, this was not found in BAL or bronchial intra-epithelial CD8 T-cell subsets, suggesting that the same level of immunosuppression may not occur in the lung of transplant recipients (table 5 and 6). This study shows that there is no difference in the percentage of bronchial intra-epithelial CD8 T-cells that produce pro-inflammatory cytokines between stable lung transplant patients and control subjects (tables 5-8) indicating that current immunosuppression protocols are ineffective at reducing pro-inflammatory T-cell cytokines in transplant grafts.

In contrast, the same authors have previously shown a decrease in CD4+ T-cell pro-inflammatory cytokine production in blood of stable transplant patients compared with control subjects consistent with immunosuppression protocol strategy [10] and the current study confirms these findings. They have also previously shown non-compartmentalisation of inflammatory T cells cytokines between blood and BAL in stable lung transplant patients compared with control group [56], results also consistent with the current findings. However, both studies showed a failure to suppress CD8+T-cell pro-inflammatory cytokine production, results consistent with the current findings in BB T cells from stable transplant patients. Transplant patients showed a CD4:CD8 inversion in BAL and BB consistent with a previous report [61] in contrast to control subjects who showed a CD4:CD8 inversion only in the BB compartment. The relative increase in CD8 T cells in BB may be due to an increase in proliferation of these cytotoxic cells and/or an increase in migration of these cells via specific Th1 chemokine receptors [62]. The percentage of CD8+ T cells producing IFNγ and TNFα in BB was increased compared with blood and BAL.

Representative dot plots showing IFNγ production by CD8+ and CD8- (CD4+) T cells from blood, BAL and BB in a lung transplant patient are shown in figure 6.

As IL-4 and TGFβ are negative regulators of Th1 inflammatory cytokines [25, 26], the findings of decreased IL-4 and TGFβ in some bronchial intra-epithelial T-cell subsets compared with blood and BAL may help explain these latter findings. Conversely, chronic rejection or OB is associated with an increase in TGF-β production [4], indicating that current immunosuppression protocols may be effective in reducing OB in lung transplant patients via this pathway.

Others have suggested that studies of intragraft immune cells may be more relevant in terms of effecting graft injury than analysis of peripheral circulating cells [63]. All transplant patients in this study had plasma levels of CsA or Tac within their therapeutic range. Our findings therefore suggest that analysis of T-cell cytokine production may provide a more accurate assessment of immunosuppression in the various compartments than systemic drug levels and show that these patients are inadequately immunosuppressed especially in the lung compartment.

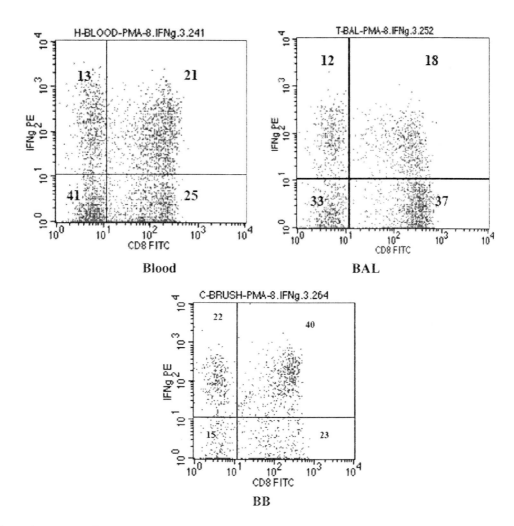

Figure 6. Representative dot plots showing IFNγ production by CD8+ and CD8- (CD4+) T cells from blood, BAL and BB in a lung transplant patient. T cells were identified by CD3 PC5 versus side scatter characteristics. Transplant patients showed an increase in the percentage of CD8+ T cells producing IFNγ in BB compared with blood. Transplant patients showed an increase in IFNγ in both CD4+ and CD8 T cells in BB compared with BAL. Note the decrease in CD4+ and increase in CD8+ T cells in BB compared with blood and BAL.

A longitudinal surveillance of cell phenotypes in individuals has been suggested to identify a preclinical state of rejection [57]. Monitoring intracellular T-cell cytokine profiles may be a more appropriate indicator of patient immunosuppression and transplant status than cell phenotypes. This study demonstrates that it is possible to monitor intracellular cytokines in bronchial intra-epithelial T cells and that there is compartmentalisation of pro-and anti-inflammatory CD8+ T-cell cytokine production in BB compared with blood and BAL. Drugs that effectively reduce bronchial intra-epithelial CD8+ T-cell pro-inflammatory cytokines may improve current protocols for prolonging graft survival in these patients. The clinical relevance of this work is being further pursued with longitudinal follow-up of this patient group as comparison of T-cell cytokine levels between the three compartments may show important changes during rejection episodes.

Airway Infection Is Associated with Decreased Intracellular Th1 Cytokines in Bronchoalveolar Lavage CD8+ T Cells of Stable Lung Transplant Patients

Current immunosuppression protocols to reduce lung transplant rejection include drugs to reduce pro-inflammatory Th1 cytokines. However, Th1 cytokine production is important in host defense against microbial infection in the lungs, particularly *Aspergillus* and *Pseudomonas spp.*, organisms shown to be leading causes of mortality in immunocompromised patients [64, 65] Excessive immunosuppression of these cytokines may leave patients susceptible to infection. To investigate whether infection is associated with reduced Th1 cytokines, whole blood and BAL from a group of 13 lung transplant patients with "culture negative" BAL, and a group of 13 lung transplant patients with "culture positive" BAL were stimulated *in vitro* and cytokine production by T cell subsets studied.

Table 9. Predisposing pathology and organisms isolated from "culture positive" transplant patient group

Patient	Predisposing pathology	Cultured organism	CsA / Tac levels
1	Bronchiecstasis	*Asp. Pseud.*	Tac 14.5
2	Congenital bronchial webbs	*Pseud.*	Tac 11.4
3	Cystic fibrosis	MRSA. *Pseud*	Tac 9
4	Pulmonary hypertension	*Asp. Pseud.*	CsA 276
5	Cystic Fibrosis	*Asp. Pseud.*	CsA 258
6	Emphysema	*Pseud.*	CsA 300
7	Emphysema	*Pseud.*	CsA 260
8	Emphysema	*Pseud.*	Tac 6
9	Pulmonary fibrosis	*Asp.*	CsA 349
10	Pulmonary hypertension	*E. coli*	CsA 152
11	Cystic fibrosis	*Asp.*	CsA 205
12	Emphysema	*Asp.* MRSA	CsA 235
13	Agammaglobulinaemia	*Pseud.*	CsA 185

Therapeutic range for CsA (80-250 µg/L) and Tac (5-20 µg/L).
Asp. (Aspergillus spp.), Pseud. (Pseudomonas spp.), MRSA (Methicillin resistant *Staphylococcus aureus*), *E. coli (Escherichia coli).*

Table 10. The percentage of T-cells producing intracellular cytokines in blood of the 13 BAL culture-negative (N) and 13 culture-positive (P) lung transplant groups (mean ± SD). There were no significant differences in intracellular cytokine production by T-cell subsets between either patient group

	IFNγ			IL-2			IL-4			TNFα		
	CD4	CD8	CD3	CD4	CD8	CD3	CD4	CD8	CD3	CD4	CD8	CD3
N	10±6	24±17	34±12	14±12	6±5	20±9	1.4±1	.9±.6	2±4	20±15	15±10	35±12
P	9±6	16±11	25±8	15±14	2.4±2	17±8	.9±.7	1.4±.1	2±4	15±10	18±16	33±12
P	.965	.265	.348	.935	.284	.728	.765	.785	.820	.690	.560	.889

Table 11. The percentage of T-cells producing intracellular cytokines in BAL of the 13 BAL culture-negative (N) and 13 culture-positive (P) lung transplant groups (mean ± SD) . There was a significant decrease in the percentage of CD3+ T cells producing IL-2 and CD8+ T cells producing TNFα in BAL of the culture-negative compared to the culture-positive transplant group (bold)

	IFNγ			IL-2			IL-4			TNFα		
	CD4	CD8	CD3	CD4	CD8	CD3	CD4	CD8	CD3	CD4	CD8	CD3
N	9±6	22±12	31±9	5±4	5±4	10±4	6±4	11±4	17±4	12±9	15±11	27±9
P	7±6	11±8	18±8	2±2	1.7±1.1	3.7±2	6±2	6±5	12±4	12±8	8±6	20±8
P	.765	.165	.248	.218	.104	**.031**	.898	.157	.657	.890	**.038**	.200

Intracellular Th1/Th2 cytokines in BAL and blood T cells from clinically stable lung transplant patients in whom potentially pathogenic organisms were isolated from BAL were compared with a culture-negative group. The predisposing pathology, cultured organsim and plasma drug levels in these patients is shown in table 9.

We showed that Th1 cytokines were significantly higher in BAL from stable, non-infected transplant recipients compared with culture-positive patients. All transplant patients in this study had plasma levels of CsA or Tac within therapeutic range (table 9). There was no change in T cell cytokines in the blood of infected and non-infected patients (table 10). Importantly the investigations showed that the majority of patients with the greatest degree of immunosuppression, as judged by intracellular Th1 cytokine production in BAL, were infected with pathogenic microorganisms (table 11).

These organisms have been shown to be the leading cause of mortality in immunocompromised patients [64, 65]. In the mouse model, lung challenge with *P. aeriginosa* resulted in significantly less severe lung pathology, bacterial loads and mortality in mice that responded with a Th1-like response [66]. Transient over-expression of IFNγ within the lungs augmented host immunity against *Aspergillus* [64]. Hence excessive suppression of Th1 cytokines may leave patients susceptible to infection. There was no correlation between type of infective organism cultured, predisposing patient pathology and BAL or blood cytokines, although these findings need confirmation in a larger study. Although levels of BAL Th1 cytokines differed between patient groups, there was no difference in Th1 cytokines in blood, suggesting that reduced BAL Th1 cytokines were only associated with localised lung infection and not systemic disease. There has been a report of cytokine modulatory activity of CD4+ splenic T cells in the mouse model by Pseudomonas aeruginosa quorum-sensing signal molecules [67] suggesting that infection with this organism may inhibit the patient's immune response. However, there have been no reports of cytokine modulatory activity of CD8+ T cells or by other organisms isolated from the BAL of these patients other than immunostimulatory, [64, 66, 67] suggesting that the reduced Th1 response by these patients is more likely due to treatment with immunosuppressants.

The data shows that a cut-off value of greater than 8% CD3+ T cells producing IL-2 or 20% CD8+ T cells producing TNFα is associated with culture negative results and hence would be protective of infection in the lungs of these patients. In the ongoing study it would be of interest to investigate whether patients with the lowest levels of these BAL Th1 cytokines have the highest morbidity. Whether reducing immunosuppression in the culture-positive group would improve morbidity and mortality rates also remains to be investigated. Of further interest is whether protection from infection is afforded by subsets of T cells that produce combinations of Th1 cytokines eg., TNFα+IL2. The percentages of BAL T cells producing IL-4, an important Th2 cytokine that negatively regulates Th1 response [25] was unchanged between patient groups in this study, suggesting that the differences in Th1 cytokines observed was not due to altered levels of this regulatory cytokine. Potent immunosuppressive drugs such as tacrolimus and cylclosporin A cause significant toxic side effects [38]. Reducing levels of these drugs in culture-positive patients that have low Th1 cytokines would also have benefits associated with reduced organ toxicity. However, a reduction of immunosuppression due to infection must be balanced with appropriate immunosuppression of proinflammatory Th1 cytokines that have been reportedly increased in the lungs of patients undergoing graft rejection [1-3]. The degree to which transplant recipients are immunosuppressed influences their risk of infection and rejection [68]. The restoration of Th1 responses has been shown to be an important predictor of fungal infection outcome in stem cell transplantation patients [69]. Monitoring the balance of intracellular Th1 cytokines between levels associated with infection and rejection may improve morbidity in our patient group.

In conclusion, this study demonstrates that lung infection is associated with decreased intracellular Th1 cytokines in BAL T cell subsets of stable lung transplant patients. Modifying immunosuppression by monitoring intracellular Th1 cytokines in BAL T cells may improve morbidity and infection rates in this patient group. The clinical relevance of this work is being further pursued with longitudinal follow-up of this group and a much larger patient cohort.

Longitudinal Monitoring of Intracellular T Cell Cytokines in Transplant Patients

Analysis of intracellular T cell cytokines in blood from lung transplant patients and controls showed a broad range of cells producing individual cytokines (figure 1). To determine longitudinal changes in intracellular cytokines/chemokines in patients and controls, whole blood from several stable, non-infected lung transplant patients and control volunteers was stimulated *in vitro* and intracellular T cell cytokine production determined on several occasions over a three year period. Samples from transplant patients were collected following routine surveillance assessment and histology of bronchial biopsies showed no evidence of acute or chronic rejection. All BAL cultures were negative, as were serology for mycoplasma and CMV.

The percentage of T cell subsets producing intracellular cytokines from 5 healthy control (C) volunteers on 3-8 occasions (N) (mean ± SD) are shown in table 12. The SD of cytokines from individual subjects was significantly less compared with the overall SD of cytokines from 14 control subjects (*overall mean ± SD*), suggesting that intracellular T cell cytokines are relatively stable over time from healthy individual subjects.

The percentage of T cell subsets producing intracellular cytokines from 4 stable non-infected transplant patients (P) on 3-4 occasions (mean ± SD) are shown in table 13. The SD of cytokines from individual patients was significantly less compared with the overall SD of cytokines from 12 transplant patients (*12P*) (*overall mean ± SD*), suggesting that intracellular T cell cytokines from individual stable transplant patients are relatively stable over time.

Analysis of intracellular T cell cytokines in BAL and BB from lung transplant patients and controls also showed a broad range of cells producing individual cytokines (table 3 and 4). Intracellular cytokine analyses were performed on one stable, non-infected transplant patient on three occasions and again during one occasion when the patient was undergoing acute rejection as determined by bronchial biopsy histology (A2B0). Results of the intracellular T cell cytokines from blood, BAL and BB from this patient are shown in table 14, 15 and 16 respectively.

Table 12. The percentage of T cell subsets producing intracellular cytokines from 5 healthy control (C) volunteers on 3-8 occasions (N) (mean ± SD). The SD of cytokines from individual subjects was significantly less compared with the overall SD of cytokines from 14 control subjects (*overall mean ± SD*), suggesting that intracellular T cell cytokines are relatively stable over time from healthy individual subjects

	N	CD3		IFNγ		IL-2		IL-4		TGFβ		TNFα	
		CD4	CD8	CD4	CD8	CD4	CD8	CD4	CD8	CD4	CD8	CD4	CD8
C1	8	61±2	39±2	17±2	25±2	38±3	6±1	.6±.1	.4±.1	4±.8	3±1.1	44±4	26±2
C2	4	64±3	36±2	19±2	20±2	36±3	10±1	.4±.1	.6±.1	6±1.9	2±1.2	42±4	22±3
C3	3	58±2	42±2	23±3	15±2	28±2	8±1	.3±.1	.5±.1	3±.1.1	2±1.0	36±2	24±2
C4	5	60±3	40±2	22±2	22±3	25±2	9±2	.5±.1	.3±.1	7±1.2	4±1.4	38±3	18±2
C5	3	56±2	34±2	18±2	24±2	37±3	5±2	.4±.1	.4±.1	4±1.4	5±1.5	50±4	29±2
14C		*62±7*	*37±8*	*19±5*	*21±8*	*36±16*	*8±4*	*0.4±3*	*.5±3*	*5±3*	*3±2*	*43±11*	*24±11*

Table 13. The percentage of T cell subsets producing intracellular cytokines from 4 stable non-infected transplant patients (P) on 3-4 occasions (mean ± SD). The SD of cytokines from individual patients was significantly less compared with the overall SD of cytokines from 12 transplant patients (*12P*) (*overall mean ± SD*), suggesting that intracellular T cell cytokines from individual stable transplant patients are relatively stable over time

	N	CD3		IFNγ		IL-2		IL-4		TGFβ		TNFα	
		CD4	CD8	CD4	CD8	CD4	CD8	CD4	CD8	CD4	CD8	CD4	CD8
P1	4	36±4	64±4	12±3	25±8	8±4	6±2	.6±.2	.9±.2	5±1.5	6±1.2	9±5	9±6
P2	3	53±2	47±2	10±4	23±11	9±5	5±2	.8±.3	.6±.3	6±2.1	5±1.3	11±6	15±7
P3	3	64±3	36±3	9±1	17±5	6±3	3±1	.5±.3	.8±.1	4±1.2	7±1.8	15±4	14±5
P4	3	48±2	42±2	7±2	16±6	25±2	7±2	.5±.1	.7±.3	7±1.9	4±1.1	12±5	18±4
12P		*55±18*	*44±18*	*7±5*	*17±15*	*6±5*	*5±4*	*1±1*	*1±1*	*4.9±2*	*5±2.5*	*12±7*	*14±12*

Table 14. T cell subsets and the percentage of intracellular blood T cell cytokines from a stable transplant patient (S) on three occasions (mean ± SD) and on one occasion during an episode of acute rejection (AR). There was no significant change in CD4+ or CD8+ T cell subsets or cytokine production during the acute rejection episode

	CD3		IFNγ		IL-2		IL-4		TNFα	
	CD4	CD8	CD4	CD8	CD4	CD8	CD4	CD8	CD4	CD8
S	53±2	47±2	12±4	23±8	9±4	3±1	.8±.3	1.1±.2	11±6	15±8
AR	60	40	10	15	2	2	.6	.9	2	2

Table 15. T cell subsets and the percentage of intracellular BAL T cell cytokines from a stable transplant patient (S) on three occasions (mean ± SD) and on one occasion during an episode of acute rejection (AR). There was a significant increase in IFNγ, IL-2 and TNFα by both CD4+ and CD8+ T cell subsets during the acute rejection episode (bold)

	CD3		IFNγ		IL-2		IL-4		TNFα	
	CD4	CD8	CD4	CD8	CD4	CD8	CD4	CD8	CD4	CD8
S	55±8	45±8	5±4	4±3	3±2	1±1	12±.4	12±.7	9±6	5±3
AR	60	40	40	31	17	4	4	6	38	24

Table 16. T cell subsets and the percentage of intracellular BB T cell cytokines from a stable transplant patient (S) on three occasions (mean ± SD) and on one occasion during an episode of acute rejection (AR). There was a significant decrease in CD4:CD8 and a significant increase in IL-2 by CD8+ T cells during the acute rejection episode (bold)

	CD3		IFNγ		IL-2		IL-4		TNFα	
	CD4	CD8	CD4	CD8	CD4	CD8	CD4	CD8	CD4	CD8
S	36±5	64±5	14±6	36±13	5±4	4±2	.3±.3	1.5±1.4	18±4	36±11
AR	20	80	14	50	4	50	.3	1.5	13	54

The results from this study show that during an episode of acute rejection, there was no discernable change in blood T cell subsets or intracellular cytokines. Although plasma levels of CsA and Tac were within therapeutic range, there were significant increases in pro-inflammatory Th1 cytokines in BAL T cells and CD8 T cells and IL-2 production by CD8+ T cells in BB. These results suggest that immunosuppression therapy may be effective in the blood compartment but not in the lungs during an episode of rejection. Whether the drugs are not reaching the lungs or do enter the lungs but are ineffective in reducing pro-inflammatory T cell cytokines remains to be determined. These data suggest that analysis of intracellular cytokines in the lung compartment, particularly in BAL T cells may be an effective, relatively non-invasive technique in the diagnosis of acute rejection episodes in lung transplant patients. Although these are results from one case of acute rejection in one patient and must be viewed with caution, they are nonetheless exciting and it will be of great interest to follow the results of these longitudinal studies on a larger cohort of lung transplant patients. It will also be of interest to observe changes associated with chronic rejection as these have been reported to be associated with moderate increases in pro-inflammatory cytokines and the profibrotic cytokines TGFβ and IL-4 [1-4].

Future of Intracellular Cytokines to Improve Therapeutic Monitoring Following Lung Transplantation

It is clear that no single compartmental approach to intracellular cytokine analysis is sufficient to produce simple valid diagnostic or prognostic data at every stage during rejection of lung transplant. Results of intracellular cytokine analysis of multiple immune cell subsets within the blood may provide physiological evidence of systemic levels of immunosuppression that may be more relevant than drug plasma levels. Using these techniques, identification of specific cell subsets producing cytokines/chemokines associated with graft rejection may allow targeting of these subsets or mediators to improve the morbidity of these patients. However, direct examination of biopsy tissue still provides the "gold-standard" measure of allograft rejection, it is likely that analysis of intracellular cytokine expression within or immediately adjacent to the graft (BAL) will be of diagnostic and prognostic value. Longitudinal monitoring of cytokines in both BAL and blood in individual patients may offer early signs of episodes associated with infection (and possibly rejection). Maintaining intracellular cytokines within stable (non-infection, non-rejection) levels by regulating doses of immunosuppression drugs may lead to less adverse drug toxicity. Targeting local perturbations in pro-inflammatory cytokines/chemokines within the lung compartment may also further reduce systemic effects of therapeutics and reduce morbidity in this patient group.

Although the potential role of monitoring immunosuppression using intracellular cytokines as opposed the pharmacokinetic dose is very promising, further research is required before it is likely to become of practical value in clinical lung transplantation.

References

[1] Boehler A and Estenne M. Post-transplant bronchiolitis obliterans. *Eur. Respir. Mon,* 2003, 26, 158-178.

[2] Sundaresan S, Alevy YG, Steward N, Tucker J, Trulock EP, Cooper JD, Patterson GA, Mohanakumar T. Cytokine gene transcripts for tumor necrosis factor-alpha, interleukin-2, and interferon-gamma in human pulmonary allografts. *J. Heart Lung. Transplant.* 1995 14(3):512-8.

[3] Neuringer IP, Walsh SP, Mannon RB, Gabriel S, Aris RM. Enhanced T cell cytokine gene expression in mouse airway obliterative bronchiolitis. *Transplantation.* 2000 69(3):399-405.

[4] El-Gamel A, Sim E, Hasleton P, Hutchinson J, Yonan N, Egan J, Campbell C,Rahman A, Sheldon S,Deiraniya A, Hutchinson RV. Transforming growth factor beta (TGF-beta) and obliterative bronchiolitis following pulmonary transplantation. *J. Heart Lung Transplant.* 1999 18(9):828-37.

[5] Duncan MD, Wilkes SD. Transplant-related immunosuppression. *Proc. Am. Thor. Soc.* 2005 2:449-455.

[6] Haberal M, Emiroglou R, Dalgic A, Karakayli H, Moray G, Bilgin N. The impact of cyclosporin on the development of immunosuppressive therapy. *Tranplant. Proc.* 2004 36:143S-147S.

[7] Norman D, Turka L. Pimer on transplantation, 2nd ed. Mt. Laurel, NJ: American Society of Transplantation. 2001.

[8] Baan CC, Balk AH, van Riemsdijk IC, Vantrimpont PJ, Maat AP, Niesters HG, Zondervan PE, van Gelder T, Weimar W. Anti-CD25 monoclonal antibody therapy affects the death signals of graft-infiltrating cells after clinical heart transplantation. *Transplantation.* 2003 75:1704-1710.

[9] Levy GA. C2 monitoring strategy for optimising cyclosporin immunosuppression from the Neoral formulation. *BioDrugs.* 2001 15:279-290.

[10] Hodge G, Hodge S, Reynolds P, Holmes M. Intracellular cytokines in blood T cells in lung transplant patients- a more relevant indicator of immunosuppression than drug levels. *Clin. and Exp. Immunol.* 2005 139, 159-164.

[11] Jordan SC, Kondo T, Prehn J, Marchevsky A, Waters P. Cytokine gene activation in rat lung allografts: analysis by Northern blotting. *Transplant. Proc.* 1991 23:604-606.

[12] Rondeau E, Cerrina J, Delarue F et al. Tumor necrosis alpha (TNF-alpha) production by cells of bronchiolar lavage (BAL) and peripheral blood mononuclear cells (PBMC) in cardiopulmonary transplant patients. *Transplant. Proc.* 1990 22:1855-1856.

[13] Sundaresan S, Alevy YG, Steward N, Tucker J, Trulock EP, Cooper jd, Patterson GA, Mohanakumar T. Cytokine gene transcripts for tumor necrosis factor-alpha, interleukin-2, and interferon-gamma in human pulmonary allografts. *J. Heart Lung Transplant.* 1995 14(3):512-8.

[14] Hodge G, Hodge S, Haslam R, McPhee A, Sepulveda H, Morgan E, Nicholson I, Zola H. Rapid detection of neonatal sepsis by simultaneous measurement of multiple cytokines using 100μL sample volumes. *Clin. and Exp. Immunol.* 2004 137: 402-407.

[15] Hodge G, Osborn M, Hodge S, Nairn J, Tapp H, Kirby M, Sepulveda H, Morgan E, Zola H, Revesz T. Rapid simultaneous measurement of multiple cytokines in childhood oncology patients with febrile neutropenia: increased IL-8 or IL-5 correlates with culture-positive infection. *Brit. J. Haem.* 2005 132, 247-248.

[16] Corti A, Poiesci C, Merli S, Cassani G. Tumour necrosis factor (TNF) alpha quantification by ELISA and bioassay: effects of TNF alpha-soluble TNF receptor (p55) complex dissociation during assay incubations. *J. Immunol. Methods.* 1994 177:191-198.

[17] Muirhead KA, Wallace PK, Schmidt TC, Frescatore RL, Franco JA, Horan PK: Methodological considerations for implementation of lymphocyte subset analysis in a clinical reference laboratory. *Ann. NY Acad. Sci.* 1986 468:113-127.

[18] Hodge G, Hodge S, Han P. Increased levels of apoptosis of leucocyte subsets in PBMCs compared to whole blood as shown by Annexin V binding- relevance to cytokine production. *Cytokine.* 2000 12, 1763-1768.

[19] Heeger PS, Grenspan NS, Kuhlenschmidt S, Dejelo C, Hricik DE, Schulak JA, Tary-Lehmann M. Pretransplant frequency of donor-specific, IFNgamma-producing lymphocytes is a manifestation of immunologic memory and correlates with the risk of posttransplant rejection episodes. *J. Immunol.* 1999 163:2267-2275.

[20] Sharrock CE, Kaminski E, Man S. Limiting dilutional analysis of human T cells: a useful clinical tool. *Immunol. Today.* 1990 11:281-286. 1990

[21] Han and G. Hodge (1999) Intracellular cytokine production and cytokine receptor interaction of cord mononuclear cells: relevance to cord blood transplantation. *British Journal of Haematology.* 107, 450-457.

[22] Hodge G, Hodge S, Han, P. Allium sativum (Garlic) suppresses leucocyte inflammatory cytokine production in vitro: potential therapeutic use in the treatment of inflammatory bowel disease. *Cytometry.* 2002 48, 209-215.

[23] Lehman C, Wilkening A, Lieber N, Markus R, Krug N, Pabst R, Tschernig T. Lymphocytes in the bronchiolar space reenter the lung tissue by means of the alveolar epithelium, migrate to regional lymph nodes, and subsequently rejoin the systemic immune system. *Anat. Rec.* 2001 264:229-236.

[24] Stadler M, Birsan T, Holme B, Haririfar M, Scandling J, Morris R. Quantification of immunosuppression by flow cytometry in stable renal transplant patients. *Therap. Drug. Monit.* 2003 22:22-7.

[25] Romagnani S. The Th1 / Th2 paradigm. *Immunology Today.* 1997; 18: 263-6.

[26] Kehrl JH Transforming growth factor-β: An important mediator of immunoregulation. *Int. J. Cell Clon.* 1991 9:438-50.

[27] Chan SY, Goodman RE, Szmuszkovicz JR, Roessler B, Eichwald EJ, Bishop DK. DNA-liposome versus adenoviral mediated gene transfer of TGF beta1 in vascularised cardiac allografts: differential sensitivity of CD4+ and CD8+ T cells to TGF beta1. *Transplantation.* 2000 70:1292-301.

[28] Hodge S, Hodge G, Flower R, Han P. Methyl prednisolone upregulates monocyte IL-10 production in stimulated whole blood. *Scand. J. Immunol.* 1999 49:548-553.

[29] Andersson J, Nagy S, Groth CG, Andersson U. Effects of FK506 and cyclospotin A on cytokine production studied in vitro at a single-cell level. *Immunol.* 1992 75:136-42.

[30] Snijdewint FG, Kapsenberg ML, Warben-Penris PJ, Bos JD. Corticosteroids class-dependently inhibited in vitro Th1 and Th2-type cytokine production. *Immunopharm.* 1995; 29(2): 93-101.

[31] Berthou C, Legros-Maida S, Soulie A, Wargnier A, Guillet J, Lafaurie C, Stern M, Sasportes M, Israel-Biet D. Expansion of peripheral blood perforin+ CD8+ T-cell subset in long term survival lung transplant patients. *Transplant. Proc.* 1996; 28(3):1964-7.

[32] Lee HM and Rich S. Differential activation of $CD8^+$ T-cells by transforming-β. *J. Immunol.* 1993; 151:668-677.

[33] Widmer MB and Grabstein KH. Regulation of cytolytic T-lymphocyte generation by B-cell stimulatory factor. *Nature.* 1987; 326:795-98.

[34] Hu H, Dong Y, Feng P, Fechner J, Hamawy M, Knechtle SJ. Effect of immunosuppressants on T-cell subsets observed in vivo using carboxy-fluorescein diacetate succinimidyl ester labelling. *Transplant.* 2003; 75(7):1075-7.

[35] Sempowski M, Sakiyama S, Tanida N, Fukumoto T, Monden Y, Uyama T. Interleukin-4 and interferon-gamma discordantly regulate collagen biosynthesis by functionally distinct lung fibroblast subsets. *J. Cell Physiol.* 1996; 167(2):290-6.

[36] El-Gamel A, Awad M, Sim E, Hasleton P, Yonan N, Egan J *et al*. Transforming growth factor beta (TGF-beta) and obliterative bronchiolitis following pulmonary transplantation. *Eur. J. Cardiothorac. Surg.* 1998; 13(4):424-30.

[37] Kuypers DR, Claes K, Evenpoel P, Maes B, Vanrenterghem Y. Clinical efficacy and toxicity profile of tacrolimus and mycophenolic acid in relation to combined long-term phermacokinetics in de novo renal allograft recipients. *Clin. Pharmacol. Ther.* 2004, 75:434-47.

[38] Shapiro R. Low toxicity immunosuppressive protocols in renal transplantation. *Keio J. Med.* 2004; 53:18-22.

[39] Taub DD, Proost P, Murphy WJ, et al. Monocoyte chemotactic protein-1 (MCP-1), -2, and –3 are chemotactic for human T lymphocytes. *J. Clin. Invet.* 1995; 95: 1370.

[40] Reynaud-Gaubert M, Marvin V, Thirion X, et al. Upregulation of chemokines in bronchiolar lavage fluid as a predictor of post-transplant airway obliteration. *J. Heart Lung Transplant.* 2002; 21: 721.

[41] Belperio JA, Keane MP, Burdick MD, et al. Critical role for the chemokine MCP-1/CCR2 in the pathogenesis of bronchiolitis obliterans syndrome. *J. Clin. Invet.* 2001; 108: 547.

[42] Hodge G, Hodge S, Reynolds P, Holmes M. Upregulation of IL-8, IL-10, MCP-1 and MCP-3 in peripheral blood monocytes in stable lung transplant patients- are immunosuppression regimes working? *Transplantation.* 2004 79:387-391.

[43] Ong VH, Evans LA, Shiwen X, et al. Monocyte chemoattractant protein 3 as a mediator of fibrosis: Overexpression in systemic sclerosis and the type 1 tight-skin mouse. *Arthritis Rheum.* 2003; 48:1979.

[44] Franci C, Wong LM, van Damme J, Proost P, Charo F. Monocyte chemotactic protein-3, but not monocyte chemotactic protein-2 is a functional ligand of the monocyte chemoattractant protein-1 receptor. *J. Immunol.* 1995; 154: 6511.

[45] Boehler A. The role of interleukin-10 in lung transplantation. *Transpl. Immunol.* 2002; 9: 121.

[46] Gonnella PA, Kondali D, Weiner HL. Induction of low dose tolerance in monocyte chemotactic protein-1 and CCR2 deficient mice. *J. Immunol.* 2003; 170: 2316.

[47] Rose CE, Sund SS, Fu SM. Significant involvement of CCL2 (MCP-1) in inflammatory dissorders of the lung. *Microcirculation.* 2003; 10: 273.

[48] Tsiavou A, Degiannis D, Hatzigelaki E, Raptis S. Flow cytometric detection of intracellular IL-12 release: in vitro effect of widely used immunosuppressants. *Int. Pharmacol.* 2002; 12: 1713.

[49] Kitayama T, Hayamizu K, Egi H, Ohmori I, Yoshimitsu M, Asahara T. Facilitation of tracolimus-induced heart-allograft acceptibility by pretransplant host treatment with granulocyte colony-stimulating factor: interleukin-12-restricted suppression of intragraft monokine mRNA expression. *Transplantation.* 2003; 75: 553.

[50] Brach MA, Gruss HJ, Riedel D, Asano Y, De Vos S, Herrmann F. Effect of antiinflammatory agents on synthesis of MCP-1/JE transcripts by human blood monocytes. *Mol. Pharmacol.* 1992; 42: 63.

[51] Wong PK, Cuello C, Bertouch JV, et al. Effects of pulse methylprednisolone on macrophage chemotactic protein-1 and macrophage inflammatory protein-1alpha in rheumatoid synovium. *J. Rheumatol.* 2001; 28: 2634.

[52] Slebos DJ, Schloma J, Boezen HM, Koeter GH, van der Bij W, Postma DS, Kauffman HF. Longitudinal profile of bronchoalveolar lavage cell characteristics in patients with good outcome after lung transplantation. *Am. J. Crit. Care Med.* 2002 165(4):501-7.

[53] Reynard-Gaubert M, Thomas P, Gregoire R, Badier M, Cau P, Sampol J, Giudicelli R, Fuentes P. Clinical utility of bronchoalveolar lavage cell phenotype analyses in the postoperative monitoring of lung transplant recipients. *Eur. J. Cardiothorac. Surg.* 2002 21:60-66.

[54] Chang S, Hsu H, Perng R, Shiao G, Lin C. Significance of biochemical markers in early detection of canine allograft rejection. *Transplantation.* 1991 51:579-584.

[55] Tayebi H, Lienard A, Billot M, Tiberghien P, Herve P, Robinet E. Detection of intracellular cytokines in citrated whole blood or marrow samples by flow cytometry. *J. Immunol. Methods.* 1999 229:121-30.

[56] Hodge G, Hodge S, Reynolds P, Holmes M. Increased intracellular pro- and anti-inflammatory cytokines in bronchoalveolar lavage T cells of stable lung transplant patients. *Transplantation.* 2005 80:1040-1045.

[57] Slebos DJ, Schloma J, Boezen HM, Koeter GH, van der Bij W, Postma DS, Kauffman HF. Longitudinal profile of bronchoalveolar lavage cell characteristics in patients with good outcome after lung transplantation. *Am. J. Crit. Care Med.* 2002 165(4):501-7.

[58] Scott LJ, McKeage K, Keam SJ, Plosker G. Tacrolimus: a further update of its use in the management of organ tranplantation. *Drugs.* 2003 63(12):1247-97.

[59] Keenan RJ, Zeevi A, Iacono AT, Spichty KJ, Cai JZ, Yousem SA, Ohori NP, Paradis IL, Kawai A, Griffith BP. Efficacy of inhaled cyclosporin in lung transplant recipients with refactory rejection: correlation of intragraft cytokine gene expression with pulmonary function and histologic characteristics. *Surgery.* 1995 118(2):385-91.

[60] Hodge G, Hodge S, Reynolds P, Holmes M. Compartmentalisation of intracellular proinflammatory cytokines in bronchial intraepithelial T cells of stable lung transplant patients. *Clin. and Exp. Immunol.* 2006 145:413-419.

[61] Erle DJ, Brown T, Christian D, Aris R. Lung epithelial lining fluid T cell substes defined by distinct patterns of beta 7 and beta 1 integrin expression. *Am. J. Respir. Cell. Mol. Biol.* 1994; 10: 237-44.

[62] Neuringer IP, Chalermskulrat W, Aris R. Obliterative bronchiolitis or chronic lung allograft rejection: a basic science review. *J. Heart Lung Transplant.* 2005; 24:3-19.

[63] Corris PA and Kirby JA. A role for cytokine measurement in therapeatic monitoring of immunosuppressive drugs following lung transplantation. *Cin. Exp. Imunnol.* 2004; 139:176-178.

[64] Shao C, Qu J, He L et al. Transient expression of γ interferon promotes *Aspergillus* clearance in invasive pulmonary aspergillosis. *Clin. Exp. Immunol.* 2005; 142: 233.

[65] Zuercher AW, Imboden MA, Jampen S et al. Cellular immunity in healthy volunteers treated with an octavalent conjugate *Pseudomonas aeruginosa* vaccine. *Clin. Exp. Immunol.* 2005; 142: 381.

[66] Moser C, Johansen HK, Song Z et al. Chronic *Pseudomonas aeruginosa* lung infection is more severe in Th2 responding BALB/c mice compared to Th1 responding C3H/HeN mice. *APMIS.* 1997; 105: 838.

[67] Ritchie AJ, Jansson A, Stallberg J, Nilsson P, Lysaght P, Cooley MA. The *Pseudomonas aeruginosa* quorum-swensing molecule N-3-(oxododecanoyl)-L-homoserine lactone inhibits T-cell differentiation and cytokine production by a mechanism involving an early step in T-cell activation. *Infect. Immun.* 2005; 73(3):1648.

[68] Blazik M, Hutchinson P, Jose MD, et al. Leucocyte phenotype and function predicts infection risk in renal transplant recipients. *Nephrol. Dial Transplant.* 2005; 20(10): 2226.

[69] Safdar A, Rodriguez G, Ohmagari N, et al. The safety of interferon-gamma-1b therapy for invasive fungal infections after haemopoietic stem cell transplantation. *Cancer.* 2005; 103(4): 731.

In: Transplantation Immunology Research Trends   ISBN: 978-1-60021-578-0
Editor: Oliver N. Ulricker, pp. 147-158   © 2007 Nova Science Publishers, Inc.

Chapter V

Polyoma BK Virus Nephropathy in Renal Transplant Recipients

Henkie P. Tan, *Zebulon Z. Spector, Parmjeet Randhawa,*
Abhay Vats, Amit Basu, Amadeo Marcos and Ron Shapiro
Thomas E. Starzl Transplantation Institute;
University of Pittsburgh Medical Center; Pittsburgh, PA USA

I. BK Virus History and Characteristics

Polyomavirus (BK virus, BKV) is currently the leading cause of viral infection in the allograft of renal transplant patients. BKV was first described in 1971 by Gardner et al. in a Sudanese renal graft recipient with ureteric stricture [1]. However, the first case of BKV nephropathy (BKVN) was diagnosed by a needle biopsy in 1993 at the University of Pittsburgh [2]. The delay from first viral description to first reported case of BKVN may be attributed to the change from less potent immunosuppressive agents, such as azathiorine (AZA) and the original formulation of cyclosporine (CyA), to more potent agents such as mycophenolate mofetil (MMF), microemulsion cyclosporine, and tacrolimus (TAC) [3,4].

BKV is a non-encapsulated, icosahedral virus with a circular 5,300 base pair genome made up of double-stranded DNA. The genome contains a non-coding region, which contains the origin of replication and an enhancer region; an early-coding region, which codes for small tumor antigen (tAg) and large tumor antigen (TAg); and a late coding region, which codes for capsid proteins VP1, VP2, VP3, and for agnoprotein. TAg and tAg are thought to bind to and stabilize the tumor suppressor proteins p53 and retinoblastoma (Rb) [4, 5]. This interaction disrupts normal protein function and prevents their ubiquination and degradation, causing aggregation of p53 within cells, promoting cell entry into the cell cycle and possibly rendering cells immortal [6].

---

* Contact Author: Henkie P Tan, MD, PhD, FACS; Thomas E. Starzl Transplantation Institute; University of Pittsburgh Medical Center; Tel: 412-692-4552; Email: tanhp@upmc.edu; MUH N758, UPMC; 3459 5th Ave, Pittsburgh, PA 15213

VP1 is involved in heterogeneity among various subtypes of BKV, specifically genotypes I, II, III, and IV. It is also the protein involved with binding and entry into host cells. VP1 is thought to bind to N-linked glycoproteins on the surface of host cells, from where the virus is endocytosed by non-clathrin-coated vesicles. After endocytosis, it interacts with the endoplasmic reticulum and microtubules, before gaining entry into the cell's nucleus. VP2 and VP3 are thought to be involved with virus transport across the nuclear membrane [5]. In the nucleus, BKV DNA may incorporate into host cell DNA [7]. Agnoprotein is thought to be involved in cell cycle progression, capsid assembly, and virion release [5]. BKV is in the same family as JC virus and simian virus SV40. The BKV genome shares approximately 72% homology with JC virus, and both share about 70% homology with SV40 [4,8].

II. Epidemiology

BKV is latent in the general population, existing asymptomatically in nearly all children and up to 90% of adults [4,5]. In the renal transplant population, 10-60% of patients are reported to have BKV viruria, and approximately 45% of patients are seropositive for BKV [5,8]. Studies report anywhere from 1-9% prevalence of actual symptomatic BKVN among renal transplant patients, with an increase to 7-34% when renal allograft donors are seropositive for BKV [4, 8-12]. Of these symptomatic BKVN patients, 35-67% reportedly loses their kidney graft within one year [9]. Gupta and colleagues compared the incidence of BKVN among kidney-alone transplants and simultaneous pancreas kidney transplant (SPK) patients. In 1,492 kidney-alone transplants, they found an incidence of BKVN of 2.5%, whereas among 243 SPK patients, they found an incidence of 2.9%. Other studies have shown higher rates of BKVN among SPK patients (6.2-7.5%), closer to the higher end of the reported spectrum for kidney transplant patients [13-15].

Nolte reported on the cost benefit of screening for BKVN in the renal transplant population [10]. To periodically test for viral load, it cost $1,640 per patient and $120,000 to retransplant a lost kidney graft. The authors estimated that viral load testing prevented loss of four allografts per year, and assumed that all patients who lost their original grafts were retransplanted. With these estimates and assumptions, they calculated a cost benefit of $760 per patient of periodic viral load testing. If the incidence of BKVN in a renal transplantation program was greater than 2.1%, then periodic screening for BKV was cost effective.

III. Risk Factors

Certain factors are suspected of increasing a renal transplant recipient's chance of acquiring BKVN. These factors include number of HLA mismatches, donor seropositivity and recipient seronegativity for the virus, degree of immunosuppression, age, sex, race, length of cold ischemia time, presence of delay graft function, coinfection with CMV, and other causes of renal tubular injury, such as acute rejection [3-5, 8, 11, 16-19]. While studies have shown some of the above factors to significantly affect risk of BKVN, other factors have had a poorer association with BKVN risk. Still other factors have been shown to be associated with a higher rate of failure of BKV clearance from the allograft—donor source of virus, interstitial fibrosis, proportion of tubules infected with BKV, and plasma viral load above a certain threshold [17]. Randhawa and Brennan have noted that among all possible risk factors, immunosuppression is the most modifiable, and thus an appropriate target for current study [5].

Awadalla et al. examined the nature and extent of HLA mismatch between donor and recipient as a risk factor for BKVN [16]. They examined HLA-A, B, and DR mismatch in 444 kidney transplant patients, 40 of whom suffered from BKVN post-transplant. All patients were treated with TAC, and 67% of patients were additionally treated with MMF. They found that by univariate analysis, an increased incidence of BKVN was associated with HLA-B, DR mismatch and with combined HLA-A, B, and DR mismatch (p=0.001). By multivariate analysis, they found that 3 or more HLA-A, B, and DR mismatches were associated with increased risk of BKVN—3 to 4 mismatches was associated with an odds ratio of 4.6 and 5 to 6 mismatches with an odds ratio of 7.6 (p=0.02). No specific allele was found to be associated with BKVN risk, however. Similar to the above study, Bohl et al. found no association between specific HLA alleles and risk of BKVN [19]. However, in contrast to the above study, they also found no significant association between number of HLA mismatches and risk of BKVN. In the Bohl study, donor origin was most closely associated with risk of BKVN—recipients receiving grafts from the same donor showed similar rates of infection (p=0.017), and of note, absence of HLA-C7 in both donors and recipients was associated with sustained BKV viremia.

Rocha et al. examined co-occurrence of BKVN and acute rejection in a series of 286 patients, and looked for any factors associated with increased risk of BKVN [11]. Acute rejection was thought to lead to ongoing cellular division as the renal tubules were taxed by cell injury and repair. Associated with this cell proliferation is a simultaneous proliferation of BKV. With an increase in immunosuppression in response to acute rejection, the patient's immune system is less able to fight the BKV, and BKVN can develop. However, the authors diagnosed BKVN in only 3.1% and acute rejection in 62% of the study population. Moreover, none of the patients with BKVN were diagnosed with comorbid acute rejection. The mean trough TAC level in patients with BKVN was 11.7 ± 0.5 ng/ml, and in patients with acute rejection, it was 6.5 ± 0.6 ng/ml (p<0.001). Interestingly, authors found that there was an increased incidence of BKVN in Caucasians (p=0.05) and in males (p=0.04). The cold ischemia time and incidence of delayed graft function were found to be similar between patients who acquired BKVN and those who remained free of the disease. Of note, TAC was decreased to 5 ng/ml and MMF decreased or eliminated from immunosuppression regimen in all patients diagnosed with BKVN. At 2-year follow-up, 89% of BKVN patients had functioning grafts.

Brennan et al. compared TAC, CyA, AZA, and MMF as risk factors for BKVN in renal transplant patients [3]. While none of the 200 patients progressed to BKVN, 70 patients were found to have BK viruria by PCR. Those with a urine viral level greater than 7.0 $\log_{10}$ copies/ml were found to be at a 3-fold higher risk to proceed to viremia. None of the four drugs were found to individually increase the risk of BKV viruria. Interestingly, combined regimens of either TAC with MMF (p=0.002) or CyA with AZA (p=0.038) were found to significantly raise the risk of viruria when compared to TAC with AZA and CyA with MMF regimens. In a separate study, Nickeleit [4] reported a 10-13% increase in risk of BKVN in renal transplant patients maintained at TAC trough levels greater than 8 ng/ml and with high doses of MMF.

In addition to certain factors increasing the risk of acquiring BKVN, other factors have been studied that affect likelihood of clearing the virus once diagnosed. Wadei et al. followed 55 renal transplant patients with BKVN for 20 ± 11 months [17]. Patients were treated with low dose cidofovir, IVIG, conversion to CyA, or some combination of these therapies. Of a number of possible risk factors examined, only a combined interstitial fibrosis and tubular atrophy score greater than 2 on diagnostic biopsy predicted graft functional decline (p=0.05). Failure of viral clearance was significantly associated with the above combined fibrosis/atrophy score (odds ratio = 8.2), deceased donor source of graft (odds ratio = 8.25), more than 5% of renal tubules positive for BKV on diagnostic biopsy (odds ratio = 5.4), viral load greater than 150,000 copies/ml at diagnosis (odds ratio = 18.0), and diagnosis by non-surveillance biopsy (odds ratio = 4.48) [17]. Male gender was an adverse prognostic factor for viral clearance, with an odds ratio of 0.24 (p=0.03) of not clearing the virus once diagnosed with BKVN.

While the focus of most studies of BKVN is in renal transplant recipients, some interest has been shown and occasional cases published regarding risk of BKVN in native kidneys following transplant of an extrarenal organ. Schwarz and colleagues reported one case of BKVN in a native kidney 15 months after lung transplantation [18]. The patient was maintained on a regimen of TAC and MMF, along with steroids following several rejection episodes. The patient had also earlier been treated with cisplatin for metastatic seminoma, and the authors theorized that the cisplatin may have led to renal damage prior to the onset of BKVN, perhaps predisposing the patient. The patient was treated with three doses of 2-3 mg/kg cidofovir and leflunomide, and a marked decrease in serum and urine viral load was observed. Unfortunately, multiple further rejection episodes led to further steroid use and a subsequent rise in the viral load.

IV. Clinical Picture

The clinical picture of BKVN encompasses clinical and laboratory presentation, histological and pathologic features and staging of disease, immunological changes associated with disease, and possible sequelae. Primary infection with BKV occurs early in life, and is associated with upper respiratory tract infection or flu-like symptoms [4]. The highest rates of infection may be found in those between one and six years old, and a possible fecal-oral route for virus transmission is suggested [5,8]. During an ensuing period of increased serum viral load, the virus spreads to and becomes latent in typical cell types, especially in the kidney and urinary tract, reproductive tract, and possibly peripheral mononuclear cells. Reactivation of the virus generally only occurs in conditions of decreased immune response, such as old age, diabetes, HIV infection, and with potent immunosuppression regimens following organ transplantation [5]. This secondary infection is

BKVN, and generally occurs within the first few months following transplant although later onset has also been reported.

BKVN often presents without major clinical symptoms, usually without fever, and the presenting sign is frequently a rising serum creatinine [8,10]. Celik and Randhawa reported serum creatinine levels of 4.3 ± 2.9 mg/dL 73.5 weeks following the diagnosis of BKVN [20]. Microscopic examination of the urine will reveal "decoy cells"—cells with enlarged nuclei and basophilic "ground glass" nuclear inclusion bodies typical of disease [21]. Kwak and colleagues [8] point out that decoy cells can often be mistaken for the byproduct of CMV or adenovirus infection, and the differential diagnosis must include these viral infections, in addition to HSV infection, acute rejection, drug toxicity, or possibly malignancy. Randhawa, in a series of 22 BKVN patients, showed the viral infection to mimic acute rejection in 19 patients, chronic rejection in two patients, and drug toxicity in one patient [21].

BKVN is a focal disease of the renal tubular epithelium, more often in the renal medulla than in the cortex, and histologically is characterized by intranuclear inclusions in tubular epithelial cells and epithelial cell injury, sometimes leading to sloughing of epithelial cells from an intact basement membrane. In rare cases, tubular rupture and granulomatous disease has been seen [4]. Unlike CMV, no cytoplasmic inclusion bodies have been reported in BKVN [8]. Biopsy of the renal medulla is the gold standard for diagnosis of BKVN, with demonstration of cytopathology, and demonstrated intranuclear viral inclusions with immunohistochemical staining BKV or SV40 TAg [10]. Because of the focal nature of the disease, Nickeleit et al. suggest examination of at least two biopsy cores, including both the cortex and the medulla for proper diagnosis and monitoring of BKVN [4]. Randhawa [22] found that 58/115 renal transplant patients with measured BKV viruria failed to yield biopsy confirmation of (mainly) the renal cortex alone. Celik and Randhawa [20] described histological changes observed in 124 biopsies in 83 patients diagnosed with BKVN. More common features included ischemic glomerulopathy in 62% and mild chronic transplant glomerulopathy in 62% of biopsies. Less common features included viral cytopathology seen in the parietal Bowman's capsule epithelium in 17% of biopsies, with immunohistochemical staining revealing this feature in an additional 12% of biopsies. Increased mesangial matrix was seen in 23% of biopsies. Aneurysmal dilatation of glomerular capillaries was seen in 28% of biopsies. Some isolated crescents were observed in infected glomeruli, without rapidly progressive glomerulonephritis.

The clinical course of BKVN is divided into three stages. Stage A involves mild cytopathology and low to non-existent inflammatory infiltrate or interstitial fibrosis. Stage B involves mild to moderate cytopathology and marked inflammatory infiltrate with mild fibrosis. Stage C involves marked atrophy of renal tubules and significant interstitial fibrosis with less histologically observable cytopathology and variable levels of inflammatory infiltrate [5]. Stage A and B carry a better prognosis and are potentially reversible. However, damage in stage C BKVN is typically irreversible and carries a poor prognosis [4].

With regard to the immune response, Randhawa et al. at the University of Pittsburgh [23] demonstrated in a study of six healthy blood donors and seven kidney transplant recipients that CD8+ T-cells target BKV TAg protein. They further postulate that cytotoxic T-cells specific to this early viral protein circulate in healthy individuals with latent BKV. This allows for maintenance of a population of CD8+ T-memory cells specific to BKV in the serum of individuals unaffected by the latent virus. In a second study [24], Randhawa et al. examined the response of IgA, IgG, and IgM to BKV in renal transplants. They found a positive correlation between urine viral load and IgM titer, and a negative correlation between urine viral load and IgG and IgA titer. IgG was found to be elevated in donors and recipients. IgA levels were found elevated in 72-81% of patients who were positive for BKV DNA, and in 0-24% of those found to be negative for BKV DNA (p<0.001).

Various algorithms have been proposed for monitoring and diagnosis of BKVN [5,25,26]. Randhawa et al. proposed that in renal transplant patients, an unexplained rise in serum creatinine concentration should lead to PCR for BKV DNA to establish the true viral load and to distinguish between BKV and other polyomavirus strains [5]. They note that definitive diagnosis is made only by biopsy, with confirmation by immunohistochemistry and *in situ* hybridization. Gupta et al. reported their algorithm for BKV monitoring [25]. They developed real-time PCR (rtPCR) for BKV DNA in the late 1990's, and note that it has been clinically available since 2001. They suggested that all renal transplant patients with a renal biopsy and urine PCR positive for BKV DNA or suspicious by light microscopy should have their biopsy stained with anti-polyoma virus Ab's. A positive stain should lead to routine blood and urine PCR follow-up monitoring. Patients with a urine viral load and altered renal function should also receive routine blood and urine PCR testing. Finally, routine blood PCR screening should be performed in patients with a urine viral load greater than 10,000,000 copies/ml [25].

Aside from the typical presentation and ramifications of BKVN, some authors have investigated the association between BKV and renal cell/bladder carcinoma in immunocompetent individuals and in renal transplant patients as a sequelae to BKVN and have sought to uncover an underlying mechanism for oncogenesis by BKV [6,7,27]. Weinreb et al. followed a series of 3,782 immunocompetent patients, 133 of whom were found to have polyomavirus infected cells by urine cytology analysis. They found that the odds ratio of bladder carcinoma in the group with infected cells was 4.8 when compared to the uninfected group (p<0.001) [27]. In a separate study [6], they examined the role of p53 in renal cells infected with BKV as a possible cause of oncogenesis. Biopsy prior to BKV infection showed no expression of TAg or p53. However, following diagnosis of BKVN, anti-p53 staining was found in biopsy cells shown to be associated with BKV by nuclear staining with anti-SV40 TAg Ab. The authors theorized that TAg binding to p53 disrupts the function of the tumor suppressor gene. At the same time TAg protects p53 from ubiquination, thus avoiding degradation and allowing build-up of p53 within the cell to be detected by staining of the biopsy. Oncogenesis could then be related to survival of abnormal cells that have avoided apoptosis pathways.

V. Treatment

Treatment regimens for BKVN are controversial, and as of yet there is no definitive treatment for this complication. At this time, the standard of care is to decrease immunosuppression. However, not all studies have demonstrated improved outcomes associated with decreasing immunosuppression [3,5,17,28]. Studies have also examined the use of intravenous immunoglobulin (IVIG) [12, 17], cidofovir with and without probenecid [25, 28-30], leflunomide [9, 30], and interferon (IFN)-gamma [31], with varied results. It has further been argued (and is almost certainly true) that prevention is the best form of treatment in BKVN [3,5].

Brennan et al. in their study of 200 renal transplant patients on either TAC or CyA combined with MMF or AZA described a 35% rate of BKV viruria and 11.5% rate of BKV viremia by one year post-transplantation [3]. In patients in whom BKV viremia was detected, MMF or AZA were initially discontinued. If viremia persisted after four weeks, TAC dose was reduced to approximately 3-5 ng/ml, and the CyA dose was reduced to 100-200 ng/ml. Following this reduction in immunosuppression, BKV was eliminated from serum in 95% of affected patients. No allograft dysfunction or loss was observed, and no cases of BKVN occurred, supporting a strategy of preemptive reduction in immunosuppression based on monitoring for viruria/viremia.

IVIG has previously been used in the treatment of both acute rejection and viral infection in transplant patients, and thus if shown to be successful in the treatment of BKVN, could obviate some of the danger imposed by the immunosuppression-based balance between graft rejection and spread of viral illness. Sener et al. examined the use of 2g/kg IVIG given over 2-5 days in a series of 8 patients with BKVN [12]. All patients also had their immunosuppression decreased by half. They concluded that the decreased immunosuppression and IVIG regimen allowed for salvage of the kidney, although without improvement in renal dysfunction. The mean serum creatinine prior to diagnosis was 120 ± 16 micromoles/L; at the time of diagnosis, it was 293 ± 32 micromoles/L); three months following initiation of therapy, it was 280 ± 23 micromoles/L); and at final follow-up between 3-36 months following initiation of therapy, it was 309 ± 46 micromoles/L). At most recent follow-up, all but one patient remained off hemodialysis, 50% of patients tested negative for BKV DNA in their serum, and four of five biopsies performed showed no lingering acute rejection or evidence of BKV.

Cidofovir is a nucleoside analogue with broad-spectrum effect against DNA viruses, including herpesviruses, iridoviruses, papovaviruses, and poxviruses. Its use has been tempered, however, by the risk of drug-induced nephrotoxicity. In BKVN, the risk of toxicity may be even greater, as cidofovir is excreted through the kidneys, and the effect of BKV-induced nephropathy on its elimination has not yet been adequately studied. Accumulation of cidofovir-phosphocoline complexes within cells is thought to interfere with cellular function and lead to eventual apoptosis. Probenecid has been used in pretreatment of patients taking cidofovir, as it inhibits hOAT1, the molecule responsible for transport of cidofovir-phosphocoline complexes into renal cells [28,29]. Anecdotal evidence has shown that the EC50 of cidofovir may occur at doses that are too high to attain clinically. However, when cidofovir is modified with hexadecyloxypropyl, octadecyloxyethyl, or oleyloxyethyl groups, the possibility exists for affecting a 3 log decrease in the drug's EC50 [5].

Kuypers et al. in a series of 21 patients diagnosed with BKVN compared the outcome of low-dose cidofovir and decreased immunosuppression to decreased immunosuppression alone [28]. Eight of 21 patients received a 0.5-1.0 mg/kg regimen of cidofovir. All 21 patients had their immunosuppression decreased following the diagnosis of BKVN. The authors found that all patients suffered an irreversible loss of allograft kidney function, but that allograft survival in the group receiving cidofovir stabilized. At 8-41 months follow-up, none of the eight patients who received cidofovir had lost their grafts, BKV DNA had been eliminated from the serum of 6/8, and none had suffered nephrotoxicity as a side effect of the antiviral medication. Interestingly, urine viral load remained effectively unchanged in all eight of these patients. In comparison, at 4-40 months follow-up, nine of the 13 patients treated with reduction of immunosuppression alone had lost their allograft.

Araya et al. examined similar doses of cidofovir (0.75-1.0 mg/kg/dose) in three younger patients (8, 19, and 20 years old) [29]. Patients were not pretreated with probenecid, but, no nephrotoxicity was reported. One patient had complete elimination of virus from her blood and a serum creatinine concentration of 1.3 mg/dL at most recent follow-up. The second patient had not completely eliminated the virus from her serum, but had improved renal function. The third patient had eliminated the virus from her serum and had a serum creatinine concentration of 1 mg/dL at last follow-up.

Gupta et al. at the University of Pittsburgh examined BKVN in a series of 243 consecutive SPK patients [25]. They reported less favorable outcomes with the use of cidofovir. Concern was raised for the effect of decreased immunosuppression on the pancreas allograft in patients with affected kidneys. Patients were divided into two groups based on immunosuppressive regimen used. The first group contained all patients through August 2001, and involved immunosuppression without antibody induction, with TAC, MMF, and steroids. There was a 3.5% incidence of BKVN in this group. The second group consisted of all patients from August 2001 to December 2004, and involved immunosuppression with 10 ng/ml TAC or 7-8 ng/ml TAC and addition of MMF. Alemtuzumab or antithymocyte globulin (ATG) was used for induction, and steroids were avoided. There was a 1.4% (one patient) incidence of BKVN in this group. Six of the seven patients with BKVN received low dose cidofovir (0.20-0.50 mg/kg) every 2-4 weeks over 1-6 months. All seven patients with BKVN had their TAC dose reduced to 5 ng/ml and MMF either decreased or completely eliminated from their immunosuppressive regimen. Three of the seven patients lost their renal allograft within 8-22 months of diagnosis of BKVN. Four of the seven patients had a functioning renal allograft at most recent follow-up. Five of seven had good pancreas graft function, while one lost his pancreas from complications shortly after transplantation, and one patient retained partial function of his pancreas allograft.

Wadei et al. in a series of 55 patients, examined the effect of low dose cidofovir, IVIG, and/or conversion of immunosuppressive regimen to cyclosporine on the outcome of BKVN [17]. Cidofovir was used in 55% of patients. The authors started patients at 0.25 mg/kg in 100 ml of normal saline given every two weeks. If there was persistence of BKVN, the dose was increased to 0.5 mg/kg. IVIG was given in 20% of patients, at a dose of 1.25 g/kg for two total doses. Conversion to cyclosporine from tacrolimus or sirolimus was used in 55% of patients with target trough levels of 125-175 ng/ml. MMF was reduced in all 55 patients to 250 mg bid or eliminated completely. The authors concluded that no individual intervention significantly improved disease outcome—low dose cidofovir (p=0.60), IVIG (p=0.75), or conversion to cyclosporine (p=0.90).

Leflunomide is an anti-inflammatory arthritic agent that has immunosuppressive properties and has been shown to act as an antiviral agent in animal and *in vitro* trials. More recently, it has been used in acute and chronic rejection episodes as well as in CMV infections. Its immunosuppressive properties are likely attributable to inhibition of enzymes in the signaling pathways for T- and B-lymphocytes, vascular smooth muscle cells, and fibroblasts. Leflunomide is metabolized to its active form A77 1726 [9,30]. Josephson et al. studied individual therapy with leflunomide versus combined therapy with leflunomide and low dose cidofovir (0.25 mg/kg every two weeks) in 26 patients with BKVN [9]. In all patients, the TAC dose was kept relatively constant, and MMF was eliminated. An IC50 of 40 micromoles and IC90 of 300 micromoles for leflunomide versus BKV were established in *in vitro* experiments prior to commencement of the clinical study. At target leflunomide levels, a significant decrease in serum and urine BKV viral load was observed in 22/26 patients (p < 0.001). The serum creatinine remained stable through 12 months follow-up. Fifteen percent of patients experienced renal allograft loss. No significant difference was found between the leflunomide alone versus leflunomide plus cidofovir groups. Rash and an elevation of serum alkaline phosphatase were seen as side effects of the antiviral regimens.

Farasati [30] studied the effect of leflunomide and of cidofovir on the growth of BKV *in vitro* as detected by PCR. The drugs were tested for EC50, the concentration at which BKV DNA yield in the cell culture system was reduced by 50%; IC50, the concentration at which the drug is 50% cytotoxic; and selectivity index (SI), which is the ratio of IC50 to EC50, and defines the level of toxicity of the drug. The authors noted that an SI greater than 10.0 is usually required before a drug is pursued actively for clinical use. Results showed that leflunomide had an EC50 of 11.3 ± 2.8 micrograms/ml, an IC50 of 39.7 ± 6.9 micrograms/ml, and an SI of 3.8 ± 0.8 micrograms/ml. Cidofovir had an EC50 of 36.3 ± 11.7 micrograms/ml, an IC50 of 63.9 ± 17.2 micrograms/ml, and an SI of 2.3 ± 0.8 micrograms/ml. It was concluded that the drugs were modestly active against BKV, but that their respective SI's were not optimal.

Abend et al. in an *in vitro* study showed that IFN-gamma expresses dose-dependent inhibition of TAg and VP1 in renal proximal tubule epithelial cells, while not affecting BKV replication kinetics [31]. TAg is inhibited at a concentration of 50 U/ml, whereas VP1 is inhibited at a concentration of 250 U/ml. This response was similar between the three strands of BKV studied. They observed a 1.6-fold decrease in TAg at 48 hours and a 12-fold decrease in TAg at inhibitory concentrations of IFN-gamma at 96 hours following administration. A 50-fold decrease in viral progeny level was seen at a multiplicity of infection (MOI) of 0.5 and an 80-fold decrease in viral progeny level was seen at an MOI of 0.1. Some possible inhibition of TAg and VP1 was also seen with IFN-alpha and IL-6 administration, however, the effect of IFN-alpha, IL-6, IL-8, MCP-1, RANTES, and TNF-alpha on BKV did not reach significance.

A final consideration is retransplantation in a kidney transplant recipient with BKVN in the original renal allograft. Womer et al. attempted retransplantation in two patients with active viremia prior to graft loss and a return to dialysis [32]. The thought was that waiting until the patient had lost the original allograft would decrease the chances for long-term survival and function in the second allograft, and that replacement during active viremia might not increase the risk in the patient of infection of the second allograft. The authors removed the original graft simultaneously with transplant of the new graft. In the two patients with follow-ups of 12 and 21 months, both allografts showed stable function and no evidence of active BKV replication. However, it is best that BK viremia be cleared before retransplantation. In a multi-center study of 5 transplant centers, 10 patients with graft loss caused by BK virus-associated nephropathy underwent retransplantation successfully [33]. The risk of recurrence does not seem to be increased in comparison with the first graft after a mean follow-up of 35 months.

VI. Conclusion

While the transplantation community has come a long way in understanding the risks, pathogenesis, molecular mechanisms, clinical manifestations, and treatment of BKVN, much work remains to be done. The next major step must involve large randomized, controlled trials, especially in evaluating novel treatments for BKVN. To date, much of the evidence is anecdotal or hindered by small study size, lack of control groups, or conflicting results among clinical trials and between animal and *in vitro* studies and human patient series. Despite the increasing frequency of BKVN in the renal transplant population, the total number of patients available for trials is low. Additional efforts may also focus on developing appropriate algorithms in monitoring for viral disease and possible preemptive intervention.

References

[1]   Gardner SD, Field AM, Coleman DV, Holme B. New human paapovavirus (B.K.) isolated from urine after renal transplantation. *Lancet.* 1971; 1: 1253.

[2]   Purighalla R, Shapiro R, McCauley J, et al. BK Virus infection in a kidney allograft diagnosed by needle biopsy. *Am. J. Kidney Dis.* 1995; 26: 671.

[3]   Brennan DC, Agha I, Bohl DL, et al. Incidence of BK with tacrolimus versus cyclosporine and impact of preemptive immunosuppression reduction. *Am. J. Transplant.* 2005; 5: 582-594.

[4]   Nickeleit V, Mihatsch MJ. Polyomavirus nephropathy in native kidneys and renal allografts: An update on an escalating threat. *Transplant. International.* 2006; 19: 960-973.

[5]   Randhawa P, Brennan DC. BK virus infection in transplant recipients: An overview and update. *Am. J. Transplant.* 2006; 6: 2000-2005.

[6]   Weinreb DB, Desman GT, Burstein DE, et al. Expression of p53 in virally infected tubular cells in renal transplant patients with polyomavirus nephropathy. *Human Pathology.* 2006; 37: 684-688.

[7]   Kausman JY, Somers GR, Francis DM, Jones CL. Association of renal adenocarcinoma and BK virus nephropathy post transplantation. *Pediatr. Nephrol.* 2004; 19: 459-462.

[8]   Kwak EJ, Vilchez RA, Randhawa P, et al. Pathogenesis and management of polyomavirus infection in transplant recipients. *Clinical Infectious Diseases.* 2002; 35: 1081-1087.

[9]   Josephson MA, Gillen D, Javaid B, et al. Treatment of renal allograft polyoma BK virus infection with leflunomide. *Transplantation.* 2006; 81: 704-710.

[10] Nolte FS. Case studies in cost effectiveness of molecular diagnosis for infectious disease: Pulmonary TB, enteroviral meningitis, and BK virus nephropathy. *Medical Microbiology.* 2006; 43: 1463-1467.

[11] Rocha PN, Plumb TJ, Miller SE, et al. Risk factors for BK polyomavirus nephritis in renal allograft recipients. *Clin. Transplant.* 2004; 18: 456-462.

[12] Sener A, House AA, Jevnikar AM, et al. Intravenous immunoglobulin as a treatment for BK virus associated nephropathy: One-year follow-up of renal allograft recipients. *Transplantation.* 2006; 81: 117-120.

[13] Lipshutz GS, Mahanty H, Feng S, et al. Polyomavirus-associated nephropathy in simultaneous kidney-pancreas transplant recipients: A single center experience. *Transplant. Proc.* 2004; 36: 1097.

[14] Lipshutz GS, Mahanty H, Feng S, et al. BKV in simultaneous pancreas-kidney transplant recipients: a leading cause of renal graft loss in the first two years post-transplant. *Am. J. Transplant.* 2005; 5: 366.

[15] Trofe J, Gaber LW, Stratta RJ, et al. Polyomavirus in kidney and kidney-pancreas transplant recipients. *Transpl. Infect. Dis.* 2003; 5: 21.

[16] Awadalla Y, Randhawa P, Ruppert K, et al. HLA mismatching increases the risk of BK virus nephropathy in renal transplant recipients. *Am. J. Transplant.* 2004; 4: 1691-1696.

[17] Wadei HM, Rule AD, Lewin M, et al. Kidney transplant function and histological clearance of virus following diagnosis of polyomavirus-associated nephropathy (PVAN). *Am. J. Transplant.* 2006; 6: 1025-1032.

[18] Schwarz A, Mengel M, Haller H, Niedermeyer J. Polyoma virus nephropathy in native kidneys after lung transplantation. *Am. J. Transplant.* 2005; 5: 2582-2585.

[19] Bohl DL, Storch GA, Ryschkewitsch C, et al. Donor origin of BK virus in renal transplantation and role of HLA C7 in susceptibility to sustained BK viremia. *Am. J. Transplant.* 2005; 5: 2213-2221.

[20] Celik B, Randhawa PS. Glomerular changes in BK virus nephropathy. *Human Pathology.* 2004; 35: 367-370.

[21] Randhawa PS, Finkelstein S, Scantlebury V, et al. Human polyoma virus-associated interstitial nephritis in the allograft kidney. *Transplantation.* 1999; 67(1): 103-109.

[22] Randhawa P, Shapiro R, Vats A. Quantitation of DNA of polyomaviruses BK and JC in human kidneys. *JID.* 2005; 192: 504-509.

[23] Randhawa PS, Popescu I, Macedo C, et al. Detection of Cd8+ T-cells sensitized to BK virus large T antigen in healthy volunteers and kidney transplant recipients. *Human Immunology.* 2006; 67: 298-302.

[24] Randhawa PS, Gupta G, Vats A, et al. Immunoglobulin G, A, and M responses to BK virus in renal transplantation. *Clin. Vaccine Immunol.* 2006; 13(9): 1057-1063.

[25] Gupta G, Shapiro R, Thai N, et al. Low incidence of BK virus nephropathy after simultaneous kidney pancreas transplantation. *Transplantation.* 2006; 82: 382-388.

[26] Nickeleit V, Klimkait T, Binet IF. Testing for polyomavirus type BK DNA in plasma to identify renal-allograft recipients with viral nephropathy. *N. Engl. J. Med.* 2000; 342: 1309-1315.

[27] Weinreb DB, Desman GT, Amolat-Apiado MJ, et al. Polyomavirus infection is a prominent risk factor for bladder carcinoma in immunocompetent individuals. *Diagn. Cytopathol.* 2006; 34: 201-203.

[28] Kuypers DRJ, Vandooren AK, Lerut E, et al. Adjuvant low-dose cidofovir therapy for BK polyomavirus interstitial nephritis in renal transplant recipients. *Am. J. Transplant.* 2005; 5: 1997-2004.

[29] Araya CE, Lew JF, Fennell RS, et al. Intermediate-dose cidofovir without probenecid in the treatment of BK virus allograft nephropathy. *Pediatr. Transplantation.* 2006; 10: 32-37.

[30] Farasati NA, Shapiro R, Vats A, Randhawa P. Effect of leflunomide and cidofovir on replication of BK virus in an *in vitro* culture system. *Transplantation.* 2005; 79: 116-118.

[31] Abend JR, Low JA, Imperiale MJ, et al. Inhibitory effect of IFN-gamma on BK virus gene expression and replication. *J. Virol.* 2006; October 11, E-publication ahead of print.

[32] Womer KL, Meier-Kriesche H-U, Patton PR. Preemptive retransplantation for BK virus nephropathy: Successful outcome despite active viremia. *Am. J. Transplant.* 2006; 6: 209-213.

[33] Ramos E, Vincenti F, Lu WX, et al. Retransplantation in patients with graft loss caused by polyoma virus nephropathy. *Transplantation.* 2004; 77: 131-133.

In: Transplantation Immunology Research Trends
Editor: Oliver N. Ulricker, pp. 159-182

ISBN: 978-1-60021-578-0
© 2007 Nova Science Publishers, Inc.

Chapter VI

Evidence in Maintenance Immunosuppression after Kidney Transplantation

Domingo Hernández*, Germán Pérez, Domingo Marrero-Miranda,
Aurelio Rodríguez and José Manuel González-Posada
Nephrology Section. University Hospital of the Canary Islands.
Ofra s/n. 38200. La Laguna. Tenerife. Spain.

Abstract

Renal transplant recipients have benefited from short-term graft survival due to the introduction of new immunosuppressants. Despite this, long-term survival has improved only marginally during recent years. Chronic allograft nephropathy, cardiovascular disease, older donors, emerging new viruses and malignancies, among other factors, may be responsible for this situation. In addition, immunosuppression remains the cause of most morbidity following organ transplantation. Thus, minimization or, at least, tailoring of immunosuppression is an issue of great concern in this field. Minimization of immunosuppression is not itself a primary goal in organ transplantation, but it helps to reduce the risk of drug toxicity, as long as there is no compromise of immunosuppressive efficacy. In this respect, some strategies to achieve this goal may be: a) To minimize corticosteroid regimens, b) To minimize calcineurin inhibitor regimens, c) To tailor anticalcineuric drugs in order to optimize cardiovascular risk profile and renal function d) To use mammalian target-of-rapamycin inhibitors or purine synthesis inhibitors in order to prevent or reverse renal allograft dysfunction e) To establish therapeutic strategies against new viruses and malignancies, and f) To optimize immunosuppressive therapy in elderly patients. This review outlines several strategies for minimizing or tailoring the use of immunosuppressants in order to attain these objectives. The arguments for the various strategies are based on clinical trial data which suggest that

* Corresponding author: Domingo Hernández; Urbanization San Diego, 51; 38208. La Laguna. Tenerife. Canary Islands. Spain. Phone: (34) 922678545; FAX: (34)922644313; E-mail:dhmarrero@hotmail.com.

most patients can be transplanted with less immunosuppression than is currently standard.

Key words: Maintenance immunosuppression, kidney transplantation.

Introduction

During the last few years spectacular advances in the field of renal transplantation have occurred mainly due to the advent of new immunosuppressants that have optimized short and medium term results of this therapy. Despite this, long-term graft survival has not shown a corresponding improvement and we are still faced with the old problems inherent to renal transplantion that condition its viability[1,2]. Cardiovascular disease (CVD) is highly prevalent in these patients, chronic allograft nephropathy (CAN) is the main cause of graft loss and other clinical challenges have emerged, such as the presence of new viruses or the rise in the number of tumorous processes, within the context of an increasingly aged population (figure 1). Simultaneously, immunosuppressant drugs are contributing to the development of these complications[3]. All in all, the final consequence is the inexorable loss of renal allografts and high rates of morbidity and mortality over time, even under the best clinical conditions.

Prolonging patient and graft survival thus constitutes a clinical priority. From this perspective we may infer that tailoring immunosuppression to the individual is a vital long-term clinical objective, adapting immunosuppressant therapy to the donor/patient characteristics in order to improve survival and patient quality of life as far as possible. But, is it possible to avoid the toxicity of steroids and calcineurin inhibitors (CNIs)? Can we prevent post-transplant CVD? Is it possible to delay or avoid the appearance of chronic nephropathy? Are there therapeutic strategies to reduce the appearance of BK virus or tumorous processes? Can we optimize immunosuppression in the elderly who receive grafts from aged donors? There may be no definitive answer to each of these questions given the lack of sufficient scientific evidence in maintenance immunosuppression. However, in recent years therapeutic strategies have emerged seeking a balance between efficacy and low toxicity based on the following precepts: 1) Suspension of steroids, 2) Minimization or withdrawal of CNIs, 3) Tailoring the CNIs according to its efficacy and the vascular risk profile, 4) Optimization of renal function and/or prevention of chronic nephropathy, 5) Implementation of immunosuppressive strategies for patients with BK virus or neoplasia, and 6) Investigation of immunosuppressive regimens for the elderly.

This review outlines the evidence in support of tailored regimens that offer potential longer-term benefit without compromising immunosuppressive efficacy.

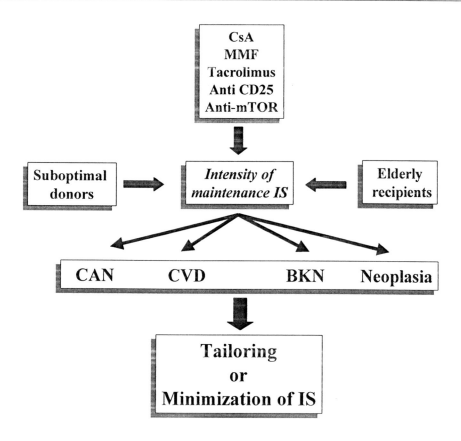

Figure 1. Clinical situations that may justify tailoring maintenance immunosuppression in renal transplantation. CsA: cyclosporine; MMF: mycophenolate mofetil; IS: immunosuppression; CAN: chronic allograft nephropathy; CVD, cardiovascular disease; BKN: BK virus nephropathy.

Suspension or Avoidance of Steroids

The use of steroids to prevent acute rejection has long been a mainstay of immunosuppression, but there is no doubt about the serious side effects that contribute to postransplant morbidity and mortality. The advent of new immunosuppressants has stimulated interest in the policy of avoiding these drugs, but has not been generally implemented. A meta-analysis by Kasiske et al[4] showed that the suspension of steroids was only safe in selected patient with low immunologic risk - white race and no history of rejection - given the increase in the number of rejections and the loss of renal grafts. However, in most of the studies included in the meta-analysis, the patients received double therapy with prednisone and cyclosporine (CsA) or triple therapy with azathioprine, treatments that do not reflect current immunosuppressive practice at most centres. A subsequent meta-analysis showed that steroid suspension in patients on triple therapy - prednisone, a CNI and mycophenolate mofetil (MMF)- was associated with a global increase in acute rejection (8%), but this had no negative impact on graft survival[5]. In this respect, a controlled trial with early withdrawal of steroids (4th day) using basiliximab, CsA and MMF showed a similar rate of acute rejection and graft survival as those of the control group[6]. Similar results have been observed with tacrolimus and MMF, short and medium-term[7-8], as well as in the pediatric population[9]. More recently a multicentre European study, with patients randomized to one of three therapeutic options, compared the efficacy of combined treatment with steroids, tacrolimus and MMF versus withdrawal of either steroids or MMF. Acute rejection rates were similar between the groups, with a lower incidence of adverse effects in those patients without steroids or without MMF[10]. Similarly, another multicentre controlled trial (*CARMEN Study Group*), comparing tacrolimus, MMF and steroids versus a conventional steroid-free therapy with daclizumab (2 doses), showed similar rates of acute rejection in the two groups, but also found improved lipid and metabolic profile in the group who did not receive steroids[11].

Finally, the combination of tacrolimus and sirolimus has been little explored in steroid-free therapy. A non-controlled multicentre pilot study has shown that treatment with basiliximab, tacrolimus and sirolimus without steroids offered an acceptable rate of rejection (<20%) and minimal adverse effects[12]. In this respect Kumar et al studied the effect of early withdrawal of steroids (2nd day) versus its use, in four groups of maintenance immunosuppression, one of which included tacrolimus plus sirolimus. Medium-term patient and graft survival, rates of acute clinical and subclinical rejection, and the incidence of CAN were similar in the different treatment groups[13]. Obviously long-term follow up is required to confirm these findings, but combining a CNI with MMF, or sirolimus, may offer greater safety for the withdrawal of steroids.

At present, there is sufficient evidence that steroid suspension is associated with a reduction of post-transplant metabolic disorders and improved anthropometric parameters related with cardiovascular risk[14]. Steroid withdrawal also diminishes arterial pressure values[15] and, presumibly, left ventricular hypertrophy, undoubtedly contributing to reduced cardiovascular risk.

Therefore, current recommendations in clinical practice, documented by a high level of evidence (Grade of recommendation A), include a) Suspension of steroids in selected patients (low immunologic risk) on triple therapy with an CNI and MMF, and b) Suspension or avoidance of steroids for optimizing cardiovascular risk profile.

Minimization or Withdrawal of Calcineurin Inhibitors

Although the immunosuppressive efficacy of CNIs drugs has been demonstrated[16,17], they paradoxically contribute to long-term graft loss because of their nephrotoxic effects. This is currently under debate in the field of renal transplantion. Transplant recipients of other solid organs present disturbingly high accumulative rates of renal dysfunction associated with the use of these drugs[18]. In renal transplantation, Solez et al[19] some years ago observed a high proportion of chronic nephropathy (70%) and nephrotoxicity (24%) after two years of treatment with CsA or tacrolimus, which increased in patients with previous rejection. Likewise, therapeutic regimens without CsA or with its early withdrawal show a significant reduction in the rate of graft loss compared to other treatments with CNIs [20,21].

Recently, protocol biopsies in pancreas-kidney recipients showed that CNIs-related chronic nephrotoxicity is a practically universal finding, even in grafts with excellent initial clinical conditions[22].

These arguments support the strategy of CNIs reduction or withdrawal after renal transplantation to improve long-term results[23]. But what evidence is there for adopting this strategy? A meta-analysis on immunosuppressant withdrawal that evaluated over 1000 renal recipients from ten studies with a mean follow up of fifty months showed that the suspension of CsA did not increase the risk of graft loss, although a mean increase of 11% was observed in the rate of acute rejection[4]. Risk factors for acute rejection after CsA suspension include a greater number of B-DR incompatibilities, obesity and young patients[24].

Clearly, the availability of new immunosuppressants such as MMF and sirolimus has increased the possibility of employing this strategy. In fact, MMF may have a synergic action with the pharmacodynamic effects of low-dose CsA (C0<100 ng/ml)[25]. Trials combining reduced or no CNIs with these drugs have shown encouraging results for renal function and cardiovascular risk parameters[26-40] (table 1). In these studies, which included immunologically low risk patients, the common denominator was a slight increase in the rate of acute rejection (10-20%) compared to controls. However, the improvement in cardiovascular risk profile and renal function were the rule in the experimental group, and more evident in stable recipients beyond the first year of transplantation[26,27,32]. Given that post-transplant renal function in the first year predicts long-term kidney transplant survival[40-42], this strategy may favor prognosis of this population. Likewise, in some of these studies eliminating CsA and using an antimetabolite or sirolimus was associated with improved graft survival and a lower incidence and severity of CAN lesions after a long period of follow up[31,38-40]. Thus, this therapeutic option may lead to higher graft survival rates, at least in selected patients. On the same lines, the use of FTY 720 at 5mg/day in association with low-dose cyclosporine seems to offer a safe and effective immunosuppression in de novo renal transplant recipients, which may become another option supporting this strategy[45].

Along with these studies, other more ambitious therapeutic regimens have emerged. They contemplate a strategy of avoiding the use of CNIs in order to improve long-term results. In this respect, clinical trials with and without induction using (poly- or monoclonal) antilymphocyte antibodies showed better renal function in the group that did not receive CNIs and similar rates of acute rejection, but only when associated with MMF[46-52] (table 2). Recently, in a prospective randomized study, Larson et al[53] compared the use of CNI-free immunosuppression using Sirolimus, MMF and prednisone, versus Tacrolimus, MMF and prednisone (both groups with Thymoglobulin induction), and found similar rates of acute rejection, glomerular filtration and graft survival at one year. However, in protocol renal graft biopsies the renal graft lesions were less relevant in the CNIs-free group. Coestimulation blockade of T cells (with Belatacept LEA29Y)[54] may also allow CNIs-free immunosuppression with improved cardiovascular risk profile. Future studies along these lines are needed to confirm these findings.

Table 1. Clinical studies investigating elimination or reduction of CsA in renal transplantion using antimetabolite drugs (Azathioprine or MMF) or sirolimus

Suspension or reduction of CsA using MMF/Azathioprine			
Reference	Rate of Acute rejection Controls* vs. MMF/Aza	Evolution of renal function Controls* vs. MMF/Aza	Renal graft Survival Controls* vs. MMF/Aza
MacPhee I et al (26) Dubey D et al (27) Schnuelle P et al (28) Smak Gregoor P a et al. (29) Abramowicz D et al. (30) Bakker R et al (31) Pascual M et al (32). Kuypers D et al (33)	1.5-11 vs. 11-20%	Better with MMF	94-100 vs. 97-100%

Suspension or reduction of CsA using Sirolimus			
Reference	Rate of Acute rejection Controls* vs Sirolimus	Evolution of renal function Control*vs Sirolimus	Renal graft Survival Control*vs Sirolimus
Baboolal K (34) Johnson R et al. (35) Gonwa T et al. (36) Oberbauer R et al. (37) Kreis H et al. (38) Mota A et al. (39) Ruiz JC et al (40)	5-18 vs. 10-20%	Better with sirolimus	91-95 vs. 93-97%

*The control group implies treatment with CsA. Abbreviations: Aza, azathioprine; MMF, mycophenolate mofetil; CsA: Cyclosporine.

Table 2. Anticalcineurin inhibitors-free therapeutic regimens

WITHOUT INDUCTION	
Reference	Therapeutic regimen
Groth CG et al. (46)	P+SRL+Aza vs. P+CsA+Aza
Kreis H et al. (47)	P+SRL+MMF vs. P+CsA+MMF

WITH INDUCTION USING AN ANTI- CD25 OR THYMOGLOBULIN	
Reference	Therapeutic reg
Tran H et al (48)	Daclizumab+P+MMF
Vincenti F et al. (49)	Daclizumab+P+MMF
Flechner S et al. (50)	Thymoglobulin+P+MMF
Grinyo JM et al. (51)	Basiliximab+P+SRL vs. CsA
Lo A et al (52)	Thymoglobulin+ ½ Tac-SRL vs ½ SRL

Abbreviations: Aza, azathioprine; MMF, Mycophenolate mofetil; CsA, Cyclosporine; SRL, sirolimus; P, prednisona; Tac, tacrolimus.

Moreover, in this immunosuppression a lower expression of genes involved in the progression to chronic nephropathy was observed[55]. It remains to be clarified whether these interesting findings are associated with lower incidence of chronic graft dysfunction.

Alternatives to these therapeutic possibilities include monitoring plasma concentrations of CsA by measuring C2 levels (2 hours after administration) which may also constitute an effective measure to reduce doses and avoid over-exposure to the deleterious effects of this drug. In stable renal transplant recipients (>3 months after transplant), monitoring plasma concentrations of CsA by C2 levels allowed dose reduction in patients with levels higher than the established range. As expected, this conditioned better renal function renal and a reduction of blood pressure[56]. A more recent study in stable patients showed that levels of C2 >661 ng/ml were associated with better renal function and a lower rate of acute rejection after three years of follow up, although not all the patients received triple therapy with MMF[57]. This strategy may entail reduced costs during the evolution[58]. It is unclear whether all this favors long-term renal graft survival.

Given the current level of evidence, in selected patients it may be recommendable to replace the CNI with sirolimus, with or without an antimetabolite (MMF or Azathioprine), in order to improve renal function, cardiovascular risk and possibly graft survival (level of evidence A). Alternatively, monitorization of CsA plasma concentration by C2 levels may be useful to optimize long-term renal function.

Tailoring the Calcineurin Inhibitor: CsA Versus Tacrolimus

CsA and tacrolimus constitute the mainstays of current immunosuppression in renal transplantion, but there is controversy about the long-term efficacy and results of each of these CNIs. Controlled studies show that tacrolimus confers lower risk of acute rejection, better renal function and lower rates of CAN than CsA (level of evidence B), so that conversion from CsA to Tacrolimus could result in improved long-term graft survival[60-63]. Something similar has been observed on analysis of large data bases and in retrospective single-center studies[70-74]. Other authors, however, have not confirmed these differences, showing similar efficacy between these two drugs for graft survival and renal function[68-71]. It is possible that the intrarrenal expression of cytokines induced by CsA and tacrolimus, as well as their vasoactive properties, result in similar degrees of nephrotoxicity, which may explain these findings[72].

The use of tacrolimus has extended to most transplant programs, but it seems prudent to tailor the choice of CNIs according to the risk profile of each patient. Tacrolimus is associated with higher rates of diabetes, while CsA is associated with increased hyperlipidemia and blood pressure[3]. Thus the choice of maintenance immunosuppression according to the biological profile of the patient, with CNI reduction or conversion, may finally depend on the cardiovascular risk profile of these patients. Various studies support these arguments. Conversion from CsA to tacrolimus has been shown to condition a significant decline in blood pressure and plasma lipid levels measured after a short period of follow up[66-68]. In addition to these effects, a controlled study showed lower cardiovascular risk score according to the Framingham study[76]. However, this strategy has not been shown to reduce long-term cardiovascular morbidity or mortality in this population.

Given this high level evidence, in clinical practice it is recommended that: a) the CNI should be tailored to the cardiovascular risk profile of the patient, or changed in the event of severe side effects (level of evidence A); b) Tacrolimus may offer greater long-term efficacy, at least in patients with previous immunologic dysfunction (level of evidence B).

Prevention or Modification of the Course of Chronic Allograft Nephropathy

CAN is the most frequent cause of long-term graft loss. This complication is conditioned by immunologic and non-immunologic factors. Histologically CAN is characterized by the presence of glomeruloesclerosis, hyperplasia of the intima and interstitial fibrosis. Autocrine secretion of cytokines and growth factors such as TGF-β may be involved in the patogenesis[77]. Due to their antiproliferative action, MMF and mammalian target of rapamycin (mTOR) inhibitors may therefore play a decisive role in maintenance immunosuppression, minimizing the progression to chronic nephropathy and chronic deterioration of graft function. The evidence available in favor of using these drugs is presented below.

The Importance of the Antimetabolite: MMF vs Azathioprine

In multicentre controlled studies MMF significantly reduced the risk of acute rejection compared with controls, but these studies did not show that MMF prolonged graft survival after three years of follow up[78-80]. Two retrospective analyses found that the use of MMF reduced by 27% the medium-term risk of graft loss and renal dysfunction, independently of acute rejection episodes[81,82].In agreement with these findings, a randomized study showed that the rate of CAN was significantly lower in patients receiving MMF (46%) versus azathioprine (71%)[83], indicating a potential protective effect of MMF against CAN. Likewise, the use of MMF has been associated with a lower rate of mortality and late acute rejection in renal patients with pretransplant diabetes[84]

Focusing on chronic graft dysfunction, an elegant study in rats with CNIs-induced chronic nephrotoxicity showed that after replacing CsA with MMF there was less tissue expression of profibrogenic factors and a regression of histological lesions[85]. Furthermore, in the animal model of chronic rejection, the combined use MMF and sirolimus reduced the parenchymal lesions typical of CAN, principally interstitial fibrosis[86]. In patients with CAN, the reduction or elimination of CNI and the addition of MMF not only improved renal function but also optimized the metabolic profile after various years of follow up[87,88]. In a recent prospective study by González-Molina et al[89] the administration of MMF in patients with CAN on double or triple therapy showed slower progression of renal failure, independently of CsA levels. Lastly, in a controlled study of patients with CAN where CsA was replaced by MMF, the authors observed a slower deterioration of glomerular filtration and improvement of lipid parameters, without increasing the risk of acute rejection[90]. However, it is unclear whether these functional changes are accompanied by improvement in histological lesions as has been observed in animal studies. Meanwhile, it seems reasonable to recommend the use of MMF (Grade of recommendation B) in patients with CAN in order to delay the progressive deterioration of renal function and reduce the long-term risk of graft loss.

Efficacy of mTOR Inhibitors in CAN

Sirolimus is a macrolide immunosuppressant whose level of efficacy is similar to that of CsA in preventing acute rejection[91,92]. This drug forms an intracelular complex with the FKBP12 protein to inhibit the functions of the mTOR peptide. It thereby blocks intracellular signals that activate the cell cycle generated by the action of interleukins on membrane receptors. The final result is inhibition of DNA synthesis and detention of the cell cycle between the G1 and S phases[93]. Its antiproliferative properties additionally give it an interesting role in preventing CAN and transplant vasculopathy, as has been observed in animal studies[94].

Initially, sirolimus and everolimus were developed for use in combination with CsA, but they increase the CNI-related nephrotoxicity, especially through the greater expression of TGF-β or increased renal concentration of the CNIs[95-96]. In effect, the combination of sirolimus and CsA did not improve renal function or histological lesions in patients with CAN despite the reduction of CsA levels[97]. Similarly, in patients with chronic deterioration of graft function and on triple therapy with prednisone, sirolimus and CsA, the withdrawal of sirolimus was associated with significant improvement of renal function[98]. In agreement with these findings are the conclusions of a recent systematic review of 7000 patients from 33 clinical trials analyzing the role of mTOR inhibitors as primary immunosuppression in renal transplant recipients after two years of follow up. In general, Sirolimus and Everolimus did not show improvement or worsening in graft or patient survival, but those immunosuppressive regimens that avoided or minimized the use of CNIs in combination with mTOR inhibitors were associated with improved renal function[99].

At present it is unclear whether sirolimus modifies the course of CAN, but it is possible that the use of mTOR inhibitors without CNIs may represent one of the few therapeutic therapies available to minimize the CAN-related lesions. In this respect, controlled studies have observed that CsA withdrawal in patients on triple therapy with sirolimus, was followed by a reduction of CAN-related histological lesions and optimization of renal function[39,40,100]. The greatest clinical benefit of this strategy seems to be attained when proteinuria is <1 g/day[101].

Everolimus, with pharmacologic properties similar to sirolimus, may constitute an interesting alternative for this objective. In animal models of chronic rejection, the administration of everolimus improves histologic lesions and is associated with a decrease in proteinuria by antiproliferative mechanisms or by stimulating apoptosis of cells that participate in tissue remodelling[102]. Obviously, these findings require confirmation in patients with CAN. Future studies will no doubt provide the necessary evidence in this regard.

Moreover, due to antiproliferative properties of anti-mTOR drugs, other additional effects of sirolimus observed in animal models, include regression of left ventricular hypertrophy and decrease of atheromatosis vascular lesions.[103-104] If these effects are confirmed in human studies, it would help to optimize the cardiovascular risk profile in this population. In any case, whether these potential beneficial actions are associated with lower long-term morbidity and mortality remains to be elucidated.

From this perspective, the use of anti-mTOR may be justified to avoid progression of chronic graft lesions and to improve renal function (Grade of recommendation A), provided they are not used in conjunction with CNIs. In these cases, early use is recommended given the irreversible nature of CAN lesions.

Immunosuppression in the Presence of BK Virus

The prevalence of polyomavirus BK in the renal transplant population is not well defined. BK-virus nephropathy (BKN) has been estimated at 8% of recipients [105-106], conditioning the progressive loss of grafts in 40-60% of cases. In general, the time lapse from transplantion to diagnosis oscillates from nine to fifteen months, although longer periods have been described. Habitually the course of this nephropathy is paucisymptomatic, with diagnosis being suspected after observing slow deterioration of renal function together with the finding of decoy cells in urine, and on detection of the virus (in blood, urine and/or renal tissue) or the presence of specific antibodies to BK virus. Less typical presentations include ureteral stenosis and hydronephrosis or even cystitis[107]. Definitive diagnosis is made histopathologically, with findings of intranuclear viral inclusions and lymphocyte infiltrate with tubulitis that mimic acute rejection, which is important to discern. Interstitial fibrosis and tubular atrophy are final consequences of this entity.

There is increasing evidence that intense immunosuppression is associated with the appearance of this post-transplant complication. Indeed, about 70-90% of patients with BKN were receiving tacrolimus with or without MMF[108-111]. Likewise, the use of antilymphocyte antibodies and high-dose steroids have been implicated in the development of BKN[106]. In this respect, a greater number of HLA incompatibilities has been associated with greater risk of BKN[112]. Active allogenic response plus the renal tissue lesion may favor the activation of the latent BK virus. In fact, BKN has not been clearly demonstrated in non-renal organ recipients.

At present there is no consensus as to diagnosis, optimal management and treatment of this infection in renal transplant recipients. The presence of decoy cells in urine is a sign of viral replication and constitutes the simplest method of monitoring the infection, but these cells are not specific markers of BKN (predictive value 20%). Determination of viremia by PCR may be a good guide for detection (sensitivity 100%, specificity 80%, positive predictive value 50%), but it remains to be shown whether the presence of the viral DNA predicts the development of BKN. Lately certain authors have suggested the detection of mRNA in urine[113] and the combination de PCR with quantification of specific antibodies to BK virus as alternatives for diagnosis and for monitoring response to treatment[114].

The reduction of immunosuppression seems, so far, the most prudent therapeutic strategy for patients with BKN. In recent years there has been a tendency to declining numbers of graft loss due to BKN related with improved and earlier diagnostic tests, and the reduction of immunosuppression. As a guide, a reduction of 30% in the doses of tacrolimus or sirolimus and 25-50% in MMF may suffice. In certain cases, the antimetabolite should be suspended[109], thus obtaining a significant reduction of the viral load and stabilization of renal function in a high percentage of patients (>50%). In contrast, increasing immunosuppression with a bolus of steroids or polyclonal antibodies may exacerbate the infection. Conversion from tacrolimus and MMF to a combination of sirolimus and prednisone has also been associated with reduced viremia[115]. Likewise, the use of leflunamide (immunosuppressant with antiviral properties) with low-dose CsA may produce similar results. Also, treatment with cidofovir (0.25-1.0 mg/kg/doses without probenecid every 2-3 weeks during 6 weeks) and intravenous immunoglobulin have been used in these patients with encouraging results, especially when there is concurrent acute rejection[116-117]. However, future studies are needed to confirm these results. Moreover, although treatment of the viruria or asymptomatic viremia is not established practice, some authors advocate performing PCR as protocol and reducing pre-emptively the immunosuppression when viremia is detected[118]. Lastly, in patients who have lost their grafts due to BKN, graft nephrectomy is recommended with a latency period of 3-4 months before a second transplant, although certain authors advocate an preemptive retransplantation to avoid the deleterious effect of time on dialysis[119].

Management of Tumors after Renal Transplantion

The incidence of solid tumors and lymphoproliferative disorders is significantly higher (3.5 times) in solid organ transplant recipients than in the general population, except for breast and prostate gland carcinomas. Observational studies have shown a close relationship between accumulated immunosuppression and the incidence of tumorous processes[120,121]. Other risk factors identified in this population are age, smoking, pre-transplant splenectomy, anti CD3 monoclonal antibodies (OKT3) and a history of cancer before transplantation. Likewise, certain neoplasias, especially lymphoproliferative disorders, have been related with viral infection such as Epstein-Barr. In general neoplasia may appear at any time after renal transplantation, but lymphoproliferative processes usually appear earlier. Thus these patients suffer greater mortality than those without post-transplant neoplasias.

In general, there is no definitive therapy for these patients, but it seems prudent to recommend overall reduction of immunosuppression. This is more evident in lymphoproliferative processes, especially those of polyclonal origen of recent onset, with only one organ affected, without organic dysfunction and normal levels of LDH[122] where reduction or interruption of immunosuppression is associated with partial or complete remission of the neoplasia.

Antimetabolite drugs such as azathioprine have been associated with the development of cutaneous neoplasias. Therefore their withdrawal or replacement with sirolimus may prove beneficial for the management of these tumors. Sirolimus has antiproliferative and therefore antineoplasic properties[122,123]. Conversion from CsA to sirolimus plus the suspension of MMF in patients with Kaposi's sarcoma has been shown to be associated with regression of cutaneous tumorous lesions after six months of follow up[124]. Preliminary data also indicate that treatment with sirolimus is associated with a lower incidence of de novo tumors as compared to treatment with other immunosuppressants. More recently, a multicenter randomized trial has shown that treatment with sirolimus and withdrawal of CNIs (third month), versus maintenance therapy of CsA and sirolimus, reduced the incidence of cutaneous and non-cutaneous cancer after five years of follow up[125].

Thus a tentative therapeutic option is to administer sirolimus in patients with a history of pre-transplant neoplasia. Future studies in this field will clarify these aspects.

Other measures that may improve prognosis in these patients include aggressive excision of resectable tumors and close monitoring during follow up, involving: 1) Annual chest x-ray, vaginal cytology in women and prostate tests in men, 2) Biannual breast examination in women, 3) Colonoscopy every 5 years in patients older than 50 years or in patients with positive occult fecal blood. In patients with a history of colon polyps, colonoscopy should be performed biannually, and 4) Routine examination of the skin on each visit[126].

Immunosuppression in Elderly Population

During recent years the renal transplant clinical scene has changed. Older patients are receiving grafts from older donors, which affects the results of this replacement therapy. In effect, graft survival is significantly lower in older recipients or in patients receiving grafts from older donors[127,128]. However, no additive effect of donor and recipient age has been shown for graft survival[129]. In any case, pretransplant renal biopsy and histological evaluation may be crucial for graft survival[130]. With respect to immunosuppression, it remains unclear what constitutes an optimal regimen that may prolong graft survival in elderly recipients. Given the increased cardiovascular risk in this population and potential graft lesions, CNIs-free immunosuppression or the use of antiproliferative drugs may be attractive options. In this respect, two relatively recent studies in patients receiving older or suboptimal grafts showed that CNIs avoidance was associated with optimization of renal function and acceptable medium-term graft survival[131,132]. More recently, a multicenter observational study using low-dose tacrolimus (5-8 ng/ml), two doses of daclizumab and MMF (2g/day) showed rates of acute tubular necrosis and immunologic dysfunction of 48% and 10% respectively, with excellent graft and patient survival at one year of follow up[133]. Although these results raise hopes, future controlled studies are needed to confirm these findings.

Conclusions

In short, although strategies using the new immunosuppressants reduce acute rejection, it remains to be established what immunosuppressive regimen is most indicated to prolong long-term graft and patient survival. The strategies currently being introduced include tailoring immunosuppression to the individual patient, minimization or withdrawal of steroids and CNIs, the introduction of new immunosuppressants to optimize management of chronic graft dysfunction, special treatment of infectious or neoplasias, and therapeutic combinations most appropriate for elderly recipients.

Acknowledgements

This study was supported by grants PI2003/008 from the Canary Island Government "Consejería de Education, Cultura y Deportes", FIS 02/1350 from the "Fondo de Investigaciones Sanitarias" and C03/03 from the Spanish Ministry of Health "Redes Temáticas de Transplante".

References

[1]   Pascual M, Theruvath T, Kawai T, Tolkoff-Rubin N, Cosimi AB: Strategies to improve long-term outcomes after renal transplantation. *N. Engl. J. Med.* 2002; 346: 580-590.

[2]   Meier-Kriesche HU, Schold JD, Kaplan B: Long-term renal allograft survival: have we made significant progress or is it time to rethink our analytic and therapeutic strategies. *Am. J. Transplant.* 2004;4: 1289-1295.

[3]   Boots JM, Christiaans MH, van Hooff JP: Effect of immunosuppressive agents on long-term survival of renal transplant recipients: focus on the cardiovascular risk. *Drugs.* 2004; 64: 2047-2073.

[4]   Kasiske BL, Chakkera HA, Louis TA, Ma JZ: A meta-analysis of immunosuppression withdrawal trials in renal transplantation. *J. Am. Soc. Nephrol.* 2000;11: 1910-1917.

[5]   Pascual J, Quereda C, Zamora J, Hernandez D; Spanish Group for Evidence-Based Medicine in Renal Transplantation: Steroid withdrawal in renal transplant patients on triple therapy with a Calcineurin inhibitor and mycophenolate mofetil: a meta-analysis of randomized, controlled trials. *Transplantation.* 2004;78: 1548-1556.

[6]   Vincenti F, Monaco A, Grinyo J, Kinkhabwala M, Roza A: Multicenter randomized prospective trial of steroid withdrawal in renal transplant recipients receiving basiliximab, cyclosporine microemulsion and mycophenolate mofetil. *Am. J. Transplant.* 2004;3: 306-311.

[7]   Borrows R, Loucaidou M, Van Tromp J, Cairns T, Griffith M, Hakim N, McLean A, Palmer A, Papalois V, Taube D: Steroid sparing with tacrolimus and mycophenolate mofetil in renal transplantation. *Am. J. Transplant.* 2004;4: 1845-1851.

[8]   Borrows R, Chan K, Loucaidou M, Lawrence C, Van Tromp J, Cairns T, Griffith M, Hakim N, McLean A, Palmer A, Papalois V, Taube D: Five years of Steroid Sparing in

renal transplantation with tacrolimus and mycophenolate mofetil *Transplantation.* 2006;1: 125-128.

[9]   Hocker B, John U, Plank C, Wuhl E, Weber LT, Misselwitz J, Rascher W, Mehls O, Tonshoff B. Successful withdrawal of steroids in pediatric renal transplant recipients receiving cyclosporine A and mycophenolate mofetil treatment: results after four years. *Transplantation.* 2004 Jul 27;78: 228-34.

[10]   Vanrenterghem Y, van Hooff JP, Squifflet JP, Salmela K, Rigotti P, Jindal RM, Pascual J, Ekberg H, Sicilia LS, Boletis JN, Grinyo JM, Rodriguez MA; European Tacrolimus/MMF Renal Transplantation Study Group: Minimization of immunosuppressive therapy after renal transplantation: results of a randomized controlled trial. *Am. J. Transplant.* 2005;5: 87-95.

[11]   Rostaing L, Cantarovich D, Budde K, Rigotti P, Mariat C,Margreiter R, Capdevilla L, Lang P, Vialtel P, Ortuno-Mirete J, Legendre C, Sanchez-Plumed J, Oppenheimer F, Kessler M; CARMEN Study Group. Corticosteroid-free immunosuppression with tacrolimus, mycophenolate mofetil, and daclizumab induction in renal transplantation. *Transplantation.* 2005; 79: 807-14.

[12]   Woodle ES, Vincenti F, Lorber MI, Gritsch HA, Hricik D, Washburn K, Matas AJ, Gallichio M, Neylan J: A multicenter pilot study of early (4-day) steroid cessation in renal transplant recipients under simulect, tacrolimus and sirolimus. *Am. J. Transplant.* 2005; 5: 157-166.

[13]   Kumar MSA, Heifets M, Moritz MI, Saaed MI, Khan SM, Fyfe B, Sustento-Riodeca N, Daniel JN, Kumar A: Safety and Efficacy of Steroids Withdrawal Two Days after Kidney Transplantation : Analysis of Results at Three Years. *Transplantation.* 2006; 81: 832-839.

[14]   Lemieux I, Houde I, Pascot A, Lachance JG, Noel R, Radeau T, Despres JP, Bergeron J: Effects of prednisone withdrawal on the new metabolic triad in cyclosporine-treated kidney transplant patients. *Kidney Int.* 2002; 62: 1839-1847.

[15]   Vanrenterghem Y, Lebranchu Y, Hene R, Oppenheimer F, Ekberg H: Double-blind comparison of two corticosteroid regimens plus mycophenolate mofetil and cyclosporine for prevention of acute renal allograft rejection. *Transplantation.* 2000; 70: 1352-1359.

[16]   Opelz G, Dohler B: Cyclosporine and long-term kidney graft survival. *Transplantation.* 2001; 72: 1267-73.

[17]   Hariharan S, Johnson CP, Bresnahan BA, Taranto SE, McIntosh MJ, Stablein D: Improved graft survival after renal transplantation in the United States, 1988 to 1996. *N. Engl. J. Med.* 2000; 342: 605-12.

[18]   Ojo AO, Held PJ, Port FK, Wolfe RA, Leichtman AB, Young EW, Arndorfer J, Christensen L, Merion RM: Chronic renal failure after transplantation of a nonrenal organ. *N. Engl. J. Med.* 2003; 349: 931-40.

[19]   Solez K, Vincenti F, Filo RS: Histopathologic findings from 2-year protocol biopsies from a U.S. multicenter kidney transplant trial comparing tacrolimus versus cyclosporine: a report of the FK506 Kidney Transplant Study Group. *Transplantation.* 1998; 66: 1736-40.

[20] Marcen R, Pascual J, Teruel JL, Villafruela JJ, Rivera ME, Mampaso F, Burgos FJ, Ortuno J: Outcome of cadaveric renal transplant patients treated for 10 years with cyclosporine: is chronic allograft nephropathy the major cause of late graft loss?. *Transplantation.* 2001;72: 57-62.

[21] Gallagher MP, Hall B, Craig J, Berry G, Tiller DJ, Eris J; Australian Multicenter Trial of Cyclosporine Withdrawal Study Group and the ANZ Dialysis and Transplantation Registry: A randomized controlled trial of cyclosporine withdrawal in renal-transplant recipients: 15-year results. *Transplantation.* 2004;78: 1653-60.

[22] Nankivell BJ, Borrows RJ, Fung CL, O'Connell PJ, Allen RD, Chapman JR: The natural history of chronic allograft nephropathy. N Engl J Med 2003;349: 2326-33.

[23] 23. Vincenti F: Immunosuppression minimization: current and future trends in transplant immunosuppression. *J. Am. Soc. Nephrol.* 2003; 14: 1940-8.

[24] Anjum S, Andany MA, McClean JC, Danielson B, Kasiske BL: Defining the risk of elective cyclosporine withdrawal in stable kidney transplant recipients. *Am. J. Transplant.* 2002; 2: 179-85.

[25] Grinyo JM, Cruzado JM, Millan O, Caldes A, Sabate I, Gil-Vernet S, Seron D, Brunet M, Campistol JM, Torras J, Martorell J: Low-dose cyclosporine with mycophenolate mofetil induces similar calcineurin activity and cytokine inhibition as does standard-dose cyclosporine in stable renal allografts. *Transplantation.* 2004; 78: 1400-3.

[26] MacPhee IA, Bradley JA, Briggs JD, Junor BJ, MacPherson SG, McMillan MA, Rodger RS, Watson MA: Long-term outcome of a prospective randomized trial of conversion from cyclosporine to azathioprine treatment one year after renal transplantation. *Transplantation.* 1998; 66: 1186-92.

[27] Dubey D, Kumar A, Srivastava A, Mandhani A, Sharma AP, Gupta A, Sharma RK: Cyclosporin A withdrawal in live related renal transplantation: long-term results. *Clin. Transplant.* 2001; 15: 136-41.

[28] Schnuelle P, van der Heide JH, Tegzess A, Verburgh CA, Paul LC, van der Woude FJ, de Fijter JW: Open randomized trial comparing early withdrawal of either cyclosporine or mycophenolate mofetil in stable renal transplant recipients initially treated with a triple drug regimen. *J. Am. Soc. Nephrol.* 2002; 13: 536-43.

[29] Smak Gregoor PJ, de Sevaux RG, Ligtenberg G, Hoitsma AJ, Hene RJ, Weimar W, Hilbrands LB, van Gelder T: Withdrawal of cyclosporine or prednisone six months after kidney transplantation in patients on triple drug therapy: a randomized, prospective, multicenter study. *J. Am. Soc. Nephrol.* 2002; 13: 1365-73.

[30] Abramowicz D, Manas D, Lao M, Vanrenterghem Y, Del Castillo D, Wijngaard P, Fung S; Cyclosporine Withdrawal Study Group: Cyclosporine withdrawal from a mycophenolate mofetil-containing immunosuppressive regimen in stable kidney transplant recipients: a randomized, controlled study. *Transplantation.* 2002; 74: 1725-34.

[31] Bakker RC, Hollander AA, Mallat MJ, Bruijn JA, Paul LC, de Fijter JW: Conversion from cyclosporine to azathioprine at three months reduces the incidence of chronic allograft nephropathy. *Kidney Int.* 2003; 64: 1027-34.

[32] Pascual M, Curtis J, Delmonico FL, Farrell ML, Williams WW Jr, Kalil R, Jones P, Cosimi AB, Tolkoff-Rubin N: A prospective, randomized clinical trial of cyclosporine

reduction in stable patients greater than 12 months after renal transplantation. *Transplantation.* 2003; 75: 1501-5.

[33] Kuypers DR, Evenepoel P, Maes B, Coosemans W, Pirenne J, Vanrenterghem Y: The use of an anti-CD25 monoclonal antibody and mycophenolate mofetil enables the use of a low-dose tacrolimus and early withdrawal of steroids in renal transplant recipients. *Clin. Transplant.* 2003; 17: 234-41.

[34] Baboolal K: A phase III prospective, randomized study to evaluate concentration-controlled sirolimus (rapamune) with cyclosporine dose minimization or elimination at six months in de novo renal allograft recipients. *Transplantation.* 2003; 75: 1404-8.

[35] Johnson RW, Kreis H, Oberbauer R, Brattstrom C, Claesson K, Eris J: Sirolimus allows early cyclosporine withdrawal in renal transplantation resulting in improved renal function and lower blood pressure. *Transplantation.* 2001; 72: 777-86.

[36] Gonwa TA, Hricik DE, Brinker K, Grinyo JM, Schena FP; Sirolimus Renal Function Study Group: Improved renal function in sirolimus-treated renal transplant patients after early cyclosporine elimination. *Transplantation.* 2002; 74: 1560-7.

[37] Oberbauer R, Kreis H, Johnson RW, Mota A, Claesson K, Ruiz JC, Wilczek H, Jamieson N, Henriques AC, Paczek L, Chapman J, Burke JT; Rapamune Maintenance Regimen Study Group: Long-term improvement in renal function with sirolimus after early cyclosporine withdrawal in renal transplant recipients: 2-year results of the Rapamune Maintenance Regimen Study. *Transplantation.* 2003; 76: 364-70.

[38] Kreis H, Oberbauer R, Campistol JM, Mathew T, Daloze P, Schena FP, Burke JT, Brault Y, Gioud-Paquet M, Scarola JA, Neylan JF; Rapamune Maintenance Regimen Trial: Long-term benefits with sirolimus-based therapy after early cyclosporine withdrawal. *J. Am. Soc. Nephrol.* 2004; 15: 809-17.

[39] Mota A, Arias M, Taskinen EI, Paavonen T, Brault Y, Legendre C, Claesson K, Castagneto M, Campistol JM, Hutchison B, Burke JT, Yilmaz S, Hayry P, Neylan JF; Rapamune Maintenance Regimen Trial: Sirolimus-based therapy following early cyclosporine withdrawal provides significantly improved renal histology and function at 3 years. *Am. J. Transplant.* 2004; 953-61.

[40] Ruiz JC, Campistol JM, Grinyo JM, Mota A, Prats D, Gutierrez JA, Henriques AC, Pinto JR, Garcia J, Morales JM, Gomez JM, Arias M: Early cyclosporine a withdrawal in kidney-transplant recipients receiving sirolimus prevents progression of chronic pathologic allograft lesions. *Transplantation.* 2004; 78: 1312-8.

[41] Oberbauer R, Segoloni G, Campistol JM, Kreis H, Mota A, Lawen J, Russ G, Grinyo JM, Stallone G, Hartmann A, Pinto JR, Chapman J, Burke JT, Brault Y, Neylan JF; Rapamune Maintenance Regimen Study Group: Early cyclosporine withdrawal from a sirolimus-based regimen results in better renal allograft survival and renal function at 48 months after transplantation. *Transpl. Int.* 2005; 18: 22-8.

[42] Hariharan S, McBride MA, Cherikh WS, Tolleris CB, Bresnahan BA, Johnson CP: Post-transplant renal function in the first year predicts long-term kidney transplant survival. *Kidney Int.* 2002; 62: 311-8.

[43] Siddiqi N, McBride MA, Hariharan S: Similar risk profiles for post-transplant renal dysfunction and long-term graft failure: UNOS/OPTN database analysis. *Kidney Int.* 004; 65: 1906-13.

[44] Kasiske BL, Andany MA, Hernandez D, Silkensen J, Rabb H, McClean J, Roel JP, Danielson B: Comparing methods for monitoring serum creatinine to predict late renal allograft failure. *Am. J. Kidney. Dis.* 2001; 38: 1065-73.

[45] Mulgaonkar S, Tedesco H, Oppenheimer F, Walker R, Kunzendorf U, Russ G, Knoflach A, PatelY, Fergunson R. FTYA121 study group. FTY720/Cyclosporine. Regimens in de novo renal transplantation: A 1-years dose-Finding Stady. *Am. J. Transplantation.* 2006; 6:1848-1857.

[46] Groth CG, Backman L, Morales JM, Calne R, Kreis H, Lang P, Touraine JL, Claesson K, Campistol JM, Durand D, Wramner L, Brattstrom C, Charpentier B: Sirolimus (rapamycin)-based therapy in human renal transplantation: similar efficacy and different toxicity compared with cyclosporine. Sirolimus European Renal Transplant Study Group. *Transplantation.* 1999; 67: 1036-42.

[47] Kreis H, Cisterne JM, Land W, Wramner L, Squifflet JP, Abramowicz D, Campistol JM, Morales JM, Grinyo JM, Mourad G, Berthoux FC, Brattstrom C, Lebranchu Y, Vialtel P. Sirolimus in association with mycophenolate mofetil induction for the prevention of acute graft rejection in renal allograft recipients. *Transplantation.* 2000; 69: 1252-60.

[48] Tran HT, Acharya MK, McKay DB, Sayegh MH, Carpenter CB, Auchincloss H JR, Kirkman RL, Milford EL: Avoidance of cyclosporine in renal transplantation: effects of daclizumab, mycophenolate mofetil, and steroids. *J. Am. Soc. Nephrol.* 2000; 11: 1903-9.

[49] Vincenti F, Ramos E, Brattstrom C, Cho S, Ekberg H, Grinyo J, Johnson R, Kuypers D, Stuart F, Khanna A, Navarro M, Nashan B: Multicenter trial exploring calcineurin inhibitors avoidance in renal transplantation. *Transplantation.* 2000; 71: 1282-7.

[50] Flechner SM, Goldfarb D, Modlin C, Feng J, Krishnamurthi V, Mastroianni B, Savas K, Cook DJ, Novick AC: Kidney transplantation without calcineurin inhibitor drugs: a prospective, randomized trial of sirolimus versus cyclosporine. *Transplantation.* 2002; 74: 1070-76.

[51] Grinyo JM, Gil-Vernet S, Cruzado JM, Caldes A, Riera L, Seron D, Rama I, Torras J: Calcineurin inhibitor-free immunosuppression based on antithymocyte globulin and mycophenolate mofetil in cadaveric kidney transplantation: results after 5 years. *Transpl. Int.* 2003; 16: 820-7.

[52] Lo A, Egidi MF, Gaber LW, Amiri HS, Vera S, Nezakatgoo N, Gaber AO: Comparison of sirolimus-based calcineurin inhibitor-sparing and calcineurin inhibitor-free regimens in cadaveric renal transplantation. *Transplantation.* 2004; 77: 1228-35.

[53] Larson T.S, Dean P.G, Stegall M.D, Griffin M.D,Textor.S.C, Schwab T.R,Gloor.J.M,Cosio F.G,Lund W.J, Kremwers W.K, Nyberg.S.L, Ishitani. M.B, Prieto M, Velosa J.A. Complete avoidance of calcineurin inhibitors in renal transplantation: A randomized trial comparing Sirolimus and Tacrolimus. *Am. J. Transplantation.* 2006; 6: 514-522.

[54] Vincenti F, Larsen C, Durbac A, et al for The Belatacept Study Group. Coestimulation Blockade with Belatacept in Renal Transplantation. *NEJM.* 2005; 353:770-781.

[55] Flechner SM, Kurian SM, Solez K, Cook DJ, Burke JT, Rollin H, Hammond JA, Whisenant T, Lanigan CM, Head SR, Salomon DR: De novo kidney transplantation

without use of calcineurin inhibitors preserves renal structure and function at two years. *Am. J. Transplant.* 2004; 4: 1776-85.

[56] Cole E, Maham N, Cardella C, Cattran D, Fenton S, Hamel J, O'Grady C, Smith R: Clinical benefits of neoral C2 monitoring in the long-term management of renal transplant recipients. *Transplantation.* 2003; 75: 2086-90.

[57] Di Paolo S, Teutonico A, Schena A, Infante B, Stallone G, Grandaliano G, Ditonno P, Battaglia M, Schena FP: Conversion to C2 monitoring of cyclosporine A exposure in maintenance kidney transplant recipients: results at 3 years. *Am. J. Kidney Dis.* 2004; 44:886-92.

[58] Hardinger KL, Schnitzler MA, Koch MJ, Enkvetchakul D, Desai N, Jendrisak M, Lowell JA, Miller B, Shenoy S, Brennan DC: Cyclosporine minimization and cost reduction in renal transplant recipients receiving a C2-monitored, cyclosporine-based quadruple immunosuppressive regimen. *Transplantation.* 2004; 78: 1198-203.

[59] Vincenti F, Jensik SC, Filo RS, Miller J, Pirsch J: A long-term comparison of tacrolimus (FK506) and cyclosporine in kidney transplantation: evidence for improved allograft survival at five years. *Transplantation.* 2002; 73: 775-82.

[60] Gonwa T, Johnson C, Ahsan N, Alfrey EJ, Halloran P, Stegall M, Hardy M, Metzger R, Shield C 3rd, Rocher L, Scandling J, Sorensen J, Mulloy L, Light J, Corwin C, Danovitch G, Wachs M, VanVeldhuisen P, Leonhardt M, Fitzsimmons WE: Randomized trial of tacrolimus + mycophenolate mofetil or azathioprine versus cyclosporine + mycophenolate mofetil after cadaveric kidney transplantation: results at three years. *Transplantation.* 2003; 75: 2048-53.

[61] Pascual J, Segoloni G, Gonzalez Molina M, del Castillo D, Capdevila L, Arias M, Garcia J, Ortuno J; Spanish-Italian Tacrolimus Study Group: Comparison between a two-drug regimen with tacrolimus and steroids and a triple one with azathioprine in kidney transplantation: results of a European trial with 3-year follow up. *Transplant. Proc.* 2003; 35: 1701-3.

[62] Meier M, Nitschke M, Weidtmann B, Jabs WJ, Wong W, Suefke S, Steinhoff J, Fricke L: Slowing the Progresion of Chronic Allograft Nephropathy by Conversion from Cyclosporine to Tacrolimus: A Randomized Controlled Trial. *Transplantation.* 2006; 81: 1035-1040.

[63] Kaplan B, Schold JD, Meier-Kriesche HU: Long-term graft survival with neoral and tacrolimus: a paired kidney analysis. *J. Am. Soc. Nephrol.* 14: 2980-4, 2003.

[64] Gill JS, Tonelli M, Mix CH, Johnson N, Pereira BJ: The effect of maintenance immunosuppression medication on the change in kidney allograft function. *Kidney Int.* 2004; 65: 692-9.

[65] Pascual J, Marcen R, Burgos FJ, Tenorio MT, Merino JL, Arambarri M, Villafruela JJ, Liano F, Mampaso F, Ortuno J: One-center comparison between primary immunosuppression based on neoral cyclosporine and tacrolimus for renal transplantation. *Transplant. Proc.* 2002; 34: 94-5.

[66] Neu AM, Ho PL, Fine RN, Furth SL, Fivush BA: Tacrolimus vs. cyclosporine A as primary immunosuppression in pediatric renal transplantation: a NAPRTCS study. *Pediatr. Transplant.* 2003; 7: 217-22.

[67] Jurewicz WA: Tacrolimus versus cyclosporin immunosuppression: long-term outcome in renal transplantation. *Nephrol. Dial. Transplant.* 2003; 18 (Suppl 1): 17-11.

[68] Meier-Kriesche HU, Kaplan B: Cyclosporine microemulsion and tacrolimus are associated with decreased chronic allograft failure and improved long-term graft survival as compared with sandimmune. *Am. J. Transplant.* 2002; 2: 100-4.

[69] Irish W, Sherrill B, Brennan DC, Lowell J, Schnitzler M: Three-year posttransplant graft survival in renal-transplant patients with graft function at 6 months receiving tacrolimus or cyclosporine microemulsion within a triple-drug regimen. *Transplantation.* 2003; 76: 1686-90.

[70] Margreiter R; European Tacrolimus vs Ciclosporin Microemulsion Renal Transplantation Study Group: Efficacy and safety of tacrolimus compared with ciclosporin microemulsion in renal transplantation: a randomised multicentre study. *Lancet.* 2002; 359: 741-6.

[71] Offermann G: Immunosuppression for long-term maintenance of renal allograft function. *Drugs.* 2004; 64: 1325-38.

[72] Khanna A, Plummer M, Bromberek C, Bresnahan B, Hariharan S: Expression of TGF-beta and fibrogenic genes in transplant recipients with tacrolimus and cyclosporine nephrotoxicity. *Kidney Int.* 2002; 62: 2257-63.

[73] McCune TR, Thacker LR II, Peters TG, Mulloy L, Rohr MS, Adams PA, Yium J, Light JA, Pruett T, Gaber AO, Selman SH, Jonsson J, Hayes JM, Wright FH Jr, Armata T, Blanton J, Burdick JF: Effects of tacrolimus on hyperlipidemia after successful renal transplantation: a Southeastern Organ Procurement Foundation multicenter clinical study. *Transplantation.* 1998; 65: 87-92.

[74] Ligtenberg G, Hene RJ, Blankestijn PJ, Koomans HA: Cardiovascular risk factors in renal transplant patients: cyclosporin A versus tacrolimus. *J. Am. Soc. Nephrol.* 2001; 12: 368-73.

[75] Baid-Agrawal S, Delmonico FL, Tolkoff-Rubin NE, Farrell M, Williams WW, Shih V, Auchincloss H, Cosimi AB, Pascual M: Cardiovascular risk profile after conversion from cyclosporine A to tacrolimus in stable renal transplant recipients. *Transplantation.* 2004; 77: 1199-202.

[76] Artz MA, Boots JM, Ligtenberg G, Roodnat JI, Christiaans MH, Vos PF, Blom HJ, Sweep FC, Demacker PN, Hilbrands LB: Improved cardiovascular risk profile and renal function in renal transplant patients after randomized conversion from cyclosporine to tacrolimus. *J. Am. Soc. Nephrol.* 2003; 14: 1880-8.

[77] Mas V, Alvarellos T, Giraudo C, Massari P, De Boccardo G: Intragraft messenger RNA expression of angiotensinogen: relationship with transforming growth factor beta-1 and chronic allograft nephropathy in kidney transplant patients. *Transplantation.* 2002; 74: 718-21.

[78] European Mycophenolate Mofetil Cooperative Study Group: Mycophenolate mofetil in renal transplantation: 3-year results from the placebo-controlled trial. *Transplantation.* 1999; 68: 391-6.

[79] US Renal Transplant Mycophenolate Mofetil Study Group:Mycophenolate mofetil in cadaveric renal transplantation. *Am. J. Kidney Dis.* 1999; 34: 296-303.

[80] Mathew TH: A blinded, long-term, randomized multicenter study of mycophenolate mofetil in cadaveric renal transplantation: results at three years. Tricontinental Mycophenolate Mofetil Renal Transplantation Study Group. *Transplantation.* 1998; 65: 1450-4.

[81] Ojo AO, Meier-Kriesche HU, Hanson JA, Leichtman AB, Cibrik D, Magee JC, Wolfe RA, Agodoa LY, Kaplan B: Mycophenolate mofetil reduces late renal allograft loss independent of acute rejection. *Transplantation.* 2000; 69: 2405-9.

[82] Meier-Kriesche HU, Steffen BJ, Hochberg AM, Gordon RD, Liebman MN, Morris JA, Kaplan B: Mycophenolate mofetil versus azathioprine therapy is associated with a significant protection against long-term renal allograft function deterioration. *Transplantation.* 2003; 75: 1341-6.

[83] Merville P, Berge F, Deminiere C, Morel D, Chong G, Durand D, Rostaing L, Mourad G, Potaux L: Lower incidence of chronic allograft nephropathy at 1 year post-transplantation in patients treated with mycophenolate mofetil. *Am. J. Transplant.* 2004; 4: 1769-75.

[84] David KM, Morris JA, Steffen BJ, Chi-Burris KS, Gotz VP, Gordon RD. Mycophenolate mofetil vs. azathioprine is associated with decreased acute rejection, late acute rejection, and risk for cardiovascular death in renal transplant recipients with pre-transplant diabetes. *Clin. Transplant.* 2005; 19:279-85.

[85] Yang CW, Ahn HJ, Kim WY, Li C, Kim HW, Choi BS, Cha JH, Kim YS, Kim J, Bang BK: Cyclosporine withdrawal and mycophenolate mofetil treatment effects on the progression of chronic cyclosporine nephrotoxicity. *Kidney Int.* 2002; 62: 20-30.

[86] Jolicoeur EM, Qi S, Xu D, Dumont L, Daloze P, Chen H: Combination therapy of mycophenolate mofetil and rapamycin in prevention of chronic renal allograft rejection in the rat. *Transplantation.* 2003; 75: 54-9.

[87] Weir MR, Ward MT, Blahut SA, Klassen DK, Cangro CB, Bartlett ST, Fink JC: Long-term impact of discontinued or reduced calcineurin inhibitor in patients with chronic allograft nephropathy. *Kidney Int.* 2001; 59: 1567-73.

[88] Ducloux D, Motte G, Billerey C, Bresson-Vautrin C, Vautrin P, Rebibou JM, Saint-Hillier Y, Chalopin JM: Cyclosporin withdrawal with concomitant conversion from azathioprine to mycophenolate mofetil in renal transplant recipients with chronic allograft nephropathy: a 2-year follow-up. *Transpl. Int.* 2002; 15: 387-92.

[89] Gonzalez Molina M, Seron D, Garcia del Moral R, Carrera M, Sola E, Jesus Alferez M, Gomez Ullate P, Capdevila L, Gentil MA: Mycophenolate mofetil reduces deterioration of renal function in patients with chronic allograft nephropathy. A follow-up study by the Spanish Cooperative Study Group of Chronic Allograft Nephropathy. *Transplantation.* 2004; 77: 215-20.

[90] Dudley C, Pohanka E, Riad H, Dedochova J, Wijngaard P, Sutter C, Silva HT JrMycophenolate mofetil substitution for cyclosporine in a renal transplant recipients with chronic progressive allograft dysfunction: the "creeping creatinine" stady. *Transplantation.* 2005; 79: 466-75.

[91] Kahan BD: Efficacy of sirolimus compared with azathioprine for reduction of acute renal allograft rejection: a randomised multicentre study. The Rapamune US Study Group. *Lancet.* 2000; 356:194-202.

[92] Kahan BD, Julian BA, Pescovitz MD, Vanrenterghem Y, Neylan J: Sirolimus reduces the incidence of acute rejection episodes despite lower cyclosporine doses in caucasian recipients of mismatched primary renal allografts: a phase II trial. Rapamune Study Group. *Transplantation.* 1999; 68: 1526-32.

[93] Halloran PF: Immunosuppressive drugs for kidney transplantation. *N. Engl. J. Med.* 2004; 351: 2715-29.

[94] Ikonen TS, Gummert JF, Hayase M, Honda Y, Hausen B, Christians U, Berry GJ, Yock PG, Morris RE: Sirolimus (rapamycin) halts and reverses progression of allograft vascular disease in non-human primates. *Transplantation.* 2000; 70: 969-75.

[95] Shihab FS, Bennett WM, Yi H, Choi SO, Andoh TF: Sirolimus increases transforming growth factor-beta1 expression and potentiates chronic cyclosporine nephrotoxicity. *Kidney Int.* 2004; 65: 1262-71.

[96] Podder H, Stepkowski SM, Napoli KL, Clark J, Verani RR, Chou TC y cols: Pharmacokinetic interactions augment toxicities of sirolimus/cyclosporine combinations. *J. Am. Soc. Nephrol.* 2001; 12: 1059-1071.

[97] Saunders RN, Bicknell GR, Nicholson ML: The impact of cyclosporine dose reduction with or without the addition of rapamycin on functional, molecular, and histological markers of chronic allograft nephropathy. *Transplantation.* 2003; 75: 772-80.

[98] Kaplan B, Schold J, Srinivas T, Womer K, Foley DP, Patton P, Howard R, Meier-Kriesche HU: Effect of sirolimus withdrawal in patients with deteriorating renal function. *Am. J. Transplant.* 2004; 4: 1709-12.

[99] Webster AC, Lee VWS, Chapman JR, Craig JC: Target of Rapamycin Inhibitors (Sirolimus and Everolimus) for Primary Immunosuppression of Kidney Transplant Recipients: A Systematic Review and Meta-Analysis of Randomized Trials. *Transplantation.* 2006; 81: 1234-1248.

[100] Stallone G, Di Paolo S, Schena A, Infante B, Grandaliano G, Battaglia M, Gesualdo L, Schena FP: Early withdrawal of cyclosporine A improves 1-year kidney graft structure and function in sirolimus-treated patients. *Transplantation.* 2003; 75: 998-1003.

[101] Diekmann F, Budde K, Oppenheimer F, Fritsche L, Neumayer HH, Campistol JM: Predictors of success in conversion from calcineurin inhibitor to sirolimus in chronic allograft dysfunction. *Am. J. Transplant.* 2004; 4: 1869-75.

[102] Lutz J, Zou H, Liu S, Antus B, Heemann U: Apoptosis and treatment of chronic allograft nephropathy with everolimus. *Transplantation.* 2003; 76: 508-15.

[103] McMullen JR,Sherwood MC, Tarnavski O, Zhang L, Dorfman AL, Shioi T, Izumo S. Inhibition of mTOR signaling with rapamycin regresses established cardiac hypertrophy induced by pressure overload._*Circulation.* 2004;109:3050-5.

[104] Elloso MM, Azrolan N, Sehgal SN, Hsu PL, Phiel KL, Kopec CA, Basso MD, Adelman SJ. Protective effect of the immunosuppressant sirolimus against aortic atherosclerosis in apo E-deficient mice. *Am. J. Transplant.* 2003; 3:562-9.

[105] Nickeleit V, Klimkait T, Binet IF, Dalquen P, Del Zenero V, Thiel G, Mihatsch MJ, Hirsch HH: Testing for polyomavirus type BK DNA in plasma to identify renal-allograft recipients with viral nephropathy. *N. Engl. J. Med.* 2000; 342: 1309-15.

[106] Hirsch HH, Knowles W, Dickenmann M, Passweg J, Klimkait T, Mihatsch MJ, Steiger J: Prospective Study of Polyomavirus Type BK Replication and Nephropathy in Renal-Transplant Recipients. *N. Engl. J. Med.* 2002; 347: 488-96.

[107] Gupta M, Miller F, Nord EP, Wadhwa NK. Delayed renal allograft dysfunction and cystitis associated with human polyomavirus (BK) infection in a renal transplant recipient: a case report and review of literature. *Clin. Nephrol.* 2003; 60:405-414.

[108] Nickeleit V, Hirsch HH, Zeiler M, Gudat F, Prince O, Thiel G, Mihatsch MJ: BK-virus nephropathy in renal transplants-tubular necrosis, MHC-class II expression and rejection in a puzzling game. *Nephrol. Dial. Transplant.* 2000; 15:324-32.

[109] Barri YM, Ahmad I, Ketel BL, Barone GW, Walker PD, Bonsib SM, Abul-Ezz SR: Polyoma viral infection in renal transplantation: the role of immunosuppressive therapy. *Clin. Transplant.* 2001; 15:240-6.

[110] Ramos E, Drachenberg CB, Papadimitriou JC, Hamze O, Fink JC, Klassen DK, Drachenberg RC, Wiland A, Wali R, Cangro CB, Schweitzer E, Bartlett ST, Weir MR: Clinical course of polyoma virus nephropathy in 67 renal transplant patients. *J. Am. Soc. Nephrol.* 2002; 13:2145-51.

[111] Brennan DC, Agha I, Bohl DL, Schnitzler MA, Hardinger KL, Lockwood M, Torrence S, Schuessler R, Roby T, Gaudreault-Keener M, Storch GA: Incidence of BK with tacrolimus versus cyclosporine and impact of preemptive immunosuppression reduction. *Am. J. Transplant.* 2005; 5:582-94.

[112] Awadalla Y, Randhawa P, Ruppert K, Zeevi A, Duquesnoy RJ: HLA mismatching increases the risk of BK virus nephropathy in renal transplant recipients. *Am. J. Transplant.* 2004; 4:1691-6.

[113] Ding R, Medeiros M, Dadhania D, Muthukumar T, Kracker D, Kong JM, Epstein SR, Sharma VK, Seshan SV, Li B, Suthanthiran M: Noninvasive diagnosis of BK virus nephritis by measurement of messenger RNA for BK virus VP1 in urine1 *Transplantation.* 2002; 74: 987-994.

[114] Hariharan S, Cohen EP, Vasudev B, Orentas R, Viscidi RP, Kakela J, DuChateau B: BK Virus-Specific Antibodies and BKV DNA in Renal Transplant Recipients with BKV Nephritis. *Am. J. Transplant.* 2005; 5;2719-2724.

[115] Wali RK, Drachenberg C, Hirsch HH, Papadimitriou J, Nahar A, Mohanlal V, Brisco MA, Bartlett ST, Weir MR, Ramos E: BK virus-associated nephropathy in renal allograft recipients: rescue therapy by sirolimus-based immunosuppression. *Transplantation.* 2004; 78: 1069-73.

[116] Farasati NA, Shapiro R, Vats A, Randhawa P: Effect of leflunomide and cidofovir on replication of BK virus in an in vitro culture system. *Transplantation.* 2005; 79: 116-8.

[117] Senner A, House AA, Jevnikar AM, Boudville N, McAlister VC, Muirhead N, Rehman F, Luke PPW: Intravenous Immunoglobulin as a Treatment for BK Virus Asociated Nephropathy: One Year Follow Up of Renal Allograft Recipients. *Transplantation.* 2006; 81: 117-120.

[118] Brennan DC, Agha I, Bohl DL,Schnitzler MA, Hardinger KL, Lockwood M, Torrence S, Schuessler R, Roby T, Gaudreault-Keener M, Storch GA: Incidence of BK with Tacrolimus Versus Cyclosporine and Impact of Preemptive Immunosuppression Reduction. *Am. J. Transplant.* 2005; 5:582-594.

[119] Womera KL, Meier-Kriesche HU, Patton PR, Dibadj K, Bucci CM, Foley D,Fujita S, Croker BP, Howard RJ, Srinivas TR, Kaplan B: Preemptive Retransplantation for BK Virus Nephropathy: Successful Outcome Despite Active Viremia. *Am. J. Transplant.* 2006; 6:209-213.

[120] Kasiske BL, Snyder JJ, Gilbertson DT, Wang C: Cancer after kidney transplantation in the United States. *Am. J. Transplant.* 2004; 4:905-13.

[121] Morath C, Mueller M, Goldschmidt H, Schwenger V, Opelz G, Zeier M: Malignancy in renal transplantation. *J. Am. Soc. Nephrol.* 2004; 15: 1582-8.

[122] Koehl GE, Andrassy J, Guba M, Richter S, Kroemer A, Scherer MN, Steinbauer M, Graeb C, Schlitt HJ, Jauch KW, Geissler EK: Rapamycin protects allografts from rejection while simultaneously attacking tumors in immunosuppressed mice. *Transplantation.* 2004; 77: 1319-26.

[123] Campistol JM, Gutierrez-Dalmau A, Torregrosa JV: Conversion to sirolimus: a successful treatment for posttransplantation Kaposi's sarcoma. *Transplantation.* 2004; 77: 760-2.

[124] Stallone G, Schena A, Infante B, Di Paolo S, Loverre A, Maggio G, Ranieri E, Gesualdo L, Schena FP, Grandaliano G. *N. Engl. J. Med.* 2005;352:1317-23.

[125] Campistol JM, Eris J, Oberbauer R, Friend P, Hutchinson B, Morales JM, Claesson K, Stallone G, Russ G, Rostaing L, Kreis H, Burke JT, Brault Y, Scarola JA, Neylan JF: Sirolimus therapy after Early Cyclosporine Withdrawal Reduces the Risk for Cancer in Adult Renal Transplantation. *J. Am. Soc. Nephrol.* 2006; 7:581-589.

[126] Kasiske BL, Cangro CB, Hariharan S, Hricik DE, Kerman RH, Roth D, Rush DN, Vazquez MA, Weir MR; American Society of Transplantation: The evaluation of renal transplantation candidates: clinical practice guidelines. *Am. J. Transplant.* 2001;1 (Suppl 2):3-95.

[127] Moreso F, Ortega F, Mendiluce A. Recipient age as a determinant factor of patient and graft survival. *Nephrol. Dial. Transplant.* 2004; 19 (Suppl 3): iii16-20.

[128] Meier-Kriesche HU, Ojo AO, Cibrik DM, Hanson JA, Leichtman AB, Magee JC, Port FK, Kaplan B. Relationship of recipient age and development of chronic allograft failure. *Transplantation.* 2000; 70:306-10.

[129] Kasiske BL, Snyder J. Matching older kidneys with older patients does not improve allograft survival. *J. Am. Soc. Nephrol.* 2002; 13: 1067-72.

[130] Remuzzi G, Cravedi P, Perna A, Dimitrov BD, Turturro M, Locatelli G, Rigotti P, Baldan N, Beatini M, Valente U, Scalamogna M, Ruggenenti P; Dual Kidney Transplant Group: Long-term outcome of renal transplantation from older donors. *N. Engl. J. Med.* 2006; 354: 343-52.

[131] Lo A, Egidi MF, Gaber LW, Amiri HS, Vera S, Nezakatgoo N, Gaber AO. Comparison of sirolimus-based calcineurin inhibitor-sparing and calcineurin inhibitor-free regimens in cadaveric renal transplantation. *Transplantation.* 2004; 77: 1228-35.

[132] Grinyo JM, Gil-Vernet S, Cruzado JM, Caldes A, Riera L, Seron D, Rama I, Torras J. Calcineurin inhibitor-free immunosuppression based on antithymocyte globulin and mycophenolate mofetil in cadaveric kidney transplantation: results after 5 years. *Transpl. Int.* 2003; 16: 820-7.

[133] Osuna A, Gentil MA, Capdevila L, Cantarell C, Mazuecos A, Periera P, Rodriguez-Algarra G, Alarcón A, Sánchez-Plumed J, González-Molina M. Delayed introduction of low dose tacrolimus with daclizumab and mycophenolate mofetil in elderly recipients of cadaveric renal transplant from donors over 55 years of age. *Am. J. Transplant.* 2005; 5 (Suppl. 11): 460.

In: Transplantation Immunology Research Trends   ISBN: 978-1-60021-578-0
Editor: Oliver N. Ulricker, pp. 183-201   © 2007 Nova Science Publishers, Inc.

Chapter VII

Study of Proliferation Response of the HLA-DQB1*0302 Molecule Associated to Acute Rejection Development in Liver Transplant and Soluble HLA Class I Depletion

Manuel Muro, Luis Marin, Rosa Moya,
Alfredo Minguela and Rocío Álvarez-López
Immunology Service, University Hospital Virgen Arrixaca, Murcia 30120, Spain.

Abstract

Previous studies including those of our group have demonstrated that pre-transplant serum soluble HLA (sHLA-I) class I levels and the presence of HLA-DQB1*0302 allele in liver recipients are different factors implicated in acute rejection development. Indeed, this HLA allele is related to several autoimmune diseases and could be implicated in an increased alloreactivity state in determined individuals.

Our objective was to investigate the proliferation response of different HLA-DQB1 molecules with and without allogeneic sera sHLA depletion.

We examined the primary (MLR-I, mixed lymphocyte reaction) and secondary (MLR-II) proliferation response from individuals with different matching and mismatching HLA-DQ combinations in situations of sHLA molecules depletion in cellular cultures.

Sera soluble HLA class I molecules depletion was performed by ligation of the HLA class I antibody (IgG2a isotype, w6.32 clone) to Sepharose 4B gel and treatment of human sera samples, as previously published. Cellular cultures were performed by unidirectional primary MLR-I (5 days) and secondary MLR-II (re-stimulated at 5 days) by using allogeneic and autologous responder cells and irradiated stimulator cells (EBV-transformed lymphoblastoid lines) in allogeneic and autologous HLA-DQB1 specific combinations (presence or absence of HLA-DQB1*0302).

The relative response of HLA-DQB1*0302$^+$ lymphocytes in primary MLR-I, when the stimulator cells were semiallogeneic or incompatibles, did not show an increased proliferation, in situations of absence or presence of sHLA-I molecules.

However, in secondary MLR-II (primed responder cell against stimulator cell), we detected an increased relative response in situation of absence of allogeneic sHLA and using semiallogeneic HLA-DQB1*0302$^+$ cells. This result was not obtained with HLA-DQB1*0302$^-$ cells were used.

In conclusion, these data indicate that, in a primary response the different tested combinations show a similar manner to respond, but in the secondary response, when the responder cells have been primed and sensibilized, sHLA molecules plays a different role in proliferation response depending to specific HLA-DQ molecules constitution.

Introduction

Both cellular and humoral immunologic mechanisms are involved in the spontaneous tolerance observed in liver allograft transplant [Gonwa et al., 1988; Mor et al., 1992; Rassmussen et al., 1995], among them the functional inactivation of donor-reactive cells and the blockage of donor specific cytotoxic T lymphocytes (CTL) [Alters et al., 1991; Dalman et al., 1991, 1993]. Some studies have also found that the liver is the major producer of soluble HLA class-I (sHLA-I) and liver recipients present an increased quantity in the post-transplant evolution [Rhynes et al., 1993; Mcdonald et al., 1994, 1998]. Indeed, it could exist an association of serum concentrations of sHLA-I molecules with HLA allotypes [Chauchan et al., 1995; Adamashvili et al., 1996]. However, the function of sHLA antigens in the process of immunoregulation and especially in graft tolerance versus rejection has not been established, as appointed in other soluble markers [Weimer et al., 2006; Filg et al., 1990]. These molecules appear to be important natural immunoregulatory factors in vivo capable of inducing donor specific tolerance by inhibiting recipient cytotoxic response [Krensky et al., 1994]. In this sense, it has been suggested that donor-derived sHLA may exert an immunotolerant influence on the allograft [Chudyk et al., 2006]. In addition, it has also been suggested that acute rejection process induces a strong up-regulation of membrane HLA class-I both on hepatocytes and bile duct epithelia of the grafted liver [Steinhoff et al., 1988; Rouger et al., 1990; Nocera et al., 1991] and also that there is considerable increase in serum sHLA-I molecules levels [Puppo et al., 1994, 1995].

On the other hand, the genetic status of liver recipient could also play a role in the capacity to respond against allograft, as suggested in several solid organ transplants [Hendricks et al., 1983; Dyer et al., 1985; Cook et al., 1989] and in liver allograft transplants in particular [Superina et al., 1989; Doran et al., 1992, 2000]. In this sense, HLA-DQ molecules have also been implicated on organ transplant outcome [Matsuno et al., 1990; Tong et al., 1993].

Indeed, previous studies including those of our research group have demonstrated that pre-transplant sHLA-I molecules levels and the presence of the HLA-DQB1*0302 allele in liver allograft recipients are different factors implicated on acute rejection episodes development [Muro et al., 1997, 2001; Minguela et al., 1999, 2000]. Indeed, this HLA class II allele is widely related to several viral, autoimmune and inflammatory diseases and could be implicated in an increased alloreactivity state in determined susceptible individuals [Sairinji *et al.*, 1991; Thorsby *et al.*, 1993; Todd *et al.*, 1993; Lundin *et al.*, 1994; Rowe *et al.*, 1994; She *et al.*, 1996; Zhang *et al.*, 1998; Sollid, 2000). This observed association was not demonstrated for other HLA class I and class II genes (HLA-A, -B, -C and HLA-DRB1, -DQA1 and –DPB1) [Muro *et al.*, 1997, 2002; Ontañón *et al.*, 1998; Moya-Quiles *et al.*, 2003]. Indeed, it was also independent of linkage disequilibrium with other neighbouring or close genes [Muro *et al.*, 1997] and the genetic polymorphism found and analyzed in its promoter region [Muro *et al.*, 2001], whose Collaborative International Study was also performed by our group [Reichstetter *et al.*, 1997]. In this sense, our hypothesis was that whether HLA class I peptides could be recognised by indirect pathway preferently on HLA-DQB1*0302 molecules. This indirect allorecognition of MHC allopeptides has been reported in other solid organ transplants [Benichou *et al.* 1992; Vella *et al.*, 1997].

Thus, our objective was to investigate the proliferation response of different HLA-DQB1 molecules with and without allogeneic sera sHLA molecules depletion.

Materials and Methods

We intend to establish an *in vitro* model of study stimulating allogenecally positive HLA-DQB1*0302 cells in cultures supplemented with human pool sera and this same sera with depleted sHLA class I molecules. Thus, we examined the primary (MLR-I, mixed lymphocyte reaction) and secondary (MLR-II) proliferation responses from individuals with different matching and mismatching HLA-DQB1 combinations in situations of sHLA molecules depletion in cellular proliferation cultures.

Donors gave written informed consent to the collection and storage of blood, isolation of DNA, and determination of HLA polymorphisms and cellular cultures. Indeed, the study was approved by the local medical committee.

HLA Typing

HLA class I and class II typing was performed by using a standard complement dependent cytotoxicity (CDC) assay and also DNA-based methods [Muro *et al.*, 2002, Marin *et al.*, 2005, 2006; Botella *et al.*, 2006]. Briefly, subjects were typed for HLA-A and –B antigens and the sera used for antigen determination were either generated in our centre (well-defined local antisera), supplied by participant laboratories of Spanish Histocompatibility Workshops and well-defined commercial sera, or commercial typing trays (One Lambda Inc, Los Angeles, CA). Genomic DNA was extracted from peripheral blood leukocytes with standard techniques based on digestion with proteinase K (Boehringer Mannheim, Mannheim, Germany), as previously published [Muro *et al.*, 1997]. HLA-DRB1 and -DQB1 alleles were typed by PCR-sequence-specific oligonucleotide probing, which involves genomic amplification of DRB1 and DQB1 gene sequences and a panel of digoxigenin-labeled oligonucleotide probes for allelic definition, as previously published

[Muro *et al.*, 1997, 2001]. The amplification reactions were carried out in a Thermal Cycler 9700 (Perkin-Elmer, Cetus Instruments, Norwalk, CT).

Serum sHLA Depletion

Sera soluble HLA class I molecules depletion was performed by binding of the HLA class I antibody to sepharose 4B gel and treatment of human sera samples, as previously published [Brieva *et al.*, 1990; Ferreira *et al.*, 1991]. Briefly, a monomorphyc anti-HLA class I antibody (IgG2a isotype, w6.32 clone) was linked to sepharose 4B gel (Amershan Pharmacia Biotech, Buckinghamshire, UK). Working concentration was 5 mg of the HLA antibody w6.32/mililiter of sepharose 4B [Escobar *et al.*, 1996; Nocito *et al.*, 1997]. This antibody was gently given by our colleagues from the University Hospital 'Ramon y Cajal' from Madrid (Spain).

One mililiter of target sera containing sHLA molecules was diluted ½ with phosphate buffer solution (BioMériux, Marci l'Etoile, France), and mixed to 5 µl of sepharose 4B+antibody w6.32 in continuous orbital shaking for 2 hours at 4°C. Later, treated samples were centrifuged at 5000 G for 2 minutes at 4°C. Supernatants were recovered to continue our cellular experiments. Autologous and allogeneic sera (pool of 50 donors from Blood Bank of our university hospital) were used on proliferation cultures.

EBV-Transformation of Stimulator Cells

Stimulator cells were transformed by Einsptein-Barr virus (EBV), using derived supernatants of the cellular line B95-8 (EBV particles releasing). B95-8 line was cultured for 7 days in 24-well plates (Costar, Cambridge, MA) (0.5×10^6 cells in 1 ml/well) (Coulter T-540, Northwell Drive, UK) in a humidified atmosphere in the presence of 5% CO_2 on medium HT containing DMEM medium buffered with hepes at 20 mM (Biochrom, Cambridge, UK) and supplemented with NCTC135 at 10% (Flow Laboratories, Irvine, UK), fetal calf sera at 20% (GibcoBRL, Life Technologies, Scotland), gentamicine at 50 µg/ml (Biochrom), L-glutamine at 4 mM (Biochrom), hypoxanthine (Flow Laboratories), at 100 µM and thymidine at 16 µM (Sigma Chemical, St Louis, MO). EBV supernatants were centrifuged at 700 G for 10 minutes and filtered on 0.45 µm filters. These EBV-supernatants were diluted at 1/3 in culture medium and mixed with the target lymphocytes in HT medium supplemented with 2 µg/ml of cyclosporine (CsA, Sandoz, Basel, Switzerland) at 0.75×10^6 cells/ml. Cultures were incubated for 8 days and adding fresh HT+CsA medium each 3-4 days until colonies formation was patent [Muro *et al.*, 2002]. Two lines were selected corresponding to spleen cells of liver allograft donors with the following HLA phenotype: B98 (A23, -; B44, 61; DRB1*04, -; DQB1*0302, -) and B249 (A29, 30; B8, 18; DRB1*15, -; DQB1*0602, -). The first line being DQB1*0302 homozygous and the second line being non-DQB1*0302 homozygous.

Mixed Lymphocyte Cultures

Our objective was to study the proliferation capacity of negative and positive HLA-DQB1*0302 cells in response to different stimulation and, with and without allogeneic sHLA molecules. Cellular proliferation cultures were performed by primary (MLR-I, mixed lymphocyte reaction) and secondary (MLR-II) responses. The used protocol in these cultures is described on figure 1. Several responder cells of different HLA phenotypes were used, between these, as type example and indicated in the figures 2 and 3, the following cells are shown: JM cell (A3, 24; B38, -; DRB1*03, *04; DQB1*0201, *0302) and RM cell (A1, 29; B8, 44; DRB1*04, *07; DQB1*0202, *0302). Cellular cultures were performed by unidirectional primary MLR-I (5 days) and secondary MLR-II (re-stimulated at 5 days) by using allogeneic and autologous responder cells and irradiated stimulator cells (EBV-transformed lymphoblastoid lines, B98 and B249) in allogeneic and autologous HLA-DQB1 specific combinations (presence or absence of HLA-DQB1*0302).

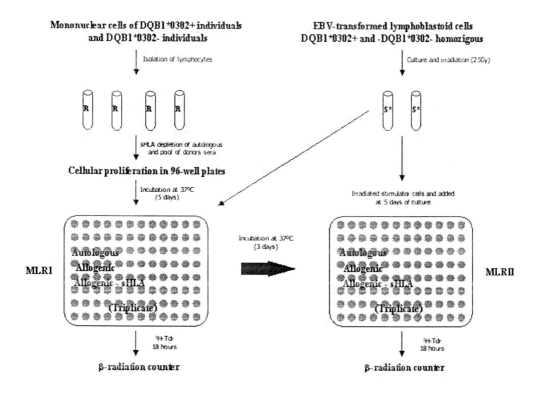

Figure 1. Protocol of assayed cellular proliferation cultures with and without sHLA molecules depletion and using HLA-DQB1*0302 negative and positive cells. Mononuclear cells of healthy individuals were used as responder cells (R) and EBV-transformed lymphoblastoid lines from liver allograft donor as stimulator cells (S). MLR-I (mixed lymphocyte reaction) and MLR-II are showed in this scheme.

Briefly, peripheral blood mononuclear cells (PBMCs) were isolated from heparinized whole blood of normal healthy donors by standard gradient centrifugation with Ficoll-Hypaque (Lymphoprep, Nicomed Pharma, Norway). PBMCs were harvested from the interface, washed twice, and resuspended in complete culture medium (CCM) with

RPMI1640 (GibcoBRL) supplemented with inactivated human AB sera at 10% (Sigma), L-glutamine 2 mM (Gibco) and antibiotics [penicillin at 50 U/ml and streptomycin at 50 µg/ml (Flow Laboratories)]. These cells were grown in 96-well-round-botton microtiter plates (Costar) (5 x 10^4 cells in 150 µl/well for each one) with sera, with and without allogeneic sHLA molecules and irradiated stimulator cells (EBV-lymphoblastoid lines) in the same concentration in a incubator with humidified atmosphere 37° in the presence of 5% CO_2. All of stimulator cells were treated with irradiation (2500 rad) to prevent DNA synthesis without killing the cell before cellular culture. In all combinations, responder cells and irradiated responder (used as stimulator cell) cells were used as autologous proliferation control. Proliferation assays were performed in two modalities: first unidirectional allogeneic stimuli *in vitro* for 5 days (MLR-I) and assays with a second allogeneic re-stimulation in similar conditions to that the primary culture, but for 3 additional days (MLR-II). All assayed experiments were performed in triplicate.

Proliferation of responder lymphocytes was monitored by measuring [^{3}H]-thymidine incorporation. Briefly, in 5th or 7th day of culture 1 µCi of the [^{3}H]-thymidine radionuclide with specific activity of 37 MBq/ml (Moravek Biochemicals, Brea, CA) was added to each well and the plates were returned to a CO_2 incubator to pulse 18-24 hours. Then, cells were transferred to nitrocellulose filters (Skatron Instruments, Lier, Norway) with a cellular harvester (Skatron Instruments), as previously published (Marin *et al.*, 2002, 2003). These filters were mixed with scintillion liquid (Optiscint Hisafe, LKB, Leics, UK) and the uptake of [^{3}H]-thymidine was measured using a *Beta* scintillation counter (LKB Wallac, Rackbetta, Turka, Finland). All values of *cpm* (counts per minute) were calculated from triplicates and indicated as mean ± SEM.

Statistical Analysis

Statistical analysis of the proliferation culture results was performed by using Sigma Plot (Richmond, CA) and SPSS v10.0 softwares (SPSS, Inc., Chicago, IL). The results of cellular proliferation cultures were estimated by relative response (RR) index with respect to the proliferation of the corresponding autologous control, as previously published [Muro *et al.*, 2002]. Briefly, the formula for RR is as follows: %RR=[(test cpm – autologous cpm / (median response cpm – autologous cpm)] x 100. Finally, student's test was used to determine whether the difference between autologous and allogeneic controls and samples were statistically significance [Garcia-Alonso *et al.*, 1997; Muro *et al.*, 1999; Minguela *et al.*, 2000].

Results

The tested experiments could be indicative, whether a proliferation response was obtained, of a priority of recognizing for allogeneic sHLA-I molecules, restricted by HLA-DQ molecules. In this sense, it is very important to remember that, in the indirect pathway, T cells recognize processed alloantigen presented as allopeptides by self APCs. This pathway can also be triggered by MHC molecules on donor cells that are shared with the recipient.

The results corresponding to primary response (MLR-I) are shown in figure 2. The relative response in the proliferation culture of the HLA-DQB1*0302[+] lymphocytes, when the stimulator cell had a matched HLA class II haplotype, does not show an increased cellular proliferation in presence of sHLA-I molecules, instead of this, the cellular proliferation response in presence of sHLA-I molecules was the same or even more decreased in all performed assays. For this primary response, the results were similar to these when stimulator cells does not present any matched HLA class II haplotype with responder lymphocytes and when a HLA class II haplotype was matched.

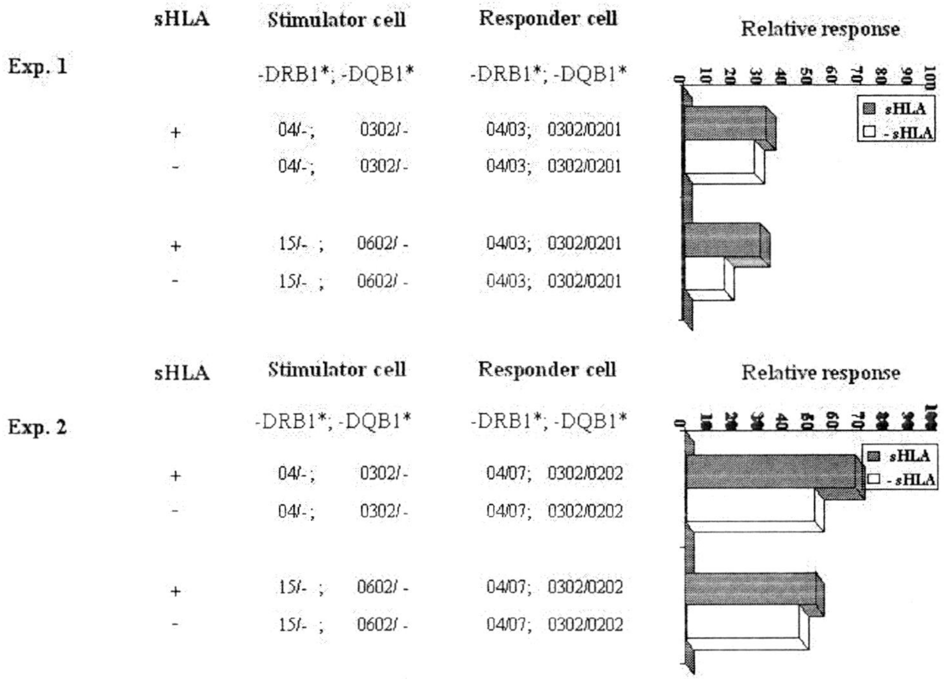

Figure 2. Example of primary culture or MLRI. The relative response of HLA-DQB1*0302+ lymphocytes, when the stimulator cells are matched HLA class II haplotype, does not show a increased proliferation in presence of sHLA-I molecules, instead of this, the response in presence of sHLA-I molecules was the same or even more decreased in all performed assays. For this primary response, the results were similar to these when stimulator cells does not present any matched HLA class II haplotype with responder lymphocytes and when a haplotype was matched.

However, in the secondary response (MLR-II) (figure 3), after responder cells have been primed against stimulator cells and allogeneic sHLA molecules, it was curiously detected an increasing of cellular proliferation in absence of allogeneic sHLA molecules, when stimulation was performed with a matched HLA-DRB1*04-HLA-DQB1*0302[+] haplotype with responder cells. This result was opposite to our hypothesis because, instead of that the HLA-DQB1*0302[+] individuals presented an increased reactivity in presence of soluble HLA-I alloantigens, we observed that when the responder cells had previously been sensitized in a primary culture, allogeneic sHLA class I molecules produced an increase in cellular proliferation response. However, this effect did not occur when the used stimuli had not a matched HLA class II haplotype with responder cell, in this case, co-existence of allogeneic soluble HLA molecules in culture medium, produced an increase of secondary response of the HLA-DQB1*0302^{+} lymphocytes, whereas this effect had not been evident in primary response (see figure 2).

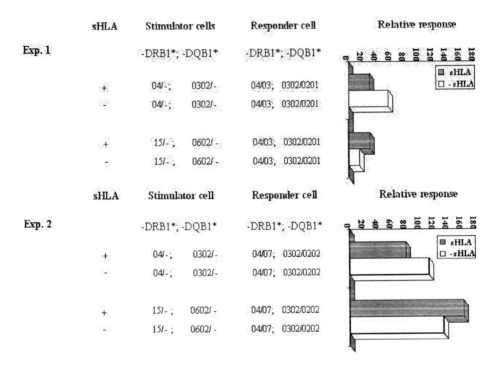

Figure 3. Example of secondary culture *or MLRII*. When responder cells had previously been primed in primary culture or MLRI, sHLA-I molecules depletion in situation of HLA-DQB1*0302 matched haplotype with stimulator cells produced an increase of cellular proliferation. However, this observed effect did not occur when the used stimuli has not a matched HLA class II haplotype with the responder cell.

Globally, these results indicate, first of all, that although in a primary response both alloreactivity models work in a similar manner, after that responder cells are primed for previous primary sensitization, their actuation seem to be dependent on compatibility, at least partial, in HLA-DRB1*04-HLA-DQB1*0302^{+} and, second, that the presence of soluble HLA-I molecules conditionate in different manner the results in both combinations. Thus, whereas in total incompatibility sHLA depletion decreased specific proliferation response, in combinations with a matched HLA class II haplotype we did not observed a decreased cellular proliferation and even in the secondary response it produce a clear increasing in cellular proliferation.

Altogether, it can suggest that the role of HLA class I antigens could be different depending on the used allogeneic combinations, even to conditionate specific antagonism responses, in relation to their capacity to induce alloreactivity or allotolerance.

Whether or not indirect allorecognition plays a significant role in allograft rejection is of fundamental importance in transplantation, since the requirements for activation and the mechanisms of regulation will be quite different from those for indirect recognition. Thus, self-restricted T cell recognition of processed alloantigens may play a critical role in transplantation. However, defining polymorphic MHC peptides able to prime allogeneic T cells is problematic, for this reason, an extensive sHLA pool was used in our experiments.

In conclusion, the relative response of HLA-DQB1*0302[+] lymphocytes in primary MLR-I, when the stimulator cells were semiallogenic or incompatibles, did not show an increased cellular proliferation, in situations of absence or presence of sHLA-I molecules. However, in secondary MLR-II (primed responder cell against stimulator cell), we detected an increased relative response in situation of absence of allogeneic sHLA molecules and using semiallogeneic HLA-DQB1*0302[+] cells. This result was not obtained when the HLA-DQB1*0302[-] responder cells were used.

Discussion

Our obtained observation showing that the peripheral blood lymphocytes of HLA-DQB1*0302[+] individuals sensitized in primary cultures in presence of allogeneic sHLA class I antigens in medium culture translate a decreasing in cellular proliferation in secondary response, could be interpreted in several manners. However, it results surprisely the different behaviour of the same responder cell when, in presence of allogeneic HLA peptides, it is stimulated with HLA class II partial or incompatible cells.

With respect to the possibility of that the HLA-DQB1*0302 molecule could be a restriction element for determined peptides, it is known that HLA-DQ8 can bind insulin B and gliadin peptides [Lundin et al., 1994; Lee et al., 2001] and that, in determined conditions, this allele can bind peptides from VP16 protein of type 2 herpes virus (HSV-2) and activate HVS-specific T cells restricted by HLA-DQB1*0302 molecules [Kwok et al., 1999]. On the other hand, it is known that other HLA class II molecules can present HLA class I peptides, particularly, it has been described that HLA-DR1 can present HLA-A2 peptides [Chicz et al., 1992] and that HLA-DQ7 can also present, between other, derived peptides of HLA class I molecules [Khalil-Daher et al., 1998], therefore the possibility of that HLA-DQB1*0302 could present these molecules is not discernable.

Other question to dilucidate could be this corresponding to whether different HLA alleles have similar or different capacity to induce alloreactive or allotolerance responses, depending to the structure of antigenic pocket and the different antigenic peptides to bind to this pocket. In this sense, HLA-DQB1*0302 allele could induce antagonism responses in diabetes [Lee et al., 2001].

On the other hand, whether the blockage effect of cellular proliferation, when allogeneic HLA peptides are presented in the context of the HLA-DQB1*0302 molecule, is demonstrated, it would be necessary to analyze the capacity to induce regulatory T cells (CD4[+]CD25[+]) or even cytotoxic T effectors or suppressors of allogeneic response, restricted by this HLA allele, whose nature and phenotypic and functional characteristics should be studied in next experiments. In this line, Lundin et al. [1994] have described the possibility of that activated T CD4[+] cells are generated in response to gliadin, whereas other studies refer the existence of HLA-DQ-restricted suppressor CD8[+] clones [Salgame et al., 1991].

However, it can not be descrambled that, besides the restriction effect mediated by determined HLA class II genotypes, it could be associated to an own effect of sHLA class I molecules to favour apoptosis of T cells for specific effector T cells [Puppo *et al.*, 1997] or for non-specific interactions with the α_3 domain of CD8 molecule, as reported [Puppo *et al.*, 2000]. However, these facts do not explain the observed increased proliferation in the cultures corresponding to secondary response and, thus, indicative of specific T cells expansion, opposite to a decreased proliferation as consequence of a hypothetical apoptosis process. Indeed, induced apoptosis for soluble HLA class I molecules seems to be mediated for monomorphic regions and, therefore, its action would not be specific, whereas that the effect described in our work, potentially dependent of the structure of presenting molecule, could have a more specific character.

Although, as in transplant situations allogeneic sHLA molecules can stay in peripheral blood circulation, it could be indication that these can produce succesive specific stimuli that could conduce to tolerogenic signals, as consequence of their presentation in the context of HLA-DQB1*0302 allele that, as suggested in this work, could conditionate states of a minor response or even adding effects of a presentation on non-professionals APCs (antigen presentig cells), conducing to a final result favourable to graft acceptation, instead of that their reactivity was involuntarily responsible to induce acute rejection development.

In the first point, it has originally been reported that preoperative appearance of serum class I and II antigen during liver allograft transplantation [Pollard *et al.*, 1990; Filaci *et al.*, 1995] and later it has been showed that serum soluble HLA antigens can be markers and modulators of an immune response [Puppo *et al.*, 1995, 1997; Mathew *et al.*, 1996]. The rapid apparition of sHLA molecules in liver recipient circulation (30 minutes post-transplant) has postulated that this fact could play a role in the hyper-acute rejection prevention and in the special immune-regulation of liver transplantation [Pollard *et al.*, 1990].

Indeed, human Vdelta1 or Vdelta2 T lymphocytes secrete FasL and undergo apoptosis upon incubation with soluble HLA-I or after cross-linking of CD8, with a kinetics different from that observed following ligation of TCR. Thus, sHLA-I can regulate gammadelta T cell survival and that activating KIR may amplify antigen-specific Vdelta2 T cell responses [Poggi *et al.*, 2005; Cortini *et al.*, 2005]. Indeed, sHLA-I molecules also induces NK cells apoptosis interacting with its ligands [Poggi *et al.*, 2005].

On the other hand, sHLA molecules releasing have been implicated in other pathologies. In this sense, during relapses in relapsing-remitting multiple sclerosis (RRMS), serum soluble HLA class I surface antigen (sHLA-I) levels are reported to either decrease or remain unchanged, whereas serum sHLA-II levels increase. Thus, monitoring of both sHLA-I and sHLA-II appears necessary if these molecules are to be developed as RRMS activity marker [Minagar *et al.*, 2005].

In the second point, HLA-DQ molecules are very important in immune processes [Kwow *et al.*, 1988; Knight *et al.*, 1996], their polymorphisms are highly selective for peptide binding interactions [Kwow *et al.*, 1995] and polymorphic DQα and DQβ interactions dictate HLA class II determinants of allo-recognition [Kwow *et al.*, 1990]. Indeed, HLA-DQB1 codon 57 is critical for peptide binding and recognition [Kwow *et al.*, 1996] and peptide binding affinity and pH variation establish functional thresholds for activation of HLA-DQ-restricted T cell recognition [Kwow *et al.*, 1999].

However, it is a little unknown of the role of HLA-DQ molecules in liver transplant. The first work was this of Doran *et al.* [1992] describing to the liver recipients bearing HLA-DQ2 molecule associated to earlier and more severe acute rejection episodes. These authors corroborate this observation in other more recent article [Doran *et al.*, 2000]. However, in kidney transplant, these class II antigens seem to play contradictory effects [Matsuno *et al.*, 1990; Sengar *et al.*, 1990; Fukuda *et al.*, 1994]. In this sense, a study firstly established that HLA-DQ mismatching could be irrelevant in kidney grafts HLA-DR matched [Bushell *et al.*, 1989], and other works have showed that HLA-DQ mismatching could even be more important than HLA-DR matching for kidney transplant survival in related individuals [Duquesnoy *et al.*, 1980; Matsuno *et al.*, 1990], whereas other groups indicate that HLA-DQ matching show a negative effect in graft survival [Fukuda *et al.*, 1994].

On the other hand, several HLA-DQ alleles have been related with a induction of immune response suppression [Nishimura *et al.*, 1990, 1991], suggesting an implication of these molecules in a active immunosuppressor system conducting to a particular tolerance state and showing a way to the study of the importance of these molecules in transplantation. Thus, several authors reported that the presence of a determined HLA-DQ phenotype could define to recipients as responder or non-responder [Altmann *et al.*, 1991]. Indeed, HLA-DQ molecules have extensively been related with susceptibility to infectious and autoimmune diseases [Nishimura *et al.*, 1991; Lundin *et al.*, 1994], based in the fact that HLA molecules determine a peptide repertoire against which individual T cells are able to respond [Brown *et al.*, 1988]. In the same manner, it has been demonstrated that *in vitro* T CD8$^+$ cells activation is restricted by HLA-DQ molecules [Salgame *et al.*, 1991]. On the other hand, specific HLA-DQ alleles, such as DQw6, is considered as a marker of high responders against renal allografts [Vereerstraeten *et al.*, 1992] and, in experimental models, this allele is able to alter positively specific immunoresponses [Nishimura *et al.*, 1990]. All these data suggest that this molecules can play an important role in allogeneic responses post transplantation.

Curiously, other authors correlationate determined diseases in recipients bearing DQB1*0302 allele, as reported in patients with protection to hepatocellular carcinoma [Donaldson *et al.*, 2001; Maciag *et al.*, 2002], and VHC infection protection [Cramp *et al.*, 1998; Tillmann *et al.*, 2001], although other authors do not show this effect [Mangia *et al.*, 1999; Barret *et al.*, 1999; Belli *et al.*, 2000; Samuel *et al.*, 2000]. Thus, the precise role of HLA-DQB1*0302 in liver is, at the moment, very variated and non completely dilucidated.

Our next experiments will be directed to perform *ex vivo* cultures with lymphocytes from liver transplant recipients with acute rejection episodes for interpretate their proliferation and the presence of cytotoxic and/or suppressor effectors by using adequate assays to respect, as possible associated anergization and apoptosis processes that contribute to establishment of tolerance state.

Conclusion

These data indicate that, in a primary response the different tested combinations show a similar manner to respond, but in the secondary response, when the responder cells have been primed and sensibilized, soluble HLA class I molecules plays a different role in proliferation response depending to specific HLA-DQ molecules constitution.

Acknowledgements

This work was supported by the Program of 'Redes Temáticas de Investigación' from the Fondo de Investigación Sanitaria. Red de Grupos de Investigación (G03/104; Inmunología del Transplante), Ministerio de Sanidad y Consumo, Spain.

References

Adamashvili, I; Fraser, PA; McDonald, JC. Association of serum concentrations of soluble class I HLA with HLA allotypes. *Transplantation.* 1996; 61: 984-987.

Alters, SE; Shizuru JA; Ackerman, J; Grossman D; Seydel KB; Fathman CG. Anti-CD4 mediates clonal anergy during transplantation tolerance induction. *J. Exp. Med.* 1991; 173: 491-498.

Altmann, DM; Sansom, D; Marsh, SGE. What is the basis for HLA-DQ associations with autoimmune disease?. *Immunol. Today.* 1991; 8: 267-272.

Barret, S; Ryan, E; Crowe J. Association of the HLA-DRB1*01 allele with spontaneous viral clearance in a Irish cohort infected with hepatitis C virus via contaminated anti-D immunoglobulin. *J. Hepatol.* 1999; 30: 979-983.

Belli, LS; Zavaglia, C; Alberti, AB; Poli, F; Rondinara, G; Silini, E; Carlis, L; Scalamogna, M; Forti, D; Pinzello, G; Ideo, G. Influence of immunogenetic background on the outcome of recurrent hepatititis C after liver transplantation. *Hepatology.* 2000; 31: 1345-1350.

Benichou, G; Takizawa, PA; Olson, CA; McMillan, M; Sercarz EE. Donor major histocompatibility complex (MHC) peptides are presented by recipient MHC molecules during graft rejection. *J. Exp. Med.* 1992; 175: 305-308.

Botella, C; Marín, L; Moya-Quiles, MR; Miras, M; Sánchez-Bueno, F; Minguela, A; Robles, R; Bermejo, J; Parrilla, P; Álvarez-López, R, Muro M. Lack of association between the promoter polymorphism in the human CCL5/RANTES chemokine gene on liver transplant outcome. *Transplant. Int.* 2006; 19: 98-104.

Brieva, JA; Villar, LM; Leoro, G; Alvarez-Cermeno, JC; Roldan, E; Gonzalez-Porque, P. Soluble HLA class I antigen secretion by normal lymphocytes: relationship with cell activation and effect of interferon-gamma. *Clin. Exp. Immunol.* 1990; 82: 390-395.

Brown, JH; Jardetzky, T; Saper, MA; Samraoui, B; Bjorkman, PJ; Wiley, DC. A hypothetical model of the foreign antigen binding site of class II histocompatibility molecules. *Nature.* 1988; 332: 845-853.

Bushell, A; Higgins, RM; Wood, KJ; Morris, PJ. HLA-DQ mismatches between donor and recipient in the presence of HLA-DR compatibility do not influence the function or outcome of renal transplants. *Human Immunol.* 1989; 26: 179-188.

Contini, P; Ghio, M; Merlo, A; Poggi, A; Indiveri, F; Puppo, F. Apoptosis of antigen-specific T lymphocytes upon the engagement of CD8 by soluble HLA class I molecules is Fas ligand/Fas mediated: evidence for the involvement of p56lck, calcium calmodulin kinase II, calcium-independent protein kinase C signalling pathways and for NF-KappaB and NF-AT nuclear translocation. *J. Immunol.* 2005; 175: 7244-7254.

Cook, DJ. Immune responsiveness. In: *Clinical. Transplants.* 1988. Terasaki, PI (ed.). UCLA Tissue Typing Laboratory. Los Angeles, 1989: 357-363.

Cramp, ME; Carucci, P; Underhill, J; Naoumov, NV; Williams, R; Donaldson, PT. Association between HLA class II genotype and spontaneous clearance of hepatitis C viraemia. *J. Hepatol.* 1998; 29: 207-213.

Chauchan, B; Mathew, JM; Shenoy, S; Flye, MW; Howard, T; Mohanakumar, T. Donor human leukocyte antigens in the circulation of liver allograft recipients. *Clin. Transplant.* 1995; 9: 14-19.

Chicz, RM; Urban, RG; Lane, WS; Gorga, JC; Stern, LJ; Vignali, DAA; Strominger, JL. Predominant naturally processed peptides bound to HLA-DR1 are derived from MHC-related molecules and are heterogeneous in size. *Nature.* 1992; 358: 764-768.

Chudyk, A; Masiuk, M; Myslak, M; Domanski, L; Sienko, J; Sulikowski, T; Machalinski, B; Giedrys-Kalemba, S. Soluble HLA class I molecules exert differentiated influence on renal graft condition. *Transplant. Proc.* 2006; 38: 90-93.

Dallman, MJ; Shiho, O; Page, TH; Wood, KJ; Morris, PJ. Peripheral tolerance to alloantigen results from altered regulation of the interleukin 2 pathway. *J. Exp. Med.* 1991; 173: 79-87.

Dallman, MJ; Wood, KJ; Bushell, AR; Morris, PJ; Wood, MJA; Chartlon, HM. Cytokines and peripheral tolerance to alloantigens. *Immunol. Rev.* 1993; 133: 5-18.

Donaldson, PT; Ho, S; Willians, R; Johnson, J. HLA class II alleles in Chinese patients with hepatocellular carcinoma. *Liver.* 2001; 21: 143-148.

Doran, TJ; Derley, L; Chapman, J; McCaughan, G; Painter, D; Dorney, M; Sheil, AG. Severity of liver transplantation rejection is associated with recipient HLA type. *Transplant. Proc.* 1992; 24: 192-193.

Doran, TJ; Geczy, AF; Painter, D; McCaughan, G; Sheil, AG; Susal, C. A large, single center investigation of the immunogenetic factors affecting liver transplantation. *Transplantation.* 2000; 69: 1232-1233.

Duquesnoy, RJ; Marrarrai, N; Chia, K. Influence of MB compatibility on survival of kidney transplant from one-haplotype mismatched related donors. En: *Histocompatibility testing 1980.* Terasaki, P. L. (ed.). UCLA Tissue Typing Laboratory Press. Los Angeles, 1980: 898.

Dyer, PA; Martin, S; Kippax, R; et al. HLA-DR3 is a marker of reduced transplant outcomes. *Transplant. Proc.* 1985; 17: 2248-2249.

Escobar-Morreale, HF; Serrano-Gotarredona, J; Villar, LM; García-Robles, R; Gonzalez-Porque, P; Sancho, JM; Varela, C. Methimazole has no dose-related effect on the serum concentrations od soluble class I major histocompatibility complex antigens, soluble interleukin-2 receptor, and beta 2 microglobulin in patients with Graves' disease. *Thyroid.* 1996; 6: 29-36.

Ferreira, A; Garcia-Rodriguez, MC; Omenaca, F; Jimenez, A; Villar, LM; Gonzalez-Porque, P; Fontan, G. Soluble class I histocompatibility antigens (s-HLA) and beta-microglobulin at delivery. *Clin. Exp. Immunol.* 1991; 84: 167-169.

Filaci, G; Contini, P; Brenci, S; Lanza, L; Scudeletti, M, Indiveri, F; Puppo, F. Increased serum concentration of soluble HLA-DR antigens in HIV infection and following transplantation. *Tissue Antigens.* 1995; 46: 117-223.

Fukuda, Y; Hoshino, S; Kimura, A; Dohi, K; Sasazuki, T. Negative effect of HLA-DQ antigen compatibility (concordance) on the survival of kidney grafts. *Transplant. Proc.* 1994; 26: 1887-1896.

García-Alonso, A; Minguela, A; Muro, M; Ontañón, J; Torío, A; Marín, L; López-Segura, P; Álvarez-López MR. CD28 expression on peripheral blood T lymphocytes after orthotopic liver transplant: upregulation in acute rejection. *Human Immunol.* 1997; 53: 64-72.

Gonwa, TA; Nery, JR; Husberg, BS; Klintman, GB. Simultaneous liver and renal transplantation in man. *Transplantation.* 1988; 46: 690-693.

Hendriks, GFJ; D´Amaro, J; Persijn, GG; et al. Excellent outcome after transplantation of renal allografts from HLA-DRw6-positive donors even in HLA-DR mismatches. *Lancet* 1983; II: 187-189.

Khalil-Daher, I; Boisgerault, F; Feugeas, JP; Tieng, V; Toubert, A; Charron, D. Naturally processed peptides from HLA-DQ7 (alpha*0501, beta*0301): influence of both alpha and beta chain polymorphism in the HLA-DQ peptide binding specificity). *Eur. J. Immunol.* 1998; 28: 3840-3849.

Knight, SW; Mijovic, C; Barnett, AH. HLA-DQB1 upstream regulatory region polymorphism and type I diabetes. *Tissue Antigens.* 1996; 47: 231-236.

Krensky, AM. T cells in autoimmunity and allograft rejection. *Kidney Int.* 1994; 45: S50.

Kwok, WW; Domeier, ME; Johnson, ML; Nepom, GT; Koelle, DM. HLA-DQB1 codon 57 is critical for peptide binding and recognition. *J. Exp. Med.* 1996; 183: 1253-1258.

Kwok, WW; Mickelson, E; Masewicz, S; Milner, ECB; Hansen, J; Nepom, GT. Polymorphic DQα and DQβ interactions dictate HLA class II determinants of allo-recognition. *J. Exp. Med.* 1990: 171: 85-95.

Kwok, WW; Nepom, GT; Raymond, FC. HLA-DQ polymorphisms are highly selective for peptide binding interactions. *J. Immunol.* 1995; 155: 2468-2476.

Kwok, WW; Reijonen, H; Falk, BA; Koelle, DM; Nepom, GT. Peptide binding affinity and pH variation establish functional thresholds for activation of HLA-DQ-restricted T cell recognition. *Human Immunol.* 1999; 60: 619-626.

Kwok, WW; Schwarz, D; Nepom, BS; et al. HLA-DQ molecules form ab heterodimers of mixed allotypes. *J. Immunol.* 1988; 141: 3123-3127.

Lee, KH; Wucherpfennig, KW; Wiley, DC. Structure of a human insulin peptide-HLA-DQ8 complex and susceptibility to type 1 diabetes. *Nature Immunol.* 2001; 2: 501-507.

Lundin, KE; Scott, H; Fausa, O; Thorsby, E; Sollid, LM. T cells from the small intestinal mucosa of a DR4, DQ7/DR4, DQ8 celiac disease patient preferentially recognize gliadin when presented by DQ8. *Human Immunol.* 1994; 41: 285-294.

Maciag, PC; Schlecht, NF; Souza, PS; Rohan, TE; Franco, EL; Villa, L. Polymorphism of the human leukocyte antigen DRB1 and DQB1 genes and the natural history of human papillomavirus infection. *J. Infect. Dis.* 2002; 186: 164-172.

Mangia, A; Gentile, R; Cascavilla, I; Margaglione, M; Rosaria, M; Stella, F; Modola, G; Agostiano, V; Gaudiano, C; Andria, A. HLA class II favors clearance of HCV infection and progression of chronic liver damage. *J. Hepatol.* 1999; 30: 984-989.

Marín, L; Minguela, A; Moya-Quiles, MR; Torío, A; Muro, M; García-Alonso, AM; Sánchez-Bueno, F; Bru, M; Parrilla, P; Álvarez-López, MR. CD95 increased expression on CD3+ and CD19+ cells is related with an increased apoptosis in response to PHA on lymphocytes from liver recipients suffering acute rejection. *Transplant. Proc.* 2002; 34: 280-282.

Marín, L; Minguela, A; Torío, A; Moya-Quiles, R; Muro, M; Montes, O; Parrado, A; García-Alonso, AM; Álvarez-López, MR. Flow cytometry quantification of apoptosis and proliferation in MLC. *Cytometry.* 2003; 51: 107-118.

Marin, L; Moya-Quiles, MR; Miras, M; Muro, M; Minguela, A; Bermejo, J; Ramírez, P; García-Alonso, AM; Parrilla, P; Álvarez-López, MR. Evaluation of CD86 gene polymorphism at +1057 position in liver transplant recipients. *Transplant. Immunol.* 2005; 15: 69-74.

Marin, L; Muro, M; Moya-Quiles, MR; Miras, M; Minguela, A; Bermejo, J; Sánchez-Bueno, F; Parrilla, P; Álvarez-López, MR. Study of Fas (CD95) and FasL (CD178) polymorphism in liver transplant recipients. *Tissue Antigens.* 2006; 67: 117-126.

Mathew, JM; Shenoy, S; Phelan, D; Lowell, J; Howard, T; Mohanakumar, T. Biochemical and immunological evaluation of donor-specific soluble HLA in the circulation of liver transplant recipients. *Transplantation.* 1996; 62: 217-223.

Matsuno, N; Inoko, H; Ando, A, et al. Importance of DQB as an indicator in living-related kidney transplant. *Transplantation.* 1990; 49: 208-217.

McDonald, JC; Adamashvili, I. Soluble HLA: a review of the literature. *Human Immunol.* 1998; 59: 387-403.

McDonald, JC; Adamashvili, I; Hayes, JM; Aultman, DF; Rhynes, VK; Gelder, FB. Soluble HLA class II concentrations in normal individuals and transplant recipients. Comparison with soluble HLA class I concentrations. *Transplantation.* 1994; 58: 1268-1272.

Minagar, A; Adamashvilli, I; Jaffe, SL; Glabus, MF; Gonzalez-Toledo, E; Kelley, RE. Soluble HLA class I and class II molecules in relapsing-remitting multiple sclerosis: acute response to interferon-beta1a treatment and their use as markers of disease activity. *Ann. N.Y. Acad. Sci.* 2005; 1051: 111-1120.

Minguela, A; Marín, L; Torio, A; Muro, M; García-Alonso, AM; Moya-Quiles, MR; Sánchez-Bueno, F; Parrilla, P; Alvarez-López, MR. CD28/CTLA-4 and CD80/CD86 costimulatory molecules are mainly involved in acceptance or rejection of human liver transplant. *Human Immunol.* 2000; 61: 658-669.

Minguela, A; Torío, A; Marin, L; Muro, M; Villar, LM; Pons, JA; Diaz, J; Parrilla, P; García-Alonso, AM; Álvarez-López, MR. Implication of soluble and membrane HLA class-I and serum IL-10 in liver graft acceptance. *Human Immunol.* 1999; 60: 500-509.

Mor, MD; Solomon, H; Gibbs, JF; Holman, MJ; Goldstein, RM; Husberg, BS; Gonwa, TA; Klintmalm, GB. Acute cellular rejection following liver transplant: clinical pathologic features and effect on outcome. *Semin. Liver. Dis.* 1992; 12: 28-39.

Moya-Quiles, MR; Muro, M; Torío, A; Sánchez-Bueno, F; Miras, M; Marín, L; García-Alonso, AM; Parrilla, P; Dausset, J; Álvarez-López, MR. Human Leukocyte Antigen-C in short- and long-term liver graft acceptance. *Liver Transplant.* 2003; 9: 218-227.

Muro, M. In: *Análisis de la región HLA en trasplante hepático: Implicación en rechazo agudo, rechazo crónico y en la supervivencia del injerto.* Universidad de Murcia, Murcia, Spain, 2002.

Muro, M; Álvarez-López, MR; Torío, A; Ontañón, J; Minguela, A; Marín, L; García-Calatayud, MC; Bermejo, J; García-Alonso, AM. HLA-DRB1 and -DQB1 polymorphism in liver recipients: relationship between HLA-DQB1*0302 allele frequency and acute rejection. *Human Immunol.* 1997; 56: 70-76.

Muro, M; Herrero, N; Marín, L; Torío, A; Minguela, A; Sánchez-Bueno, F; García-Alonso, AM; Álvarez-López, MR. Polymorphism in the upstream regulatory region of the HLA-DQB1 gene in liver graft recipients. *Human Biol.* 2001; 73: 845-854.

Muro, M; Llorente, S; Marín, L; Moya-Quiles, MR; Gonzalez-Soriano, MJ; Gimeno, L; Prieto, A; Álvarez-López, MR. Acute vascular rejection mediated by HLA antibodies in a cadaveric kidney recipient: discrepancies between FlowPRA™, ELISA and CDC *vs* luminex screening. *Nephr. Dyal. Transplant.* 2005; 20: 223-226.

Muro, M; Marin, L; Miras, M; Moya-Quiles, MR; Sánchez-Bueno, F; Minguela, A; Robles, R; Bermejo, J; Ramírez, P; García-Alonso, AM; Parrilla, P; Álvarez-López, MR. Human liver allograft recipients harbouring anti-donor preformed lymphocytotoxic antibodies exhibit a poor graft survival at the first year after transplantation. Experience of one centre. *Transplant. Immunol.* 2005; 14: 91-97.

Muro, M; Marín, L; Torío, A; Moya-Quiles, MR; Minguela, A; Rosique-Roman, J; Sanchís, MJ; Garcia-Calatayud, MC; García-Alonso, AM; Álvarez-López, MR. HLA polymorphism in the Murcia Population (Spain) in the Cradle of the Archaeologic Iberians. *Human. Immunol.* 2001; 62: 910-921.

Muro, M; Marín, L; Torío, A; Moya-Quiles, MR; Ontañón, J; Minguela, A; Alemany, JM; Sánchez-Bueno, F; García-Alonso, AM; Álvarez-López, MR. Effect of HLA matching on liver graft survival. *Transplant. Proc.* 1999; 31: 2477-2479.

Muro, M; Moya-Quiles, MR; Marín, L; Torío, A; Vallejo, C; Moraleda, JM; Álvarez-López MR. Report of recombinations between HLA locus within two families: Utility of high resolution typing. *Clin. Transplant.* 2002; 16: 329-333.

Muro, M; Sánchez-Bueno, F; Marín, L; Torío, A; Moya-Quiles, MR; Minguela, A; Ramirez, P; Alemany, JM; Miras, M; Pérez-López, MJ; García-Alonso, AM; Parrilla, P; Alvarez-López MR. DQA1 and DPB1 genes polymorphism on acute rejection development in liver transplantation. *Transplant. Proc.* 2002; 34: 3302-3303.

Muro, M; Sánchez-Bueno, F; Robles, R; Miras, M; Ramirez, R; Parrilla, P. Recipient factors analysis in long-term allograft survival of liver transplantation. *Transplant. Proc.* 2002; 34: 290-291.

Nishimura, Y; Iwanaga, T; Inamitsu, T; et al. Expression of the human, HLA-DQw6 genes alters the immune response in C57BL/6 mice. *J. Immunol.* 1990; 145: 353-362.

Nishimura, Y; Kamikawaji, N; Fujisawa, K; et al. Genetic control of immune response and disease susceptibility by the HLA-DQ gene. *Res. Immunol.* 1991; 142: 459-468.

Nocera, A; Pellicci, R; Barocci, S; Valente, U; Cantarella, S; Celada, F; Callea, F; Ceppa, P; Leprini, A. HLA antigens expression and cellular infiltrate analysis in rejected and accepted human liver allografts. *Clin. Transplant.* 1991; 5: 23-29.

Nocito, M; Montalban, C; Gonzalez-Porque, P; Villar, LM. Increased soluble serum HLA class I antigens in patients with lymphoma. *Human. Immunol.* 1997; 58: 106-111.

Ontañón, J; Muro, M; García-Alonso, AM; Minguela, A; Torio, A; Bermejo, J; Pons, JA; Campos, M; Álvarez-López, MR. Effect of partial HLA-Class I match on acute rejection in viral preinfected human liver allograft recipients. *Transplantation.* 1998; 65: 1047-1053.

Poggi, A; Contini, P; Catellani, S; Setti, M; Murdaca, G; Zocchi, MR. Regulation of gammadelta T cell survival by soluble HLA-I: involvement of CD8 and activating killer Ig-like receptors. *Eur. J. Immunol.* 2005; 35: 2670-78.

Poggi, A; Zocchi, MR. Cyclosporin A regulates human NK cell apoptosis induced by soluble HLA-I or by target cells. *Autoimmun. Rev.* 2005; 4: 532-536.

Pollard, SG; Davies, H; Calne, RY. Preoperative appearance of serum class I antigen during liver transplantation. *Transplantation.* 1990; 49: 659-670.

Puppo, F; Contini, P; Ghio, M; Brenci, S; Scudeletti, M; Filaci, G; Ferrone, S; Indiveri, F. Soluble human MHC class I molecules induce soluble Fas ligand secretion and trigger apoptosis in activated CD8+ Fas (CD95)+ T lymphocytes. *Int. Immunol.* 2000; 12: 195-203.

Puppo, F; Indiveri, F; Scudeletti, M; Ferrone, S. Soluble HLA antigens: new roles and uses. *Immunol. Today.* 1997; 18: 154-155.

Puppo, F; Pellicci, R; Brenci, S; Nocera, A; Morelli, N; Dardano, G; Bertocchi, M; Antonucci, A; Ghio, M; Scudeletti, M. HLA class-I-soluble antigen serum levels in liver transplantation. A predictor marker of acute rejection. *Human. Immunol.* 1994; 40: 166-170.

Puppo, F; Scudeletti, M; Indiveri, F; Ferrone, S. Serum HLA class I antigens: markers and modulators of an immune response?. *Immunol. Today.* 1995; 16: 124-127.

Rasmussen, A; Davies, HFFS; Jamieson, NV; Evans, DB; Calne, RY. Combined transplantation of liver and kidney from the same donor protects the kidney from rejection and improves kidney graft survival. *Transplantation.* 1995; 59: 919-921.

Reichstetter, S; Adorno, D; Alaez, C; Albert, E; Böhm, B; Canossi, A; Carrier, C; Colombo, G; Contu, L; Cuzzia, M; Dolzan, V; Fan, L; Hsu, S; Ikäheimo, I; Klitz, W; Mantovani, V; Mazzilli, M; Middleton, D; Muro, M; Per, C; Tongio, M, Wassmuth, R. DQB1 promoter polymorphism: 12th International Histocompatibility Workshop Study. In: D. Charron. ed., *Genetic Diversity of HLA: Functionnal and Medical Implications.* Sevres. France; EDK Publishers; 1997; 176-183.

Rhynes, VK; McDonald, JC; Gelder, F; Aultman, DF; Hayes, JM; McMillan, RW; Mancini, MC. Soluble HLA class I in the serum of transplant recipients. *Ann. Surg.* 1993; 217: 485-489.

Rouger, P; Gugenheim, J; Gane, P; Capran-Landereau, M; Michel, T, Reynes, M; Bismuth, J. Distribution of the MHC antigens after liver transplantation: relationship with biochemical and histological parameters. *Clin. Exp. Immunol.* 1990; 80: 404-408.

Rowe, RE; Leech, NJ; Nepom, GT; McCulloch, M. High genetic risk for IDDM in the Pacific Northwest. First Report from the Washington State Diabetes Prediction Study. *Diabetes.* 1994; 43: 87-98.

Sairenji, T; Daibata, M; Sorli, CH. Relating homology between the Epstein-Barr virus BOLF1 molecule and DQw8 beta chain to recent onset type 1 (insulin dependent) diabetes mellitus. *Diabetologia.* 1991; 34: 33-42.

Salgame, P; Convit, J; Bloom, BR. Immunological suppression by CD8+ T cells is receptor dependent and HLA-DQ restricted. *Proc. Natl. Acad. Sci. USA.* 1991; 88: 2598-2609.

Samuel, D; Feray, C. Recurrent hepatitis C after liver transplantation: Clinical and therapeutical issues. *J. Viral. Hepat.* 2000; 7: 87-92.

Sengar, DPS; Couture, RA; Raman, S; Jindal, SL. Beneficial effect of HLA-DQ compatibility on the survival of cadaveric renal allograft in cyclosporine-treated recipients. *Transplantation.* 1990; 49: 1007-1015.

She, JX. Susceptibility to type I diabetes: HLA-DQ and DR revisited. *Immunol. Today.* 1996: 17: 323-329.

Sollid, ML. Molecular basis of celiac disease. *Ann. Rev. Immunol.* 2000; 18: 53-81.

Steinhoff, G; Wonigeit, K; Pichlmayer, R. Analysis of sequential changes in major histocompatibility complex expression in human liver grafts after transplantation. *Transplantation.* 1988; 45: 394-401.

Superina, RA; Pearl, RH; Greig, PD; Levy, G; Falk, J; Langer, B. Effect of Drw6 antigen in recipients and donors on survival after liver transplant. *Transplant. Proc.* 1989; 21: 786-788.

Thorsby, E; Ronningen, KS. Particular HLA-DQ molecules play a dominant role in determining susceptibility or resistance to Type 1 (insulin-dependent) diabetes mellitus. *Diabetologia.* 1993; 36: 371-380.

Tilg, H; Vogel, W; Auliztky, WE; Herold, M; Konigsrainer, A; Margreiter, R; Huber, C. Evaluation of cytokines and cytokines-induced secondary messages in sera of patients after liver transplantation. *Transplantation.* 1990; 49: 1074-1080.

Tillmann, HL; Chen, DF; Trautwein, C; Kliem, V; Grundey, A; Berning-Haag, A; Böker, K; Kubicka, S; Pastucha, L; Stangel, W; Manns, MP. Low frequency of HLA-DRB1*11 in hepatitis C virus induced end stage liver disease. *Gut.* 2001; 48: 714-718.

Todd, JA; Bell, JI; McDevitt, HO. HLA-DQ beta gene contributes to susceptibility and resistance to insulin-dependent diabetes mellitus. *Nature.* 1993; 329: 599.

Tong, JY; Hsia, S; Parris, GL; et al. Molecular compatibility and renal graft survival-The HLA-DQB1 genotyping. *Transplantation.* 1993; 55: 390-395.

Vela, JP; Spadafora-Ferreira, M; Murphy, B; Alexander, SI; Harmon, W; Carpenter, CB; Sayegh MH. Indirect allorecognition of major histocompatibility complex allopeptides in human renal transplant recipients with chronic graft dysfunction. *Transplantation.* 1997; 64: 795-800.

Vereerstraeten, P; Andrien, M; Dupont, E; et al. Detrimental role of donor-recipient HLA-DQ$_5$ and HLA-DQ$_6$ disparities on cadaver kidney graft survival. *Transplant. Int.* 1992; 5 (Suppl 1): S143-145.

Weimer, R; Susal, C; Yildiz, S; Staak, A; Pelzl, S; Renner, F; Dietrich, H; Daniel, V; Kamali-Ernst, S; Ersnt, W; Padberg, W; Opelz, G. Post-transplant sCD30 and neopterin as predictors of chronic allograft nephropathy: Impact of different immunosuppressive regimens. *Am. J. Transplant.* 2006; 35: 63-74.

Zhang, S; Cheng, H, Fu, Z; Zhong, G; Yan, T. Contribution of the absence of aspartic acid at position 57 on HLA-DQ beta chain to predisposition to insulin-dependent diabetes mellitus in a southern Chinese population. *Chin. Med. J.* 1998; 111: 694-697.

In: Transplantation Immunology Research Trends
Editor: Oliver N. Ulricker, pp. 203-217

ISBN: 978-1-60021-578-0
© 2007 Nova Science Publishers, Inc.

Chapter VIII

Immunobiology of Xenograft Rejection

Cristina Costa

Institut d'Investigació Biomèdica de Bellvitge (IDIBELL),
L'Hospitalet de Llobregat, Barcelona, Spain

Abstract

Research in pig-to-primate xenotransplantation aims to solve the great shortage of cells and organs for transplantation. Despite some great advances in the field, the main impediment to its clinical application is the strength of the immune response triggered by the xenograft. Cell-, tissue- and organ-based xenografts are subjected to distinct rejection processes that share humoral and cellular mechanisms. Rejection of vascularized organs is the best characterized and one of the most challenging. Various types of xenograft rejection have been described in solid organs that differ in the time of onset and the immune pathways involved. Hyperacute rejection (HAR) is the first to take place (within minutes to hours after transplantation). When HAR is averted, the xenograft succumbs to acute humoral xenograft rejection (AHXR) in a period of days to months. It is the main cause of rejection, as acute cellular xenograft rejection (ACXR, which is T cell-mediated and occurs in the same time frame) is presumably controlled by immunosuppression and is less severe than AHXR. Finally, chronic rejection is only observed in a few organs, those with the longest survival times.

The main triggers of HAR are well known: natural anti-Gal α1,3-Gal antibodies and complement. Consequently, the approaches developed to express human complement regulatory proteins or removal of the Gal α1,3-Gal antigen by genetic engineering of the donor pig have successfully averted HAR. On the contrary, the process of AHXR is more complex and key molecules that trigger AHXR remain to be identified. Both complement and the Gal α1,3-Gal antigen seem to exacerbate AHXR, but their inhibition does not prevent rejection. The presence of an innate cellular component (NK cells and macrophages) indicates these cells probably participate in AHXR. In vitro, human NK cells kill porcine cells by using two triggering receptors, NKG2D and NKp44, as well as the CD28 variant that binds the porcine costimulatory molecule CD86. Human monocytes also bind and activate porcine endothelial cells, but the molecular interactions remain to be fully characterized. In vivo, both NK cells and macrophages may have an effect on the B cell antibody response that ultimately leads to AHXR. Controlling the B cell response will be key to attain long-term xenograft survival. In summary, the elucidation of the mechanisms that contribute to acute xenograft rejection may allow the development of therapeutic solutions that result in successful clinical xenotransplantation.

Introduction

There is no cure for many patients who suffer organ failure or cell/tissue dysfunction because the tissues and organs available for allotransplantation do not suffice to meet the demand [1]. Research in xenotransplantation aims to provide a therapeutic solution to these patients as xenogeneic organs and tissues could be obtained in a practically unlimited manner [2]. For multiple reasons, the pig has been chosen as the most appropriate source of xenogeneic cells, tissues and organs. It is domesticated, reproduces with large litters, has a primate-like physiology and can be genetically modified [1,2]. The main organs considered for xenotransplantation are heart, kidney and lung, whereas different cell types such as pancreatic islets, hepatocytes, chondrocytes and neural cells are also studied for cell-based therapies [1-3]. Taking into account all these advantages and potential benefits, the main impediment to the clinical application of xenotransplantation is the strength of the immune response triggered by the xenograft [2]. Transplantation of porcine organs and tissues into nonhuman primate models results in xenograft rejection by humoral and cellular mechanisms [2,3]. In solid organ xenotransplantation, three main types of rejection have been described that differ in the time of onset and the immune pathways involved.

Hyperacute rejection is the fastest rejection process and takes place within minutes to hours after xenotransplantation (figure 1A). HAR is initiated by a humoral immune response in which xenoreactive natural antibodies (XNA) (preexisting in the host) are deposited on the donor endothelium resulting in complement activation and hemorrhage [2,4]. This process also triggers the coagulation cascade leading to thrombosis, ischemia and necrosis. The major xenoepitope recognized by XNA is the carbohydrate antigen Gal α1,3-Gal, which is highly expressed in pig tissues and is synthesized by the α1,3-galactosyltransferase (α1,3-GT) [5]. Humans and Old World primates lack a functional α1,3-GT and produce anti-Gal α1,3-Gal antibodies in high titers [5,6]. Several strategies that prevent XNA reactivity and/or complement activation have successfully overcome HAR.

Acute cellular xenograft rejection occurs within days after transplantation and is predominantly a T cell-mediated response to donor antigens. The activation of T cells during transplant rejection is mediated by a primary signal through the T cell receptor and costimulatory secondary signals that are preserved crossspecies [2,9,10]. Consequently, both the direct and indirect pathways are involved in this process, although the indirect pathway is thought to play a predominant role. It is still unclear whether ACXR can be controlled using standard immunosuppression. This cannot be fully evaluated unless the fundamental triggers of AHXR are averted.

Acute humoral xenograft rejection (figure 1B), also named acute vascular rejection or delayed xenograft rejection, occurs in a period of days to months in spite of available immunosuppression [2,7]. It comprises a very strong humoral immune response elicited by the xenograft with antibody and complement deposition, as well as thrombosis. Moreover, AXHR is characterized by the presence of an innate cellular infiltrate (NK cells and macrophages) and a type II endothelial cell activation that promotes hemorrhage, intravascular thrombosis and fibrin deposition [2,7]. In a few organs that have attained prolonged survival, signs of chronic vasculopathy have accompanied AXHR [8].

Critical molecules and pathways that trigger acute xenograft rejection remain to be identified. Efforts are now directed toward elucidating the molecular mechanisms of AHXR in order to develop strategies that attain long-term xenograft survival. Cell-based transplantation studies may help to identify key pathways in simpler systems. The following sections describe the immunobiology of xenograft rejection, including the latest advances and tools used in these studies. Two main types of approaches have been developed to overcome xenograft rejection. The most elegant and with potential for long-term clinical success are those based on genetic engineering of the donor pig because they are less detrimental to the patient, minimizing the need for immunosuppression and conditioning therapies. However, they are technologically challenging and involve labor-intensive, slow and costly procedures. Systemic treatments, on the contrary, may help us to identify key molecules or pathways of the rejection process at a faster pace and accelerate the clinical use of xenotransplantation.

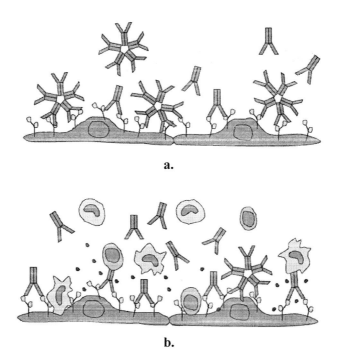

a.

b.

Figure 1. Scheme of the mechanisms of xenograft rejection. A) Hyperacute Rejection: it is produced by the deposition of xenoreactive natural antibodies (mainly IgM) that recognize the Galα1,3-Gal antigen and massive complement activation. This process leads to formation of the membrane attack complex C5b-9 resulting in cytolisis and cell death. The histopathologic features are hemorrhage, thrombosis and necrosis. B); Acute Humoral Xenograft Rejection: rejects solid organs in spite of standard immunosuppression. It is constituted by a strong elicited antibody response, type II endothelial-cell activation and an acute cellular immune infiltrate (Møs, NK cells). This results in hemorrhage and thrombotic disorders.

Immunobiology of Hyperacute Rejection

Complement activation by the classical pathway (mainly mediated by IgM deposition) is the primary mechanism leading to HAR in the pig-to-primate setting, involving formation of the membrane attack complex (C5b-9) and citolysis [4]. The key role of XNA and complement in causing HAR was confirmed in vivo by the efficacy of antibody absorption by plasmapheresis and systemic complement inhibition in primate models [11]. An appropriate tool to inhibit complement systemically is the anti-C5 monoclonal antibody which prevents the cleavage of this complement component and prolongs survival of rat and pig hearts perfused *ex vivo* with human serum [12]. In general, long-term systemic inhibition of complement upstream of C5 (targeting C3 for instance) is unadvised because it would compromise the capacity of the recipient to fight infections. The first approaches developed to counteract HAR by genetic engineering focused on inhibiting complement activation by expressing human complement regulatory proteins in transgenic pigs [2,13]. The function of complement regulatory proteins is highly restricted by the species [2,13]. It was therefore reasoned that the porcine molecules were ineffective to control human complement activation. Transgenic expression of human CD59 (hCD59) and/or human CD55 (hDAF) on porcine cells and organs increased their resistance to human serum-mediated cytolysis [2,11,12]. Most importantly, this approach has consistently prolonged survival of transgenic pig organs in the various pig-to-primate transplant models tested to date [14].

The use of complement inhibitors alone represented the first step toward the development of engineered donor cells and organs. However, these approaches did not accomplish complete protection from humoral xenograft rejection, as they did not address the massive XNA reactivity toward the donor tissue. Transgenic expression of human α1,2-fucosyltransferase (H transferase, HT) was first developed to reduce the expression of the Gal α1,3-Gal antigen by competition with α1,3-GT [15-17]. HT generates fucosylated residues (H-antigen, the O blood group antigen) that are universally tolerated and prevents the transfer of the terminal galactose residue to its main substrate N-acetyl lactosamine [15]. The reduction in the Gal α1,3-Gal epitope in HT engineered cells and organs resulted in decreased human antibody reactivity and serum-mediated cytolysis [15-17]. As HT or other competitive enzymes are unable to completely remove the Gal α1,3-Gal antigen, this approach was combined with expression of human complement inhibitors in mice and pigs [18,19]. In both cases, co-expression of HT and hCD59 had an additive protective effect from human serum-mediated lysis when compared to controls and single transgenic cells [18,19]. The combination of the α1,3-GalT knockout and hCD59 in mice also showed a better outcome than each single approach [18]. Now, the Gal α1,3-Gal antigen has been successfully eliminated from pig tissues by homologous recombination and nuclear transfer/cloning technology [20,21]. Kidneys from pigs with the null phenotype transplanted into baboons are resistant to HAR [22]. However, most human sera show some reactivity toward α1,3-GalT knockout pig cells, pointing out the existence of anti-non-Gal α1,3-Gal natural antibodies [23]. Therefore, the incorporation of a complement inhibitor to the α1,3-GalT knockout is still advised to completely prevent human serum-mediated cytotoxicity.

Immunobiology of Acute
Cellular Xenograft Rejection

Both vascular and avascular xenografts are susceptible to cellular rejection in which CD4$^+$ T cells play a major role [2,3,24-26]. Nonetheless, CD8$^+$ T cells can also reject xenografts when CD4$^+$ T cells are depleted or absent [27]. The xenogeneic T cell responses show greater intensity and diversity than the allogeneic cellular responses [28,29]. This occurs in spite of human IFN-γ inability to activate porcine cells [30]. The contribution of T cell responses to xenograft rejection is most appreciated in cell-based xenotransplantation, being pancreatic islet transplantation the best studied [24,25]. In non-immunosuppressed primates, porcine pancreatic islets infused into the liver are rejected within a few days with histopathological features of cellular rejection (dense T cell and macrophage infiltrate with sparse C4d deposition). Accordingly, immunotherapies directed to suppress T cell activation have attained long-term survival of porcine islets in diabetic monkeys (>140 days) [24,25]. Similarly to cell-based xenografts, the presence of a mononuclear cell infiltrate containing primarily CD4$^+$ T cells, fewer CD8$^+$ T cells and some macrophages (and NK cells) is observed in solid organs transplanted into nonhuman primates without immunosuppression [26,31]. However, in the case of vascularized organs, there is also widespread antibody and complement deposition, as well as thrombosis and hemorrhage [26,31]. The use of strong immunosuppression successfully averts the cellular immune infiltrate in solid xenografts and prolongs graft survival, but it does not prevent AHXR [8,31]. One possible explanation for this key difference between cell and organ xenografts may be that certain cellular immune pathway/s inherent to solid organ xenotransplantation are resistant to immunosuppression, resulting in T cell-dependent B cell activation.

The underlying mechanisms of how vascularized organs trigger ACXR are under study. Most of the work has been done using in vitro systems that co-culture PAEC with human peripheral blood mononuclear cells (PBMC) or purified lymphocyte populations. Porcine endothelial cells such as PAEC can function as authentic antigen presenting cells promoting direct activation of CD8$^+$ and CD4$^+$ T cells through respective binding of SLA I and II together with costimulatory molecules [2,9,10]. Engagement of human CD28 by porcine CD86 is the main costimulatory mechanism used by PAEC to activate human T cells, whereas the CD40-CD154 pathway (also preserved crossspecies) appears to be of secondary importance [32]. Interestingly, the CD28 pathway shows resistance to immunosuppression by calcineurin inhibitors [33] and therefore its specific inhibition may have great therapeutic value. However, combination therapies such as CD152Ig with CD154 blockade only confer a partial protection, delaying but not preventing the rejection of concordant (rat-to-mouse) xenogeneic hearts [34]. On the contrary, blockade of the CD28 and CD40 pathways achieves indefinite survival of pancreatic islets reflecting the higher requirements of solid organ xenografts for tolerance induction [34]. It is also interesting to consider whether the different mechanisms of peripheral tolerance can be induced in a xenogeneic setting. In a highly stringent discordant system in which we transplanted PAEC under the kidney capsule of BALB/c mice, we showed that blockade of porcine CD86 significantly delays xenograft rejection by different mechanisms [35]. In this model we observed diminished cellularity in the local lymph nodes, some early signs of hyporesponsiveness in secondary lymphocyte/PAEC co-culture assays and an increase in $CD4^+ CD25^+$ T cells in peripheral lymphoid organs. The generation of regulatory T cells in a xenogeneic setting is consistent with recent findings that show the ability of purified human $CD4^+ CD25^+$ T cells to suppress xenogeneic T cell responses inhibiting $CD4^+ CD25^-$ T cell proliferation, cytokine production and cytolytic activity [29]. Thus, approaches designed to promote the generation of regulatory T cells may be beneficial to prolong xenograft survival in the pig-to-primate setting. Finally, another potential target for intervention may be the T cell effector functions, which are also preserved crossspecies [36]. Both $CD4^+$ and $CD8^+$ T cells display cytotoxicity toward porcine cells involving the Fas-FasL and the perforin/granzime B pathways [26,36,37]. Expression of a decoy Fas (lacking the death domain) on porcine endothelial cells partially protects them from the human $CD8^+$ CTL activity, whereas coexpression of decoy Fas with FasL further reduces the killing of pig cells [37]. In summary, several strategies remain to be further developed, especially incorporating genetic engineering of the donor, to control the xenogeneic cellular immune response. These may allow to better understand the contribution of T cells to xenograft rejection.

Immunobiology of Acute Humoral Xenograft Rejection

Targeting its leading cause has successfully averted HAR and cellular rejection is much diminished by standard immunosuppression. However, it has proven far more difficult to address AHXR. The process of AHXR is complex and multifactorial. The humoral response is responsible for rejection of the xenografts, but a contribution of T cells, cells of the innate immune system, or even coagulation incompatibilities cannot be disregarded.

Most of the information collected to date about AHXR in preclinical (pig-to-primate) organ xenotransplantation comes from studies that utilized hDAF-transgenic pigs as donors and cynomolgus monkeys or baboons as recipients. This genetic modification, alone or combined with hCD59, not only protects from HAR, but confers some advantage in front of AHXR [38,39]. Expression of hDAF on the donor organ prolongs survival when combined with antibody immunoadsorption, CVF and immunosuppression (28.7 versus 10 days mean survival) [39]. In fact, the higher the expression level of hDAF, the longer the xenograft survives in the baboon [40]. Studies in pig-to-cynomolgus kidney transplantation further support a role of complement in AHXR, as a 3-day treatment with C1-inhibitor (C1-inh) can reverse a diagnosed AHXR and prolong the mean survival time from 11.5 to 33.7 days [41]. The inconveniency of this systemic treatment is that it renders the monkeys susceptible to infections, precluding its clinical application [41]. How complement contributes to AHXR is not completely understood, although it probably acts at multiple levels. Different complement components are known to play different roles in the course of an inflammatory response [42]. The classical pathway generates membrane-bound C4b, C3b and the complex C5b-9 in this order, as well as producing anaphylatoxins C4a, C3a and C5a. C4b, C3b and breakdown products of C3 are ligands for several complement receptors expressed on immune cells and promote immune functions such as B cell activation and phagocytosis [42]. The membrane attack complex leads to cell death and the anaphylotoxins (C5a being the most potent) recruit and activate leukocytes [42]. It is of special interest to mention the recent discovery that mouse DAF reduces T cell activation in the presence of complement [43]. Thus, all these complement-dependent mechanisms may participate in acute xenograft rejection and transgenic expression of DAF may help in unexpected ways.

Complement activation is tightly associated to antibody deposition in xenograft rejection. The characteristic anatomopathological features of AHXR are accompanied by deposition of IgM, IgG and complement components (C3, C4d and C5b-9) [8,22]. The anti-Galα1,3-Gal antibodies play a part in the elicited antibody response that leads to AHXR [44,45]. However, the role of the Gal α1,3-Gal antigen in AHXR is not completely understood. Transplant experiments with xenogeneic cartilage suggest that the presence of the Gal α1,3-Gal antigen on the donor tissue elicits an anti-Galα1,3-Gal antibody response and exacerbates rejection [3,46]. Accordingly, hearts from pigs deficient in the Gal α1,3-Gal antigen have shown the longest survival times yet when transplanted into baboons using potent immunosuppression (2-6 months with a median of 78 days) [8]. However, the α1,3-GT null organs are still rejected by AHXR [8,22]. Undoubtedly, the anti-non-Gal α1,3-Gal antibody response is now the next hurdle to attain prolonged xenograft survival [47]. Even very strong immunosuppressive protocols cannot prevent the B cell response without compromising the life of the recipient [8,22]. The first step should be to test the combination of α1,3-GalT knockout and hDAF-transgenic expression in the pig-to-baboon setting utilizing standard immunosuppression. Additional therapies may be subsequently included to assess the contribution of different pathways such as stronger T cell control or different coagulation inhibitors.

It is unclear whether the clotting abnormalities described in AHXR are reliant or independent of the deposition of xenoantibodies in the xenograft. There is evidence that counteracting some of the incompatibilities of the coagulation system may benefit the xenograft function. In fact, aspirin and/or heparin are already included in the therapeutic regimes of the most successful pig-to-primate transplant experiments [8,25]. This aspect is reviewed elsewhere in more depth [48,49]. In brief, porcine cells have an inherent tendency to spontaneously clot human plasma *in vitro* due to certain molecular incompatibilities between human and porcine regulators of coagulation [48,50]. In particular, porcine tissue factor pathway inhibitor (TFPI) does not effectively block human factor Xa and porcine thrombomodulin (a key anticoagulant expressed by endothelial cells) hardly activates human protein C relative to its human counterpart [48]. Thus, if clotting abnormalities occur independently of antibody, it could explain why AHXR has been so difficult to prevent or treat in pig-to-nonhuman primate xenotransplantation. Several approaches, including genetic engineering of the porcine organs, are currently being developed to address this problem [49,51].

Of special interest is the study of the innate immune responses in xenotransplantation, as they probably play a critical role. A direct contribution of NK cells and macrophages to AHXR has been shown in small animal models such as in the discordant guinea pig-to-rat combination [52]. In the pig-to-primate setting, the failure to control acute rejection with strong anti-T cell immunosuppression and the presence of a cellular infiltrate containing predominantly macrophages and some NK cells indicates their involvement [53]. Both NK cells and macrophages may have an effect on the B cell antibody responses that ultimately result in AHXR, but there are no good therapies at the moment to control them. Interestingly, standard immunosuppression diminishes the amount of innate cellular infiltrate delaying the time of rejection [31]. Therefore, the molecular bases for these innate immune xenogeneic responses are now the focus of active research with the ultimate goal of finding therapeutic targets.

Human NK cells recognize and kill porcine cells (effect enhanced by IL-2-mediated activation) [54]. Lysis of porcine target cells by human NK cells is mediated by antibody dependent cell-mediated cytotoxicity (ADCC) and non-ADCC mechanisms. In the absence of human serum, human NK cells lyse PAEC >2-fold more efficiently than allogeneic human counterparts [55]. The molecules involved in triggering antibody-independent NK cell-mediated cytotoxicity to porcine cells are now being defined. Two receptors in human NK cells have been identified that mediate cytotoxicity of porcine cells, NKG2D and NKp44 [56]. Porcine ULBP1 has been recognized as a ligand for human NKG2D [57]. Regarding costimulatory signals, CD86 on porcine cells also triggers human NK cell activation through a CD28 variant and enhances killing [54]. We utilized a hCD152-hCD59 chimeric molecule expressed on the porcine cells to block CD86-mediated costimulation in *cis*. PAEC and porcine fibroblasts constitutively express CD86 on the cell surface (they do not express CD80 in resting conditions). Increasing levels of hCD152-hCD59 expression in these cells correlated with a reduction in both CD86 accessibility and susceptibility to lysis mediated by human NK cells in the absence of human serum. Coexpression of high levels of HT and hCD152-hCD59 led to almost complete protection from human NK cell-mediated cytotoxicity [54].

There is controversy whether the Gal α1,3-Gal epitope is directly involved in triggering human NK cell-mediated lysis through an ADCC-independent pathway. Inverardi et al. demonstrated that carbohydrate epitopes directly mediate human NK cell adhesion to xenogeneic cells in an antibody-independent manner [58]. However, PAEC from α1,3-GalT knockout pigs show very little reduction in human NK cell-mediated lysis [59]. It is possible that the Gal α1,3-Gal residue alone engages a receptor with low affinity, sending a weak activation signal that cooperates with other triggering signals. In fact, carbohydrate remodelling by HT expression on porcine cells may be more efficient than the α1,3-GalT knockout in reducing susceptibility to human NK cell-mediated lysis [54]. In fact, expression of HT in PAEC also reduces adhesion and activation of human monocytes, suggesting a shared pathway [60].

Monocytes/macrophages are other key players in acute xenograft rejection. As mentioned previously, monocytes and macrophages are present from early on in rejecting xenografts [7,26,31,61]. Interestingly, depletion of donor macrophages from porcine lungs prolongs survival from 4 to 24 h. [62]. Moreover, macrophages contribute to xenograft rejection of solid organs in a small animal model [52]. In vitro studies show that human monocytes bind and activate porcine endothelial cells and vice versa [7,60]. In addition, human dendritic cells (DC) also bind PAEC, which results in DC activation (upregulation of CD40, CD54, CD80 and CD86 on their cell-surface and production of IL-12p70 and TNF-α) [63]. However, the ligand/receptor pairs involved in these interactions are not fully characterized. Adhesion molecules in PAEC such as VCAM-1 and ICAM-1 are known to participate in the cell binding [63,64], but these may be secondary to other pathways such as carbohydrate recognition that signal to activate both the human monocytes and the porcine endothelium. Very recently, galectin-3, a lectin expressed by various cells including monocytes/macrophages, has been shown to be responsible of monocyte binding to PAEC through the Gal α1,3-Gal antigen [65]. The relevance of this finding is still unclear and its role in NK cell-mediated lysis of PAEC remains to be assessed. The implication of the Toll-like receptors (TLR) is not fully understood either. Results from pig pancreatic islet transplantation into MyD88 (TLR signal adaptor) knockout mice, suggest they do not play a major role in that setting [66].

Cytokines and chemokines are surely involved in the rejection process too, as many function crossspecies in the pig-to-human setting. One of the most relevant is TNF-α, produced mainly by NK cells and macrophages. The contribution of TNF-α to AHXR has been shown in small-animal transplant models using inhibitory antibodies and more recently with an immunoglobulin fusion protein [67,68]. Both porcine and human TNF-α activate PAEC by elevating the cell surface expression of swine leukocyte antigens (SLA) I and II, and adhesion molecules (VCAM-1, ICAM-1 and E-selectin). As mentioned earlier, all these adhesion molecules support binding and transendothelial migration of human leukocytes [64], whereas the SLA I and II mediate direct activation of human T cells [2,9,10]. A fusion protein containing the extracellular portion of porcine TNFR1 attached to an immunoglobulin Fc portion (pTNFR1Ig) was developed to block human and porcine TNF [68]. By engineering the xenogeneic donor cell to secrete pTNFR1Ig, it was possible to avert the proinflammatory effects of TNF at the transplantation site (much preferable than systemic TNF blockade). The involvement of chemokines has been studied in a mouse model transplanted with pig pancreatic islets. In this setting, the RANTES/CCR5 pathway shows the most impact on graft survival [69].

Finally, other cellular components such as neutrophils and gamma/delta T cells have also the potential to cause damage in acute xenograft rejection [70,71]. However, their participation in vivo remains to be clarified.

Conclusion

Progress toward the clinical application of xenotransplantation depends on surmounting the massive xenogeneic immune response. Theoretically, this is an attainable goal taking into account the advancement in immunosuppressive drugs and the available tools to engineer the donor pig. Success depends on the molecular characterization of the rejection process, which is currently in progress. Strategies targeting the triggering mechanisms of HAR, natural antibody and complement, have overcome this hurdle. Control of cellular rejection through combination therapies that include T cell-costimulation blockade have led to long-term survival of pig pancreatic islets in nonhuman primates. All these results are extremely encouraging. Now, the scientific community has to persevere in further elucidating the molecular bases of AHXR to address the appropriate targets that allow the prolonged acceptance of solid organ xenografts. This should not be an insurmountable task.

References

[1]   Edge, A.S.B.; Gosse, M.E. and Dinsmore, J. (1998) Xenogeneic cell therapy: current progress and future developments in porcine cell transplantation. *Cell Transplantation.* 7:525-539.

[2]   Auchincloss Jr., H. and Sachs, D. H. (1998) Xenogeneic transplantation. *Annu. Rev. Immunol.* 16: 433-470.

[3]   Costa, C.; Brokaw, J.L.; Wang, Y. and Fodor, W.L. (2003) Delayed rejection of porcine cartilage is averted by transgenic expression of alpha1,2-fucosyltransferase. *FASEB J,* 17:109-111.

[4]   Dalmasso, A. P.; Vercelotti, G. M.; Fischel, R. J.; Bolman, R. M.; Bach, F. H. and Platt, J. L. (1992) Mechanism of complement activation in the hyperacute rejection of porcine organs in primate recipients. *Am. J. Pathol.* 140:1157-1166.

[5]   Galili, U. (1993) Evolution and pathophysiology of the human anti-α-galactosyl IgG (anti-Gal) antibody. *Springer Semin. Immunopathol.* 15:155-171.

[6]   Sandrin, M. S.; Vaughan, H. A.; Dabkowski, P. L. and McKenzie, I. F. C. (1993) Anti-pig IgM antibodies in human serum reacts predominantly with Gal(α1,3)Gal epitopes. *Proc. Natl. Acad. Sci.* USA 90:11391-11395.

[7]   Goodman, D. J.; Millan, M. T.; Ferran, C. and Bach, F. H. (1997) Mechanisms of delayed xenograft rejection. In D. K. C. Cooper and E. Kemp (Eds.), Xenotransplantation (pp 95-103). *Berlin and Heidelberg: Springer-Verlag.*

[8]   Tseng, Y. L.; Kuwaki, K.; Dor, F. J.; Shimizu, A.; Houser, S.; Hisashi, Y.; Yamada, K.; Robson, S. C.; Awwad, M.; Schuurman, H. J.; Sachs, D. H.; Cooper, D. K. (2005) alpha1,3-Galactosyltransferase gene-knockout pig heart transplantation in baboons with survival approaching 6 months. *Transplantation.* 80:1493-500.

[9]   Murray, A. G.; Khodadoust, M. M.; Pober, J. S. and Bothwell, A. L. (1994) Porcine aortic endothelial cells activate human T cells: direct presentation of MHC antigens and costimulation by ligands for human CD2 and CD28. *Immunity.* 1:57-63.

[10]   Rollins, S. A.; Kennedy, S. P.; Chodera, A. J.; Elliot, E. A., Zavoico, G.B. and Matis, L. A. (1994) Evidence that activation of human T cells by porcine endothelium involves direct recognition of porcine SLA and costimulation by porcine ligands for LFA-1 and CD2. *Transplantation.* 57: 1709-1716.

[11]   Leventhal, J. R.; Sakiyalak, P.; Witson, J.; Simone, P.; Matas, A. J.; Bolman, R. M. and Dalmasso, A. P. (1994) The synergistic effect of combined antibody and complement depletion on discordant cardiac xenograft survival in nonhuman primates. *Transplantation.* 57:974-978.

[12]   Rollins, S. A.; Matis, L. A.; Springhorn, J. P.; Setter, E. and Wolf, D. W (1995) Monoclonal antibodies directed against human C5 and C8 block complement-mediated damage of xenogeneic cells and organs. *Transplantation.* 60:1284-1292.

[13]   Fodor, W. L.; Williams, B. L.; Matis, L. A.; Madri, J. A.; Rollins, S. A.; Knight, J. W.; Velander, W. and Squinto, S. P. (1994) Expression of a functional human complement inhibitor in a transgenic pig as a model for the prevention of xenogeneic hyperacute organ rejection. *Proc. Natl. Acad. Sci. USA.* 91:11153-11157.

[14] C. Costa, and R. Mañez. (2006) State of the art in knidney xenotransplantation. In Dominick W. Mancuso (Ed.), *Progress in kidney Transplantation* (Chapter 9). Nova Science Publishers, Inc. New York.

[15] Sandrin, M. S.; Fodor, W. L.; Mouhtouris, E.; Osman, N.; Cohney, S.; Rollins, S. A.; Guilmette, E. R.; Setter, E.; Squinto, S. P. and McKenzie, I. F. C. (1995) Enzymatic remodelling of the carbohydrate surface of a xenogenic cell substantially reduces human antibody binding and complement-mediated cytolysis. *Nature Med.* 1:1261-1267.

[16] Sharma, A.; Okabe, J.; Birch, P.; McClellan, S. B.; Martin, M. J.; Platt, J. L. and Logan, J. S. (1996) Reduction in the level of Galα(1,3)Gal in transgenic mice and pigs by expression of an α(1,2)fucosyltransferase. *Proc. Natl. Acad. Sci.* USA 93:7190-7195.

[17] Costa, C.; Zhao, L.; Burton, W.; Bondioli, K. R.; Williams, B. L.; Hoaglan, T. A.; DiTullio, P. A.; Ebert, K.M. and Fodor, W.L.. (1999) Expression by α1,2-fucosyltransferase in transgenic pigs modifies the cell surface carbohydrate phenotype and confers resistance to human serum-mediated cytolysis. *FASEB J.* 13:1762-1773.

[18] Costa, C.; Zhao, L.; DeCesare, S. and Fodor, W. L. (1999) Comparative analysis of three genetic modifications designed to inhibit human serum-mediated cytolysis. *Xenotransplantation.* 6: 6-11.

[19] Costa, C.; Zhao, L.; Burton, W.; Rosas, C.; Bondioli, K.R.; Williams, B.L.; Hoaglan, T.A.; Dalmasso, A.P. and Fodor, W.L. (2002) Transgenic pigs designed to express human CD59 and H-transferase to avoid humoral xenograft rejection. *Xenotransplantation.* 9:45-57.

[20] Lai, L.; Kolber-Simonds, D.; Park, K-W.; Cheong, H. T.; Greenstein J. L.; Im, G. S.; Samuel, M.; Bonk, A.; Rieke, A.; Day, B. N.; Murphy, C. N.; Carter, D. B.; Hawley, R. J. and Prather, R. S. (2002) Production of α-1,3-galactosyltransferase knockout pigs by nuclear transfer cloning. *Science.* 295:1089-1092.

[21] Phelps, C. J.; Koike, C.; Vaught, T. D.; Boone, J.; Wells, K. D.; Chen, S. H.; Ball, S; Specht, S. M.; Polejaeva, I. A.; Monahan, J. A.; Jobst, P. M.; Sharma, S. B.; Lamborn, A. E; Garst, A. S.; Moore, M.; Demetris, A. J.; Rudert, W. A.; Bottino, R.; Bertera, S.; Trucco, M.; Starzl, T. E.; Dai, Y. and Ayares D. L. (2003) Production of alpha 1,3-galactosyltransferase-deficient pigs. *Science.* 299:411-414.

[22] Chen, G.; Qian, H.; Starzl, T.; Sun, H.; Garcia, B.; Wang, X.; Wise, Y.; Liu, Y.; Xiang, Y.; Copeman, L.; Liu, W.; Jevnikar, A.; Wall, W.; Cooper D. K.; Murase, N.; Dai, Y.; Wang, W.; Xiong, Y.; White, D. J. and Zhong, R. (2005) Acute rejection is associated with antibodies to non-Gal antigens in baboons using Gal-knockout pig kidneys. *Nat. Med.* 11:1295-11298.

[23] Hara, H.; Ezzelarab, M.; Rood P. P.; Lin, Y. J.; Busch, J.; Ibrahim, Z.; Zhu, X.; Ball, S.; Ayares, D.; Zeevi, A.; Awwad, M. and Cooper D. K. (2006) Allosensitized humans are at no greater risk of humoral rejection of GT-KO pig organs than other humans. *Xenotransplantation.* 13:357-365.

[24] Cardona, K.; Korbutt, G. S.; Milas, Z.; Lyon, J.; Cano, J.; Jiang, W.; Bello-Laborn, H.; Hacquoil, B.; Strobert, E.; Gangappa, S.; Weber, C. J.; Pearson, T. C.; Rajotte, R. V.

and Larsen, C. P. (2006) Long-term survival of neonatal porcine islets in nonhuman primates by targeting costimulation pathways. *Nat. Med.* 12:304-306.

[25] Hering, B. J.; Wijkstrom, M.; Graham, M. L.; Hardstedt, M.; Aasheim, T. C.; Jie, T.; Ansite, J. D.; Nakano, M.; Cheng, J.; Li, W.; Moran, K.; Christians, U.; Finnegan, C.; Mills, C. D.; Sutherland, D. E.; Bansal-Pakala, P.; Murtaugh, M. P.; Kirchhof, N. and Schuurman, H. J. (2006) Prolonged diabetes reversal after intraportal xenotransplantation of wild-type porcine islets in immunosuppressed nonhuman primates. *Nat. Med.* 12:301-303.

[26] Davila, E.; Byrne, G. W.; LaBreche, P. T.; McGregor, H. C.; Schwab, A. K.; Davies, W. R.; Rao, V. P.; Oi, K.; Tazelaar, H. D.; Logan, J. S. and McGregor, C. G. (2006) T-cell responses during pig-to-primate xenotransplantation. *Xenotransplantation.* 13:31-40.

[27] Uchida, T.; Tomita, Y.; Anzai, K.; Zhang, Q. W.; Yoshikawa, M.; Kishihara, K.; Nomoto, K. and Yasui, H. (1999) Roles of $CD4^+$ and $CD8^+$ T cells in discordant skin xenograft rejection. *Transplantation.* 68:1721-1727.

[28] Brouard S, Vanhove B, Gagne K, Neumann A, Douillard P, Moreau A, Cuturi C, Soulillou JP. T cell repertoire alterations of vascularized xenografts. *J. Immunol.* 1999 Mar 15;162(6):3367-77.

[29] Porter, C. M. and Bloom, E. T. (2005) Human CD4+CD25+ regulatory T cells suppress anti-porcine xenogeneic responses. *Am. J. Transplant.* 5:2052-2057.

[30] Sultan, P.; Murray, A. G.; McNiff, J. M.; Lorber, M. I.; Askenase, P. W.; Bothwell, A. L. and Pober, J. S. (1997) Pig but not human interferon-gamma initiates human cell-mediated rejection of pig tissue in vivo. *Proc. Natl. Acad. Sci. U S A* 94:8767-8772.

[31] Ashton-Chess, J.; Roussel, J. C.; Manez, R.; Ruiz, C.; Moreau, A.; Cozzi, E.; Minault, D.; Soulillou J. P.; Blancho, G. (2003) Cellular participation in delayed xenograft rejection of hCD55 transgenic pig hearts by baboons. *Xenotransplantation.* 10:446-53.

[32] Lee, R. S.; Yamada, K.; Womer, K. L.; Pillsbury, E. P.; Allison, K. S.; Marolewski, A. E.; Geng, D.; Thall, A. D.; Arn, J. S.; Sachs, D. H.; Sayegh, M. H. and Madsen, J. C. (2000) Blockade of CD28-B7, but not CD40-CD154, prevents costimulation of allogeneic porcine and xenogeneic human anti-porcine T cell responses. *J. Immunol.* 164:3434-3444.

[33] June, C. H.; Ledbetter, J. A.; Gillespie, M. M.; Lindsten, T. and Thompson, C. B. (1987) T cell proliferation involving the CD28 pathway is associated with cyclosporine resistant interleukin-2 gene expression. *Mol. Cell. Biol.* 7: 4472-4481.

[34] Lehnert, A. M.; Mottram, P. L.; Han, W.; Walters, S. N.; Patel, A. T.; Hawthorne, W. J.; Cowan, P. J. and O'Connell, P. J. (2001) Blockade of the CD40 and CD28 pathways result in acceptance of pig and rat islet xenografts but not cardiac grafts in mice. *Transpl. Immunol.* 9:51-56.

[35] Costa, C.; Pizzolato, M. C.; Shen, Y.; Wang, Y. and Fodor, W. L. (2004) CD86 blockade in genetically modified porcine cells delays xenograft rejection by inhibiting T-cell and NK-cell activation. *Cell Transplant.* 13:75-87.

[36] Yi, S.; Feng, X.; Wang, Y.; Kay, T. W.; Wang, Y. and O'Connell, P. J. (1999) CD4+ cells play a major role in xenogeneic human anti-pig cytotoxicity through the Fas/Fas ligand lytic pathway. *Transplantation.* 67:435-443.

[37] Kawamoto, K.; Tanemura, M.; Nishida, T.; Fukuzawa, M.; Ito, T. and Matsuda, H. (2006) Significant inhibition of human CD8(+) cytotoxic T lymphocyte-mediated xenocytotoxicity by overexpression of the human decoy Fas antigen. *Transplantation.* 81:789-796.

[38] Cozzi, E.; Bhatti, F.; Schmoeckel, M.; Chavez, G.; Smith, K. G.; Zaidi, A.; Bradley, J. R.; Thiru, S.; Goddard, M.; Vial, C.; Ostlie, D.; Wallwork, J.; White, D. J. and Friend P. J. (2000) Long-term survival of nonhuman primates receiving life-supporting transgenic porcine kidney xenografts. *Transplantation.* 70: 15-21.

[39] Buhler, L.; Yamada, K.; Kitamura, H.; Alwayn, I. P.; Basker, M.; Appel, J. Z. 3rd; Colvin, R. B.; White-Scharf, M. E.; Sachs, D. H.; Robson, S. C.; Awwad, M. and Cooper, D. K. (2001) Pig kidney transplantation in baboons: anti-Gal(alpha)1-3Gal IgM alone is associated with acute humoral xenograft rejection and disseminated intravascular coagulation. *Transplantation.* 72:1743-1752.

[40] Sun, H.; Chen, G.; Liu, W.; Kubelik, D.; Yang, H.; White, D. J.; Zhong, R. and Garcia, B. (2005) The influence of baseline expression of human decay accelerating factor transgene on graft survival and acute humoral xenograft rejection. *Transplantation.* 80:1331-1339.

[41] Vangerow, B.; Hecker, J. M.; Lorenz, R.; Loss, M.; Przemeck, M.; Appiah, R.; Schmidtko, J.; Jalali, A.; Rueckoldt, H. and Winkler, M. (2001) C1-Inhibitor for treatment of acute vascular xenograft rejection in cynomolgus recipients of h-DAF transgenic porcine kidneys. *Xenotransplantation.* 8:266-272.

[42] Walport, M. J. (2001) Complement at the interface between innate and adaptive immunity. *N. Engl. J. Med.* 344:1140-1144.

[43] Liu, J.; Miwa, T.; Hilliard, B.; Chen, Y.; Lambris, J. D.; Wells, A. D. and Song, W. C. (2005) The complement inhibitory protein DAF (CD55) suppresses T cell immunity in vivo. *J. Exp. Med.* 201:567-77.

[44] Lin, S. S.; Hanaway, M. J.; Gonzalez-Stawinski, G. V.; Lau, C. L.; Parker, W.; Davis, R. D.; Byrne, G. W.; Diamond, L. E.; Logan, J. S. and Platt, J. L. (2000) The role of anti-Galalpha1-3Gal antibodies in acute vascular rejection and accommodation of xenografts. *Transplantation.* 70:1667-1674.

[45] Kozlowski, T.; Shimizu, A.; Lambrigts, D.; Yamada, K.; Fuchimoto, Y.; Glaser, R.; Monroy, R.; Xu, Y.; Awwad, M.; Colvin, R. B.; Cosimi, A. B.; Robson, S. C.; Fishman J.; Spitzer, T. R.; Cooper, D. K. C. and Sachs, D. H. (1999) Porcine kidney and heart transplantation in baboons undergoing a tolerance induction regimen and antibody adsorption. *Transplantation.* 67:18-30.

[46] Stone, K. R.; Ayala, G.; Goldstein, J.; Hurst, R.; Walgenbach, A.; and Galili, U. (1998) Porcine cartilage transplants in the cynomolgus monkey. III. Transplantation of α–galactosidase-treated porcine cartilage. *Transplantation.* 65:1577-1583.

[47] Domenech, N.; Diaz, T.; Moscoso, I.; Lopez-Pelaez, E.; Centeno, A. and Manez, R. (2003) Elicited non-anti-alphaGAL antibodies may cause acute humoral rejection of hDAF pig organs transplanted in baboons. *Transplant. Proc.* 35:2049-2050.

[48] Robson, S. C.; Cooper, D. K. and d'Apice, A. J. (2000) Disordered regulation of coagulation and platelet activation in xenotransplantation. *Xenotransplantation* 7: 166-176.

[49] Banz, Y. and Rieben, R. (2006) Endothelial cell protection in xenotransplantation: looking after a key player in rejection. *Xenotransplantation.* 13:19-30.

[50] Siegel, J. B.; Grey, S. T.; Lesnikoski, B. A.; Kopp, C. W.; Soares, M.; Schulte am Esch, J. 2nd.; Bach, F. H. and Robson, S. C. (1997) Xenogeneic endothelial cells activate human prothrombrin. *Transplantation.* 64: 888-896.

[51] Chen, D.; Weber, M.; McVey, J. H.; Kemball-Cook, G.; Tuddenham, E. G.; Lechler, R. I. and Dorling, A. (2004) Complete inhibition of acute humoral rejection using regulated expression of membrane-tethered anticoagulants on xenograft endothelium. *Am. J. Transplant.* 4: 1958-1963.

[52] Xia, G.; Ji, P.; Rutgeerts, O. and Waer, M. (2000) Natural killer cell- and macrophage mediated discordant guinea pig-->rat xenograft rejection in the absence of complement, xenoantibody and T cell immunity. *Transplantation.* 70:86-93.

[53] Kobayashi. T.; Taniguchi. S.; Neethling, F. A.; Rose, A. G.; Hancock, W. W.; Ye, Y.; Niekrasz, M.; Kosanke, S.; Wright, L. J.; White, D. J. G. and Cooper, D. K. C. (1997) Delayed xenograft rejection of pig-to-baboon cardiac transplants after cobra venom factor therapy. *Transplantation.* 64: 1255-1261.

[54] Costa, C.; Barber, D. F. and Fodor, W. L. (2002) Human NK cell-mediated cytotoxicity triggered by CD86 and Galα1,3-Gal is inhibited in genetically modified porcine cells. *J. Immunol.* 168: 3808-3816.

[55] Artrip, J. H.; Kwiatkowski, P.; Michler, R. E.; Wang, S. F.; Tugulea, S.; Ankersmit, J.; Chisholm, L.; McKenzie, I. F.; Sandrin, M. S. and Itescu, S. (1999) Target cell susceptibility to lysis by human natural killer cells is augmented by alpha(1,3)-galactosyltransferase and reduced by alpha(1, 2)-fucosyltransferase. *J. Biol. Chem.* 274:10717-10722.

[56] Forte, P.; Lilienfeld, B. G.; Baumann, B. C. and Seebach, J. D. (2005) Human NK cytotoxicity against porcine cells is triggered by NKp44 and NKG2D. *J. Immunol.* 175: 5463-70.

[57] Lilienfeld, B. G.; Garcia-Borges, C. , Crew, M. D. and Seebach, J. D. (2006) Porcine UL16-binding protein 1 expressed on the surface of endothelial cells triggers human NK cytotoxicity through NKG2D. *J. Immunol.* 177:2146-2152.

[58] Inverardi, L.; Clissi, B.; Stolzer, A. L.; Bender, J. R.; Sandrin, M. S. and Pardi, R. (1997) Human natural killer lymphocytes directly recognize evolutionarily conserved oligosaccharide ligands expressed by xenogeneic tissues. *Transplantation.* 63:1318.

[59] Horvath-Arcidiacono, J. A., Porter, C. M. and Bloom, E. T. (2006) Human NK cells can lyse porcine endothelial cells independent of their expression of Galalpha(1,3)-Gal and killing is enhanced by activation of either effector or target cells. *Xenotransplantation.* 13:318-27.

[60] Kwiatkowski, P.; Artrip, J. H.; Edwards, N. M.; Lietz, K.; Tugulea, S.; Michler, R. E.; McKenzie, I. F.; Sandrin, M. S. And Itescu, S. (1999) High-level porcine endothelial cell expression of alpha(1,2)-fucosyltransferase reduces human monocyte adhesion and activation.*Transplantation.* 67:219-226.

[61] Goddard, M. J.; Dunning, J.; Horsley, J.; Atkinson, C.; Pino-Chavez, G. and Wallwork, J. (2002) Histopathology of cardiac xenograft rejection in the pig-to-baboon model. *J. Heart Lung Transplant.* 21:474-484.

[62] Cantu, E.; Gaca, J. G.; Palestrant, D.; Baig, K.; Lukes, D. J.; Gibson, S. E.; Gonzalez-Stawinski, G. V.; Olausson, M.; Parker, W. and Davis, R. D. (2006) Depletion of pulmonary intravascular macrophages prevents hyperacute pulmonary xenograft dysfunction. *Transplantation.* 81:1157-1164.

[63] Manna, P. P.; Duffy, B.; Olack, B.; Lowell, J. and Mohanakumar, T. (2001) Activation of human dendritic cells by porcine aortic endothelial cells: transactivation of naive T cells through costimulation and cytokine generation. *Transplantation.* 72:1563-1571.

[64] Holgersson, J.; Ehrnfelt, C.; Hauzenberger, E. and Serrander, L. (2002) Leukocyte endothelial cell interactions in pig to human organ xenograft rejection. *Vet. Immunol. Immunopathol.* 87: 407-415.

[65] Jin, R.; Greenwald, A.; Peterson, M. D. and Waddell, T. K. (2006) Human monocytes recognize porcine endothelium via the interaction of galectin 3 and alpha-GAL. *J. Immunol.* 177:1289-1295.

[66] Schmidt, P.; Krook, H.; Goto, M. and Korsgren, O. (2004) MyD88-dependent toll-like receptor signalling is not a requirement for fetal islet xenograft rejection in mice. *Xenotransplantation.* 11:347-352.

[67] Lin, Y.; Vandeputte, M. and Waer, M. (1997) Contribution of activated macrophages to the process of delayed xenograft rejection. *Transplantation.* 64:1677-1683.

[68] Costa, C.; Bell, N. K.; Stabel, T. J. and Fodor, W.L. (2004) Use of porcine tumor necrosis factor receptor 1-Ig fusion protein to prolong xenograft survival. *Xenotransplantation.* 11: 491-502.

[69] Yi, S.; Ouyang, L.; Ha, H.; O'Hara, J. M.; Chandra, A. P.; Akima, S.; Hawthorne, W.; Patel, A. T.; Stokes, R. and O'Connell, P. J. (2005) Involvement of CCR5 signaling in macrophage recruitment to porcine islet xenografts. *Transplantation.* 80:1468-1475.

[70] Cardozo, L. A.; Rouw, D. B.; Ambrose, L. R.; Midulla, M.; Florey, O.; Haskard, D. O. and Warrens, A. N. (2004) The neutrophil: the unnoticed threat in xenotransplantation? *Transplantation.* 78:1721-1728.

[71] Rodriguez-Gago, M.; de Heredia, A.; Ramirez, P.; Parrilla, P.; Aparicio, P. and Yelamos, J. (2001) Human anti-porcine gammadelta T-cell xenoreactivity is inhibited by human FasL expression on porcine endothelial cells. *Transplantation.* 72:503-509.

In: Transplantation Immunology Research Trends   ISBN: 978-1-60021-578-0
Editor: Oliver N. Ulricker, pp. 219-231   © 2007 Nova Science Publishers, Inc.

Chapter IX

The Role of Viruses in Allograft Rejection

Tomáš Reischig
Department of Internal Medicine I, Charles University Medical School
and Teaching Hospital, Pilsen, Czech Republic

Abstract

Increasing evidence suggests a role for viruses in allograft rejection in solid organ transplant recipients. Cytomegalovirus (CMV) disease is an independent risk factor for acute rejection in renal transplantation. CMV has also been described as a trigger for chronic rejection such as cardiac allograft vasculopathy in heart transplantation and chronic allograft nephropathy in renal transplantation. CMV may be involved in the pathology of acute rejection by several mechanisms, including up-regulation of adhesion molecules, increased expression of MHC class II antigens on allograft tissue, and release of variety of cytokines. Direct infection of arterial smooth muscle cells and endothelial cells accelerates the development of allograft vasculopathy. CMV-encoded chemokine receptor US28 has the ability to induce smooth muscle cell migration. Moreover, CMV abrogates the vascular protective effects of endothelium-derived nitric oxide system. Data on beneficial effects of antiviral prophylaxis on allograft rejection are inconsistent. Still, valacyclovir prophylaxis was associated with significant reduction of acute rejection in two randomized controlled trials in renal transplant recipients. In summary, viruses contribute importantly to the pathophysiology of acute and chronic allograft rejection. Further clinical trials are needed to determine favorable effects of antiviral prophylaxis on rejection rate.

Introduction

Immunosuppressive therapy in patients after solid organ transplantation significantly compromise cellular immunity, which has a crucial role in the control of viral infections [1].

Viral infections are a serious clinical problem limiting the success of transplantation. Cytomegalovirus (CMV) is the most frequent opportunistic pathogen in transplant recipients. Similarly to other herpes viruses, it is able to persist in the organism in a stage of latency and to reactivate under certain conditions. If the patients do not receive antiviral prophylaxis or pre-emptive therapy, the incidence of active CMV infection reaches up to 90% and occurrence of symptomatic CMV infection (CMV disease) is ranging between 20 – 60% with a typical onset within the 1st and 4th month after transplantation [2 - 8]. Since prophylaxis or pre-emptive therapy significantly decrease occurrence of CMV disease, the results still remain not optimal [11 - 13]. Up to 20% incidence of late onset CMV disease and resistance to ganciclovir are the major problems. Pre-emptive therapy does not prevent the development of asymptomatic active infection, however even with the use of prophylaxis active infection is commonly observed (14 – 49%) [5, 7, 8, 14, 15].

The risk of CMV disease is influenced by several factors [9, 10]. CMV serostatus of the donor (D) and recipient (R) prior to transplantation are extremely important in determining risk. Patients in D+/R- group endangered by primary CMV infection are at highest risk. Seropositive recipients (D+/R+ or D-/R+), in whom reactivation of the virus of the host origin or super-infection by virus of donor origin occur make up the group with moderate risk. On the other hand in D-/R- patients the occurrence of CMV infection and CMV disease is very low. The risk depends also on the type of organ transplanted with the highest risk in lung transplantation and the lowest in renal transplantation [3]. The role of immunosuppression on the development of CMV disease is well described. Since the risk is determined rather by the net state of immunosuppression than by any single immunosuppressive agent, there are some exceptions. This includes mainly induction or anti-rejection administration of depleting antilymphocyte antibodies such as antithymocyte globulin or OKT3, which is associated with several fold increased risk of CMV disease [2, 9].

The clinical picture of CMV infection after transplantation is various. Active CMV infection is defined by a culture detection of CMV in blood, urine, bronchoalveolar lavage or tissue biopsy specimens [9]. Viral culture is however low sensitive and slow. Therefore modern methods such as polymerase chain reaction (PCR) CMV DNA, PCR CMV mRNA (NASBA) or CMV pp65 antigenemia are currently successfully used for the detection of CMV. Furthermore, these tests enable quantitative determination of viral load [16, 17]. Active CMV infection may have an asymptomatic course. CMV disease is defined as a symptomatic active infection. Symptoms could include only flu-like and mononucleosis-like syndromes together with haematological abnormalities and elevation of liver enzymes (also called CMV syndrome) or tissue invasive CMV disease (pneumonitis, gastrointestinal disease, hepatitis, retinitis, and other) [9]. CMV has however also indirect effects with long term consequences. These include also a role in the pathogenesis of acute and chronic rejection.

Bidirectional Relationship between Cytomegalovirus and Acute Rejection

Despite clinical and experimental data show a significant role of CMV in the development of acute allograft rejection, it should be emphasized that the relation between CMV and rejection is more complicated. Acute rejection is a strong risk factor for the development of CMV disease [18, 19]. The reason is not only enhanced immunosuppression during anti-rejection therapy, but mainly a release of pro-inflammatory cytokines during rejection [20]. Inflammation represents the most important pathway of CMV activation from the stage of latency. Pro-inflammatory cytokines, mainly tumour necrosis factor alpha (TNF-α), activate transcription factors such as protein kinase C (PKC) or nuclear factor kappa B (NF-κB), which control expression of CMV major immediate early promoter/enhancer (MIEP). The result is a transcription of regulatory immediate early proteins and viral replication [20]. There are also other mechanisms of CMV activation (table 1). These include catecholamine-mediated pathway, which results in stimulation of CMV MIEP via cyclic adenosine monophosphate (cAMP) [20]. The last way of CMV activation is an oxidative stress with subsequent reactive oxygen species (ROS) formation [21]. ROS leads through the activation of the activator protein 1 (AP-1) to an expression of CMV MEIP.

Table 1. Mechanisms of cytomegalovirus activation

Pathway of activation	Mediators	Clinical events causing activation
Inflammation	TNF-α PKC, NF-κB	Acute rejection, bacterial sepsis, ATG or OKT3 administration, liver cirrhosis
Catecholamines	cAMP, PKA CREB, ATF	Myocardial infarction
Oxidative stress	ROS MAPK, AP-1	I/R injury during organ storage and transplantation

TNF-α = tumor necrosis factor alpha, PKC = protein kinase C, NF-κB = nuclear factor kappa B, ATG = antithymocyte globulin, OKT3 = murine anti-CD3 monoclonal antibody, cAMP = cyclic adenosine monophosphate, PKA = protein kinase A, CREB = cyclic adenosine monophosphate response element binding, ATF = activating transcription factor, ROS = reactive oxygen species, MAPK = mitogen activated protein kinase, AP-1 = activator protein 1, I/R = ischemia/reperfusion.

Clinical Evidence for Cytomegalovirus-Induced Allograft Rejection

There are several studies, which document that CMV disease and in some cases also CMV infection are independent risk factors for the development of acute rejection. In prospective studies in renal transplant recipients it has been shown that CMV disease and infection result in an increased incidence of acute rejection [22, 23]. Other authors, also with the use of prospective data however did not prove the negative effect of asymptomatic CMV infection [24 - 26]. On the other hand the effect of CMV disease was consistent and resulted in 3 – 6 fold increase of relative risk for acute rejection in multivariate analyses [25, 26]. An indirect evidence for the role of CMV in the pathogenesis of acute rejection is an observation of higher occurrence of acute rejection in CMV seromismatched patients (D+/R-), who have a higher risk of CMV activation after transplantation [27]. Similar associations were described in transplantation of other organs [28, 29].

Currently the effect of asymptomatic active CMV infection remains the main unresolved issue. From the clinical point of view this is very important information. In the case that asymptomatic infection results in an increase of acute rejection, it would mean a significant limitation of the use of pre-emptive therapy. It has been mentioned that the results of studies evaluating the effect of asymptomatic infection are controversial [22 - 26]. Furthermore several studies supporting the negative effect of CMV infection combine in the analysis patients with asymptomatic CMV infection and CMV disease [22, 23]. It seems logical to expect that the effect of CMV disease and asymptomatic CMV infection will be different. Viral load in CMV disease is significantly higher than in asymptomatic infection [30]. The levels of cytokines and adhesion molecules important in the pathogenesis of rejection correlate with viral load [31].

Chronic rejection has various patterns in transplantations of individual organs as cardiac allograft vasculopathy in heart transplantation, chronic allograft nephropathy in renal transplantation, vanishing-bile-duct syndrome in liver transplantation or bronchiolitis obliterans syndrome in lung transplantation. Nevertheless accelerated arteriosclerosis is the basis in all cases. The effect of CMV is best documented in the pathogenesis of cardiac allograft vasculopathy [32], which is characterised by diffuse and progressive thickening of arterial intima in the major and minor coronary arteries of transplanted heart. Probably in this case also the role of CMV in native atherosclerosis contributes significantly [33]. The first reports come from the late 80's when it was proved that 28% of CMV-infected patients developed severe coronary artery obstructive lesions, compared with an incidence of 10% in uninfected group [34]. It was proved in a prospective study with the utilisation of intravascular ultrasound (IVUS) that CMV infection requiring treatment negatively influences coronary-artery remodelling in the first year after heart transplantation [35]. Apart from that it was found out that CMV seropositivity in recipients is an independent predictor for the progression of cardiac allograft vasculopathy [36].

The results in studies on renal transplantation are not so definite. Some authors proved an association between CMV disease and chronic allograft nephropathy [37], nevertheless in several studies only a simultaneous occurrence of acute rejection and CMV infection and/or disease resulted in a significant increase of risk of chronic allograft nephropathy [38, 39]. In spite of that is the role of CMV in the pathogenesis of chronic allograft nephropathy probable. Not only due to the association of tissue viral DNA in biopsy samples with an increased intensity of interstitial fibrosis and tubular atrophy [40], but mainly for worsened long term survival of grafts in patients with previous CMV disease [41, 42]. Last but not least there is evidence for the association of CMV and vanishing-bile-duct syndrome in liver transplant recipients and/or bronchiolitis obliterans syndrome in lung transplantation [28, 43]. CMV therefore contributes in the pathogenesis of chronic rejection in most organs and thus represents a significant limiting factor for long term success of solid organ transplantations.

Mechanisms of Cytomegalovirus-Induced Allograft Rejection and Arteriosclerosis

There are several mechanisms described, by which CMV could induce graft impairment [20, 44]. All of them relate to chronic inflammation caused by CMV in the systemic level or locally in allograft tissue or endothelium. CMV immediate early proteins have strong transactivating properties and result in enhanced expression of adhesion molecules and their ligands. An up-regulation of vascular cell adhesion molecule 1 (VCAM-1), intercellular adhesion molecule 1 (ICAM-1), leukocyte function antigen 1 and 3 (LFA-1, LFA-3) and very late antigen 4 (VLA-4) was verified in relation with CMV infection [31, 45 - 47]. Similarly an elevation of pro-inflammatory cytokines and chemokines such as interleukin 2 and 8 (IL-2, IL-8), macrophage inflammatory protein 1 alpha (MIP-1α) or monocyte chemotactic protein 1 (MCP-1) was documented [29, 31]. Increased expression of adhesion molecules was found in infected cells as well as neighbouring non-infected cells by paracrine action of secreted interleukin 1 beta (IL-1β) [48]. A very important finding is that administration of antiviral drugs during established CMV infection does not decrease T-cell activation response to infected cells and does not prevent a possibility of rejection [45].

Major histocompatibility complex (MHC) molecules classes I and II are required for expression of alloantigen and subsequent development of acute rejection [44]. CMV infection in rats resulted in a strong upregulation of MHC class II expression on endothelial and tubular cells in the kidney [49]. Apart from that CMV immediate early gene encodes a protein that has sequence homology and immunologic cross reactivity with the HLA-DR β-chain [50]. Other CMV-encoded protein is a homologue of MHC class I molecule [51].

In the pathogenesis of chronic rejection and allograft arteriosclerosis CMV is contributing indirectly by influencing the occurrence of acute rejection. An increased expression of growth factors such as transforming growth factor beta (TGF-β), platelet-derived growth factor (PDGF) or connective tissue growth factor (CTGF) also plays a role [52]. It seems, however, that a major importance has a direct CMV infection of vascular smooth muscle cells and endothelial cells, which results in smooth muscle cell proliferation and to the impairment of the nitric oxide synthase pathway [29, 32]. Infection of smooth muscle cells results in expression of CMV-encoded chemokine receptor US28, which induces cellular migration, as verified in in-vitro as well as in-vivo studies [53, 54]. Nitric oxide is a potent endogenous anti-atherogenic molecule. Nitric oxide deficiency plays a role in cardiac allograft vasculopathy [32]. In CMV infected endothelial cells severe endothelial nitric oxide synthase disorder resulting in a deficit of nitric oxide is present [32].

The Role of Antiviral Prophylaxis in the Prevention of Allograft Rejection

Due to negative consequences of CMV disease and availability of effective oral antiviral drugs is currently a universal prophylaxis administered in many transplant centres. The most frequently used drugs for the prophylaxis include oral ganciclovir, valganciclovir, valacyclovir and acyclovir. In all of them was the efficiency proved in randomised controlled studies [4, 5, 7, 8, 14, 55]. Whereas ganciclovir, valganciclovir and valacyclovir are comparable in terms of prevention of CMV disease or active infection [8, 14, 15], the efficacy of high-dose acyclovir is significantly lower in comparison with ganciclovir [55]. Despite prophylaxis cannot fully eliminate CMV disease, it should be generally evaluated as a beneficial treatment with a good efficacy, which results in a significant decline of CMV disease incidence and active CMV infection in all types of solid organ transplantation [11, 13].

In the light of mentioned effects of CMV to allograft rejection, it could be expected that antiviral prophylaxis shall have a positive effect on the occurrence of active and chronic rejection. Indeed, in an animal model, prophylaxis with ganciclovir resulted in disappearance of aortic and cardiac allograft vasculopathy [56, 57]. Unfortunately the results of human studies are not so definite. Prophylaxis was not associated with a significant reduction of acute rejection (relative risk = 0.90, 95% confidence interval = 0.78 – 1.05) in a recently published meta-analysis of randomised controlled studies evaluating ganciclovir, valganciclovir, valacyclovir or acyclovir in comparison with placebo or a group without therapy [11]. Meta-analysis included 19 studies (totally 1981 patients), performed in patients after kidney, liver or heart transplantation. Patients with various CMV serological combinations of D/R were included. The effect of prophylaxis on acute rejection may be however different between individual groups. In the same time there may be differences between antiviral drugs as well. For example registry data reveal that in a CMV high risk D+/R- group of renal transplant recipients the prophylaxis is associated with lower incidence of acute rejection and even with the improvement of graft survival, which could indirectly prove the effect of prophylaxis on chronic allograft nephropathy [58]. The study is however limited by its retrospective character. In the same time as the aforementioned meta-analysis [11] a similar meta-analysis with a primary goal to evaluate the effect of prophylaxis on tissue invasive CMV disease [13] was published by other authors. Due to more strict selection criteria only 11 studies (totally 1582 patients) were included. In this analysis the prophylaxis was associated with a decreased risk of acute rejection (relative risk = 0.74, 95% confidence interval = 0.59 – 0.94) [13]. In a more detailed evaluation it is obvious that in liver transplantation a positive trend was observed in most studies. On the other hand a decline of acute rejection rate in renal transplant recipients was due to the results of large placebo controlled study with valacyclovir. This study included 616 patients and significantly influenced the overall results of the analysis [5, 13]. Patients treated with valacyclovir had a significantly lower incidence of acute rejection (29% vs 41%, relative risk = 0.57) mainly due to a reduction of rejection in the D+/R- group (26% vs 52%) [5]. Also another study reveals that the positive effect of valacyclovir may be greater than in ganciclovir [8]. The patients were randomised to prophylaxis with either oral ganciclovir, valacyclovir or received no prophylaxis. Since the efficiency of ganciclovir and valacyclovir in the prevention of CMV disease and CMV viremia was comparable, the group treated with valacyclovir had a significantly lower incidence of biopsy-proven acute rejection (12%) not only in comparison with patients without prophylaxis (58%, P < 0.001), but also with the group treated with ganciclovir (34%, P = 0.03) [8]. Clear explanation for these differences was not yet provided. It may be speculated that due to nephrotoxicity of ganciclovir the incidence of delayed graft function is increased, which represents a risk for subsequent acute rejection [8]. Further studies are required to determine whether valacyclovir is really advantageous than ganciclovir at least in renal transplantation.

Data on the effect of prophylaxis on chronic rejection are limited. It has been mentioned already that the role of CMV is best established in the pathogenesis of chronic cardiac vasculopathy. In a post hoc analysis of a randomised placebo controlled a decreased cardiac allograft vasculopathy in patients receiving ganciclovir prophylaxis (32% vs 62%, $P < 0.03$) was observed [59].

The Role of other Viruses

In comparison with CMV there are fewer studies, which could define the role of other viruses in the pathogenesis of allograft rejection. Nevertheless other viral infections induce immunological mechanisms and some data support their participation on the pathogenesis of rejection. Human herpesvirus 6 (HHV-6) and human herpesvirus 7 (HHV-7) belong together with CMV to the β-herpesviruses family. Their activation after transplantation is closely associated with CMV and it seems that the main effect of HHV-6 and HHV-7 infection is the increase of the risk to develop CMV infection and disease [60, 61]. Due to interactions between β-herpesviruses it is not easy to determine a separate effect of HHV-6 and HHV-7. In patients after renal transplantation, who had an episode of acute rejection, the infection with HHV-7 poses a significant risk for further rejection episode [62]. In another study HHV-6 reactivation in liver transplant recipients was associated with the risk of late acute rejection. However, even in this study the main clinical result of HHV-6 infection was a 3.6-fold increase of the risk of CMV disease [63]. Interesting findings were provided by a PCR detection of various viruses in a bronchoalveolar lavage (BAL) in lung transplantation. The results of multivariate analysis have shown that detection of HHV-6 DNA in BAL was associated with increased risk of bronchiolitis obliterans syndrome independently on acute rejection [64].

Studies of the effect of non-herpes viruses on the development of rejection are sporadic. Most information is available on influenza virus infection, which due to activation of immunological mechanisms in the graft has an ability to provoke acute cellular rejection, as documented in renal, liver and lung transplant recipients [65]. As expected, the effect of influenza is greater in lung transplantation. Influenza pneumonia is an important risk for the development of bronchiolitis obliterans syndrome [65] in these patients. In pediatric heart transplant recipients the presence of adenovirus in endomyocardial biopsies was associated with the occurrence of cardiac allograft vasculopathy [66]. On the other hand, in an extensive epidemiological study in adult patients, adenovirus infection had no serious clinical effect and did not increase the risk of acute rejection [67]. In general it is possible to claim that in solid organ transplantation is the effect of non-herpes viral infections in comparison with herpes viruses much lower. The explanation is in the ability of herpes viruses to persist in the stage of latency. An immunosuppressive therapy results in their repeated and often asymptomatic activations, which could be only within the allograft tissue. The result is a persistent T-cell activation and impairment of allograft [20].

Conclusion

There are currently many clinical and experimental data available, which document the participation of viruses (mainly CMV) in the pathogenesis of allograft rejection in solid organ transplant recipients. CMV causes T-cell activation in the region of the allograft by several mechanisms. These include increased expression of adhesion molecules and their ligands, release of pro-inflammatory cytokines and chemokines and up-regulation of MHC class II molecule. Moreover, CMV encodes proteins, which are homologues of MHC molecules. The result is an increased ability of the immune system of the host to recognize antigen structures of the graft. Direct CMV infection of smooth muscle cells with an induction of their migration and proliferation and infection of endothelial cells with an impairment of nitric oxide synthase contribute to the development of allograft ateriosclerosis. Beneficial effect of antiviral prophylaxis in prevention of acute rejection or even chronic rejection was proved only in several studies. Nevertheless the results of well designed studies with valacyclovir in renal transplantation and with ganciclovir in heart transplantation are encouraging.

Some questions still remain unanswered. It is necessary to define if an asymptomatic CMV infection and not only CMV disease have a clinically relevant significance for the development of rejection. The differences may exist between transplantations of various organs and also between various immunosuppressive regimens. Further studies should clarify the role of anti-CMV prophylaxis and choice of an optimal agent with the goal to influence the incidence of CMV infection and disease as well as rejection.

Acknowledgements

The study was supported by Research Project No. MSM0021620819 "Replacement of and Support to Some Vital Organs" awarded by the Ministry of Education, Youth, and Physical Training of the Czech Republic.

References

[1]   Radha R, Jordan S, Paliyanda D, Bunnapradist S, Petrosyan A, Amet N, Toyoda M. Cellular immune responses to cytomegalovirus in renal transplant recipients. *Am. J. Transplant.* 2005; 5: 110-117.

[2]   Fishman JA, Rubin RH. Infection in organ-transplant recipients. *N. Engl. J. Med.* 1998; 338: 1741-1751.

[3]   Sia IG, Patel R. New strategies for prevention and therapy of cytomegalovirus infection and disease in solid-organ transplant recipients. *Clin. Microbiol. Rev.* 2000; 13: 83-121.

[4]   Brennan DC, Garlock KA, Singer GG, Schnitzler MA, Lippmann BJ, Buller RS, Gaudreault-Keener M, Lowell JA, Shenoy S, Howard TK, Storch GA. Prophylactic oral ganciclovir compared with deferred therapy for control of cytomegalovirus in renal transplant recipients. *Transplantation.* 1997; 64: 1843-1846.

[5]   Lowance D, Neumayer HH, Legendre CM, Squifflet JP, Kovarik J, Brennan PJ, Norman D, Mendez R, Keating MR, Coggon GL, Crisp A, Lee IC. Valacyclovir for the prevention of cytomegalovirus disease after renal transplantation. *N. Engl. J. Med.* 1999; 340: 1462-1470.

[6]   Brennan DC, Garlock KA, Lippmann BJ, Buller RS, Gaudreault-Keener M, Lowell JA, Miller SB, Shenoy S, Howard TK, Storch GA. Control of cytomegalovirus-associated morbidity in renal transplant patients using intensive monitoring and either preemptive or deferred therapy. *J. Am. Soc. Nephrol.* 1996; 8: 118-125.

[7]   Gane E, Saliba F, Valdecasas GJC, O`Grady J, Pescovitz MD. Lyman S, Robinson CA. Randomised trial of efficacy of oral ganciclovir in the prevention of cytomegalovirus disease in liver-transplant recipients. *Lancet.* 1997; 350: 1729-1733.

[8]   Reischig T, Jindra P, Mares J, Cechura M, Svecova M, Hes O, Opatrny Jr K, Treska V. Valacyclovir for cytomegalovirus prophylaxis reduces the risk of acute renal allograft rejection. *Transplantation.* 2005; 79: 317-324.

[9]   Preiksaitis JK, Brennan DC, Fishman J, Allen U. Canadian Society of Transplantation Consensus Workshop on cytomegalovirus management in solid organ transplantation final report. *Am. J. Transplant.* 2005; 5: 216-227.

[10]   Lautenschlager I. Cytomegalovirus and solid organ transplantation: an update. *Curr. Opin. Organ. Transplant.* 2003; 8: 269-275.

[11]   Hodson EM, Jones CA, Webster AC, Strippoli GFM, Barclay PG, Kable K, Vimalachandra D, Craig JC. Antiviral medication to prevent cytomegalovirus disease and early death in recipients of solid-organ transplants: a systemic review of randomised controlled trials. *Lancet.* 2005; 365: 2105-2115.

[12]   Stripolli GFM, Hodson EM, Jones C, Craig JC. Pre-emptive treatment for cytomegalovirus viremia to prevent cytomegalovirus disease in solid organ transplant recipients. *Transplantation.* 2006; 81: 139-145.

[13]   Kalil AC, Levitsky J, Lyden E, Stoner J, Freifeld AG. Meta-analysis: the efficacy of strategies to prevent organ disease by cytomegalovirus in solid organ transplant recipients. *Ann. Intern. Med.* 2005; 143: 870-880.

[14]   Paya C, Humar A, Dominguez E, Washburn K, Blumberg E, Alexander B, Freeman R, Heaton N, Pescovitz MD. Efficacy and safety of valganciclovir vs. oral ganciclovir for prevention of cytomegalovirus disease in solid organ transplant recipients. *Am. J. Transplant.* 2004; 4: 611-620.

[15]   Pavlopoulou ID, Syriopoulou VP, Chelioti H, Daikos GI, Stamatiades D, Kostakis A, Boletis JN. A comparative randomised study of valacyclovir vs. oral ganciclovir for cytomegalovirus prophylaxis in renal transplant recipients. *Clin. Microbiol. Infect.* 2005; 11: 736-743.

[16]   Garrigue I, Boucher S, Couzi L, Caumont A, Dromer C, Neau-Cransac M, Tabrizi R, Schrive MH, Fleury H, Lafon ME. Whole blood real-time PCR for cytomegalovirus infection follow-up in transplant recipients. *J. Clin. Virol.* 2006; 36: 72-75.

[17]   Li H, Dummer S, Estes WR, Meng S, Wright PF, Tang YW. Measurement of human cytomegalovirus loads by quantitative real-time PCR for monitoring clinical intervention in transplant recipients. *J. Clin. Microbiol.* 2003; 41: 187-191.

[18] von Müller L, Schliep C, Storck M, Hampl W, Schmid T, Abendroth D, Mertens T. Severe graft rejection, increased immunosuppression, and active CMV infection in renal transplantation. *J. Med. Virol.* 2006; 78: 394-399.

[19] Razonable RR, Rivero A, Rodriguez A, Wilson J, Daniels J, Jenkins G, Larson T, Hellinger WC, Spivey JR, Paya CV. Allograft rejection predicts the occurrence of late-onset cytomegalovirus (CMV) disease among CMV-mismatched solid organ transplant patients receiving prophylaxis with oral ganciclovir. *J. Infect. Dis.* 2001; 184: 1461-1464.

[20] Reinke P, Prosch S, Kern F, Volk HD. Mechanisms of human cytomegalovirus (HCMV) (re)activation and its impact on organ transplant patients. *Transplant. Infect. Dis.* 1999; 1: 157-164.

[21] Kim SJ, Varghese TK, Zhang Z, Zhao LC, Thomas G, Hummel M, Abecassis M. Renal ischemia/reperfusion injury activates the enhancer domain of the human cytomegalovirus major immediate early promoter. *Am. J. Transplant.* 2005; 5: 1606-1613.

[22] Pouteil-Noble C, Ecochard R, Landrivon G, Donia-Maged A, Tardy JC, Bosshard S, Colon S, Betuel H, Aymard M, Touraine JL. Cytomegalovirus infection – an etiological factor for rejection? *Transplantation.* 1993; 55: 851-857.

[23] Sagedal S, Nordal KP, Hartmann A, Sund S, Scott H, Degre M, Foss A, Leivestad T, Osnes K, Fauchald P, Rollag H. The impact of cytomegalovirus infection and disease on rejection episodes in renal allograft recipients. *Am. J. Transplant.* 2002; 2: 850-856.

[24] Dickenmann MJ, Cathomas G, Steiger J, Mihatsch MJ, Thiel G, Tamm M. Cytomegalovirus infection and graft rejection in renal transplantation. *Transplantation.* 2001; 71: 764-767.

[25] Toupance O, Bouedjoro-Camus MC, Carquin J, Novella JL, Lavaud S, Wynckel A, Jolly D, Chanard J. Cytomegalovirus-related disease and risk of acute rejection in renal transplant recipients: a cohort study with case-control analyses. *Transplant. Int.* 2000; 13: 413-419.

[26] Reischig T, Jindra P, Svecova M, Kormunda S, Opatrny K Jr, Treska V. The impact of cytomegalovirus disease and asymptomatic infection on acute renal allograft rejection. *J. Clin. Virol.* 2006; 36: 146-151.

[27] McLaughlin K, Wu K, Fick G, Muirhead N, Hollomby D, Jevnikar A. Cytomegalovirus seromismatching increases the risk of acute renal allograft rejection. *Transplantation.* 2002; 74: 813-816.

[28] Zamora MR, Cytomegalovirus and lung transplantation. *Am. J. Transplant.* 2004; 4: 1219-1226.

[29] Koskinen PK, Tikkanen JM, Pulkkinen VP, Häyry PJ, Lemström KB. Cytomegalovirus-induced allograft vascular disease. *Curr. Opin. Organ. Transplant.* 2000; 5: 192-196.

[30] Emery VC, Sabin CA, Cope AV, Gor D, Hassan-Walker AF, Griffiths PD. Application of viral-load kinetics to identify patients who develop cytomegalovirus disease after transplantation. *Lancet.* 2000; 355: 2032-2036.

[31] Nordoy I, Müller F, Nordall KP, Rollag H, Aukrust P, Froland SS. Chemokines and soluble adhesion molecules in renal transplant recipients with cytomegalovirus infection. *Clin. Exp. Immunol.* 2000; 120: 333-337.

[32] Valantine HA. The role of viruses in cardiac allograft vasculopathy. Am J Transplant 2003; 4: 169-177.

[33] Smieja M, Gnarpe J, Lonn E, Gnarpe H, Olsson G, Yi Q, Dzavik V, McQueen M, Yusuf S. Multiple infections and subsequent cardiovascular events in the Heart Outcomes Prevention Evaluation (HOPE) Study. *Circulation.* 2003; 107: 251-257.

[34] Grattan MT, Moreno-Cabral CE, Starnes VA, Oyer PE, Stinson EB, Shumway NE. Cytomegalovirus infection is associated with cardiac allograft rejection and atherosclerosis. *JAMA.* 1989; 261: 3561-3566.

[35] Potena L, Grigioni F, Ortolani P, Magnani G, Marrozzini C, Falchetti E, Barbieri A, Bacchi-Reggiani L, Lazzarotto T, Marzocchi A, Magelli C, Landini MP, Branzi A. Relevance of cytomegalovirus infection and coronary-artery remodeling in the first year after heart transplantation: a prospective three-dimensional intravascular ultrasound study. *Transplantation.* 2003; 75: 839-843.

[36] Fateh-Moghamad S, Bocksch W, Wessely R, Jager G, Hetzer R, Gawaz M. Cytomegalovirus infection status predicts progression of heart-transplant vasculopathy. *Transplantation.* 2003; 76: 1470-1474.

[37] Tong CYW, Bakran A, Peiris JSM, Muir P, Herrington CS. The association of viral infection and chronic allograft nephropathy with graft dysfunction after renal transplantation. *Transplantation.* 2002; 74: 576-578.

[38] Humar A, Gillingham KJ, Payne WD, Dunn DL, Sutherland DER, Matas AJ. Association between cytomegalovirus disease and chronic rejection in kidney transplant recipients. *Transplantation.* 1999; 68: 1879-1883.

[39] Helenterä I, Koskinen P, Törnroth T, Loginov R, Grönhagen-Riska C, Lautenschlager IT. The impact of cytomegalovirus infection and acute rejection episodes on the development of vascular changes in 6-month protocol biopsy specimens of cadaveric kidney allograft recipients. *Transplantation.* 2003; 75: 1858-1864.

[40] Sebekova K, Feber J, Carpenter B, Shaw L, Karnauchow T, Diaz-Mitoma F, Filler G. Tissue viral DNA is associated with chronic allograft nephropathy. *Pediatr. Transplant.* 2005; 9: 598-603.

[41] Schnitzler MA, Lowell JA, Hmiel SP, Hardinger KL, Liapis H, Ceriotti CS, Brennan DC. Cytomegalovirus disease after prophylaxis with oral ganciclovir in renal transplantation: the importance of HLA-DR matching. *J. Am. Soc. Nephrol.* 2003; 14: 780-785.

[42] Sagedal S, Hartmann A, Nordal KP, Osnes K, Leivestad T, Foss A, Degre M, Fauchald P, Rollag H. Impact of early cytomegalovirus infection and disease on long-term recipient and kidney graft survival. *Kidney Int.* 2004; 66: 329-337.

[43] Evans PC, Soin A, Wreghitt TG, Taylor CJ, Wight DGD, Alexander GJM. An association between cytomegalovirus infection and chronic rejection after liver transplantation. *Transplantation.* 2000; 69: 30-35.

[44] Borchers AT, Perez R, Kaysen G, Ansari AA, Gershwin ME. Role of cytomegalovirus infection in allograft rejection: a review of possible mechanisms. *Transplant. Immunol.* 1999; 7: 75-82.

[45] Waldman WJ, LeClaire JD, Knight D. T-cell activation response to allogeneic CMV-infected endothelial cells is not prevented by ganciclovir or foscarnet: implications for transplant vascular sclerosis. *Transplantation.* 2002; 73: 314-318.

[46] Kloover JS, Soots AP, Krogerus LA, Kauppinen H, Loginov RJ, Holma KL, Bruggeman CA, Ahonen AJ, Lautenschlager IT. Tar cytomegalovirus infection in kidney allograft recipients is associated with increased expression of intracellular adhesion molecule-1, and their ligands leukocyte function antigen-1 and very late antigen-4 in the graft. *Transplantation.* 2000; 69: 2641-2647.

[47] Grundy JE, Downes KL. Up-regulation of LFA-3 and ICAM-1 on the surface of fibroblasts infected with cytomegalovirus. *Immunology.* 1993; 78: 405-412.

[48] Dengler TJ, Raftery MJ, Werle M, Zimmermann R, Schönrich G. Cytomegalovirus infection of vascular cells induces expression of pro-inflammatory adhesion molecules by paracrine action of secreted interleukin-1β. *Transplantation.* 2000; 69: 1160-1168.

[49] Ustinov J, Bruggeman CA, Häyry PJ, Lautenschlager IT. Cytomegalovirus-induced Class II expression in rat kidney. *Transplant. Proc.* 1994; 26: 1729.

[50] Fujinami RS, Nelson JA, Walker L, Oldstone MB. Sequence homology and immunologic cross-reactivity of human cytomegalovirus with HLA-DR beta chain: a means for graft rejection and immunosuppression. *J. Virol.* 1988; 62: 100-105.

[51] Beck S, Barrell BG. Human cytomegalovirus encodes a glycoprotein homologous to MHC class-I antigens. *Nature.* 1988; 331: 269-272.

[52] Inkinen K, Soots A, Krogerus L, Loginov R, Bruggeman C, Lautenschlager I. Cytomegalovirus enhance expression of growth factors during the development of chronic allograft nephropathy in rats. *Transplant. Int.* 2005; 18: 743-749.

[53] Streblow DN, Soderberg-Nauclear C, Vieira J, Smith P, Wakabayashi E, Ruchti F, Mattison K, Altschuler Y, Nelson JA. The human cytomegalovirus chemokine receptor US28 mediates vascular smooth muscle cell migration. *Cell.* 1999; 99: 511-520.

[54] Streblow DN, Kreklywich CN, Smith P, Soule JL, Meyer C, Yin M, Beisser P, Vink C, Nelson JA, Orloff SL. Rat cytomegalovirus-accelerated transplant vascular sclerosis is reduced with mutation of chemokine-receptor R33. *Am. J. Transplant.* 2005; 5: 436-442.

[55] Flechner SM, Avery RK, Fisher R, Mastroianni BA, Papajcik DA, O'Malley KJ, Goormastic M, Goldfarb DA, Modlin CS, Novick AC: A randomized prospective controlled trial of oral acyclovir versus oral ganciclovir for cytomegalovirus prophylaxis in high-risk kidney transplant recipients. *Transplantation.* 1998; 66: 1682-1688.

[56] Lemström KB, Bruning JH, Bruggeman CA, Koskinen PK, Aho PT, Yilmaz S, Lautenschlager IT, Häyri PJ, Cytomegalovirus infection-enhanced allograft arteriosclerosis is prevented by DHPG prophylaxis in the rat. *Circulation.* 1994; 90: 1969-1978.

[57] Lemström KB, Sihvola R, Bruggeman CA, Häyri PJ, Koskinen PK. Cytomegalovirus infection-enhanced cardiac allograft vasculopathy is abolished by DHPG prophylaxis in the rat. *Circulation.* 1997; 95: 2614-2616.

[58] Opelz G, Döhler B, Ruhenstroth A. Cytomegalovirus prophylaxis and graft outcome in solid organ transplantation: a Collaborative Transplant Study report. *Am. J. Transplant.* 2004; 4: 928-936.

[59] Valantine HA, Gao SZ, Menon SG, Renlund DG, Hunt SA, Oyer P, Stinson EB, Brown BW, Merigan TC, Schroeder JS. Impact of prophylactic immediate posttransplant ganciclovir on development of transplant atherosclerosis. *Circulation.* 1999; 100: 61-66.

[60] Mendez JC, Dockrell DH, Espy MJ, Smith TF, Wilson JA, Harmsen WS, Ilstrup D, Paya CV. Human β-herpesvirus interactions in solid organ transplant recipients. *J. Infect. Dis.* 2001; 183: 179-184.

[61] Dockrell DH, Paya CV. Human herpesvirus-6 and -7 in transplantation. *Rev. Med. Virol.* 2001; 11: 23-36.

[62] Kidd IM, Clarc DA, Sabin CA, Andrew D, Hassan-Walker AF, Sweny P, Griffiths PD, Emery VC. Prospective study of human betaherpesviruses after renal transplantation. *Transplantation.* 2000; 69: 2400-2404.

[63] Humar A, Kumar D, Caliendo AM, Moussa G, Ashi-Sulaiman A, Levy G, Mazzulli T. Clinical impact of human herpesvirus 6 infection after liver transplantation. *Transplantation.* 2002; 73: 599-604.

[64] Neurohr C, Huppmann P, Leuchte H, Schwaiblmair M, Bittmann I, Jaeger G, Hatz R, Frey L, Überfuhr P. Human herpesvirus 6 in bronchoalveolar lavage fluid after lung transplantation: a risk factor for bronchiolitis obliterans syndrome? *Am. J. Transplant.* 2005; 5: 2982-2991.

[65] Vilchez RA, Fung J, Kusne S. The pathogenesis and management of influenza virus infection in organ transplant recipients. *Transplant. Inf. Dis.* 2002; 4: 177-182.

[66] Shirali GSNJ, Chinnock RE, Johnston JK, Rosentahl GL, Bowles NE, Towbin JA. Association of viral genome with graft loss in children after cardiac transplantation. *N. Engl. J. Med.* 2001; 334: 1498-1503.

[67] Humar A, Kumar D, Mazzulli T, Razonable RR, Moussa G, Paya CV, Covington E, Alecock E, Pescovitz MD. A surveillance study of adenovirus infection in adult solid organ transplant recipients. *Am. J. Transplant.* 2005; 5: 2555-2559.

In: Transplantation Immunology Research Trends
Editor: Oliver N. Ulricker, pp. 233-246

ISBN: 978-1-60021-578-0
© 2007 Nova Science Publishers, Inc.

Chapter X

Immunosuppression for Islet Transplantation

*Hirofumi Noguchi**

Diabetes Research Institute Japan, 1-98 Dengakugakubo, Kutsukake-cho,
Toyoake, Aichi 470-1192, Japan; Department of Advanced Medicine
in Biotechnology and Robotics, Nagoya University Graduate
School of Medicine, 65 Tsurumai-cho, Showa-ku,
Nagoya 466-8550, Japan.

Abstract

Immunosuppression is critical in islet transplantation because islet grafts are prone to immune destruction not only by allorejection, but also by the recurrence of autoimmunity. In 1974, the first clinical allogeneic islet transplantation was performed at the University of Minnesota. Immunosuppressive regimens depended heavily on steroids and azathioprine because of the previous appearance of calcineurin inhibitors such as cyclosporine. Unfortunately, no patient achieved insulin independence, and only a few cases showed transient graft function, as evidenced by measurable serum C-peptide, and even when cyclosporine was available, there was not much improvement. In 2000, the Edmonton group reported extremely impressive advances in clinical islet transplantation. The development by the Edmonton group was a significant breakthrough that allowed the rate of insulin independence after islet transplantation to increase to 80% at 1 year. The design of a sirolimus-based, steroid-free, low-tacrolimus regimen has been one of the fundamentals of this progress. However, the rate is reduced to 50% at 3 years. Recently, immunosuppression agents such as cyclosporine, mycophenolate mofetil, and the novel agent FTY 720 have been used instead of tacrolimus. Lymphocyte-depleting antibodies such as anti-thymocyte globulin, alemtuzumab, and hOKT3γ1 [ala,ala] have been launched, and costimulatory blockade such as anti-CD40 monoclonal antibodies

* Address correspondence to: Hirofumi Noguchi MD, PhD.; Department of Advanced Medicine in Biotechnology and Robotics; Nagoya University Graduate School of Medicine; 65 Tsurumai-cho, Showa-ku, Nagoya 466-8550, Japan. Tel.: 81-52-719-1975; Fax: 81-52-719-1977; E-mail: noguchih@med.nagoya-u.ac.jp / noguchih@kuhp.kyoto-u.ac.jp

and CTLA4-Ig will be attempted in the near future. Moreover, the potential of novel immunosuppressing peptides/proteins could now be realized using new technology called the protein transduction system. In this review, we show some of the most recent contributions to the advancement of knowledge in this field.

Introduction

Diabetes mellitus is a devastating disease and the World Health Organization (WHO) expects that the number of diabetic patients will increase to 300 million by the year 2025. Type 1 diabetes results from autoimmune-mediated destruction of insulin-secreting β cells in the islets of Langerhans of the pancreas, whereas Type 2 diabetes is a disease of older individuals that is due to systemic insulin resistance and reduced insulin secretion by pancreatic β cells. Surgical resection of the pancreas may also cause insulin-dependent diabetes depending on the size of the remaining pancreas. It is now well established that the risk of diabetic complications is dependent on the degree of glycemic control in diabetic patients. Clinical trials such as the Diabetes Control and Complications Trial (DCCT) [1], the UK Prospective Diabetes Study (UKPDS) [2], and Kumamoto study [3] have demonstrated that tight glycemic control achieved with intensive insulin regimens can reduce the risk of developing or progressing retinopathy, nephropathy or neuropathy in patients with all types of diabetes. However, the Third National Health and Nutrition Examination Survey (NHANES III) showed that only 50% of diabetics have been able to achieve a HbA1C level of less than 7%; therefore, the only way to ensure the long-term health of diabetic patients is to maintain constant normoglycemia.

Despite intensive insulin therapy, however, most individuals with type 1 diabetes are unable to maintain a blood glucose level in the normal range at all times. Moreover, intensive glycemic control with insulin therapy is associated with an increased incidence of hypoglycemia, which is the major barrier to the implementation of intensive treatment from the perspective of both physicians and patients. The successes achieved over the last few decades by the transplantation of whole pancreas and isolated islets suggest that diabetes can be cured by the replenishment of deficient β cells. It seems logical that replacement of the islet tissue itself offers a better approach than simply replacing insulin that has been lost. Islet allotransplantation can achieve insulin independence in patients with type 1 diabetes [4-9]. Since the Edmonton protocol was announced, more than 500 type 1 diabetics in more than 50 institutions have undergone islet transplantation to cure their disease; however, the clinical benefit of this protocol is not lasting [10].

In 1974, the first clinical allogeneic islet transplantation was performed at the University of Minnesota [11]. Immunosuppressive regimens depended heavily on steroids and azathioprine because of the previous appearance of calcineurin inhibitors such as cyclosporine. Unfortunately, no patient achieved insulin independence, and only a few cases showed transient graft function, as evidenced by measurable serum C-peptide [11], and even when cyclosporine was available, there was not much improvement. In 1988, Camillo Ricordi developed an automated method for the isolation of human pancreatic islets [12]. This technique provided an opportunity for large numbers of human islets to be isolated and transplanted, leading to the first reports of insulin independence using cyclosporine-based regimens. [13, 14]

Immunosuppressive regimens in the 1990s evolved with the release of new compounds, but the rates of insulin independence reported by the International Islet Transplant Registry (ITR) culminated at a disappointing 13%. At the University of Geneva, an immunosuppression protocol consisted of cyclosporine, azathioprine, and steroids, and induction therapy was performed for a period of 14 days with anti-thymocyte globulin until 1997. From 1998 to 2000, a new protocol consisted of cyclosporine, mycophenolate mofetil, and steroids, and induction therapy with basiliximab was performed on day 0 and 4. This is the first report of the use of an anti-interleukin-2-receptor monoclonal antibody in islet transplantation [15, 16]. The protocol was used in the initial experience of the Swiss-French GRAGIL consortium from 1999 to 2000. At the completion of a 12-month follow up, 0% primary nonfunction, 50% graft survival, and 20% insulin independence were observed [17]. The Giessen group reported remarkable results in the late 1990s in which approximately 30% of transplanted patients achieved insulin independence [18, 19]. The Milan group reported that 35% of 20 consecutive patients receiving islets after kidney grafts achieved insulin independence [20]. Remarkably, the Giessen and Milan results were achieved with a conventional immunosuppressive regimen including steroids and cyclosporine, which was preferred to tacrolimus because of its alleged lower islet toxicity.

In 2000, the Edmonton group reported extremely impressive advances in clinical islet transplantation. All seven consecutive recipients of allogeneic islet grafts achieved insulin independence [4]. A subsequent update of their results reported an 80% actual rate of insulin independence at 1 year [21, 22]. This observation has led to renewed interest in islet of Langerhans transplantation as a means to cure diabetes, as clinical programs are being started at an increasing number of transplant centers throughout the world. The design of a sirolimus-based, steroid-free, low-tacrolimus regimen has been one of the fundamentals of this progress.

Currently explored alternatives to tacrolimus include cyclosporine, mycophenolate mofetil, and the novel agent FTY 720 [23, 24]. To achieve tolerance, several strategies using lymphocyte-depleting antibodies (anti-thymocyte globulin, alemtuzumab, hOKT3γ1 [ala,ala]), or costimulatory blockade (anti-CD40 antibody, CTLA4-Ig) have been performed [25-28]. Moreover, the potential of a novel immunosuppressing peptide/protein could now be realized, thanks to a new cell-delivery system [29, 30]. Here, we review some of the most recent contributions to the advancement of knowledge in this field.

Immunosuppressant of the Edmonton Protocol

The Edmonton protocol uniquely combined several strategies designed to specifically address the various obstacles encountered in the isolation, transplantation, and immunosuppression sequence. One of these strategies involved an improved immunosuppressive protocol, consisting of sirolimus (rapamycin), low-dose tacrolimus, and anti-IL2-receptor monoclonal antibody (daclizumab) induction. The immunosuppressive protocol in the Edmonton experience has also been shown to be highly effective in patients receiving islets after kidney transplantation [31]. The immunosuppressive protocol avoids the diabetrogenic effect of glucocorticoids in islet transplantation. Although the mechanisms are not fully understood, glucocorticoid-induced hyperglycemia has long been known, and its detrimental effect on islet function *in vitro* and *in vivo* is described [32, 33].

Calcineurin inhibitors such as tacrolimus have also been associated with impaired *in vitro* and *in vivo* islet graft function [33, 34]. Moreover, long-term studies have shown that short-term cyclosporine in dogs can result in the permanent loss of functionally competent islets [35]. A study of biopsies obtained from whole pancreas transplants in hosts treated with cyclosporine or tacrolimus, observed cytoplasmic swelling, vacuolization, and apoptosis as evidence of direct islet cell damage. The presence and extent of damage correlated with high serum levels of calcineurin inhibitors and pulse steroid administration. The lesions were more marked with tacrolimus than with cyclosporine therapy [36]. These observations provide a rationale for a glucocorticoid-free regime and for lowering dosages of calcineurin inhibitors in the Edomonton immunosuppressive protocol.

Sirolimus was shown to be a rather harmless agent in terms of islet toxicity. *In vitro* impairment of islet function was seen only at extremely high sirolimus concentrations. At doses 10 to 50 times the effective antirejection dosage, hyperglycemia was observed in islet-transplanted animals without histological evidence of end-organ toxicity [37]. The synergism of sirolimus and calcineurin inhibitors allows their dosage to be reduced substantially, and thus islet toxicity, without increasing the occurrence of acute rejection episodes [38, 39]. Since both sirolimus and tacrolimus bind to FKBP-12, competition for FKBP-12 would prevent synergism [40]; however, *in vivo* observations in both animal models and humans suggest a strong potentiation of the efficacy of both drugs [41-43].

Although the antirejection regimen in the Edmonton Protocol is one of the most important recent developments in making islet transplantation a clinical reality, it appears that the actual rate of insulin independence is 80% at 1 year and 50% at 3 years in Edmonton patients. The reasons for the decrease of islet function after the first year are not well understood. Although the dose of tacrolimus is low, the long-term toxicity of tacrolimus to islets is suspected. In addition to tacrolimus toxicity, relatively high doses of sirolimus (trough levels of 10–15 ng/mL for the first 3 months) have been associated with serious side effects. Although sirolimus has facilitated clinical islet transplant success through the provision of effective immunosuppression to contend with both auto- and alloimmunity, the agent is also responsible for many of the side effects, such as mouth ulceration, dyslipidemia, and myelotoxicity, encountered after islet transplantation. It is a matter of concern that such side effects are experienced by almost all patients. It has also been suggested that sirolimus could have a detrimental effect on islet engraftment and neovascularization, as well as potential detrimental direct toxicity to islets [44]; however, sirolimus has proven to be advantageous compared to former steroids and high-dose calcineurin inhibitor-based therapies. The minimization of diabetogenic agents, while maintaining adequate potency to contend with both allograft rejection and autoimmune recurrence, is a matter of tremendous importance as less toxic and more specific drugs enter the clinical area.

Progressive Immunosuppressive Protocol

After the Edmonton protocol report, several institutions consider calcineurin inhibitor-free regimens as an excellent way to avoid drug-induced diabetogenicity and to minimize the development of kidney toxicity in patients prone to develop diabetic nephropathy. The Minneapolis group has shown excellent results using tacrolimus as the initial immunosuppression, followed by the gradual replacement of tacrolimus with mycophenolate mofetil as maintenance immunosuppression beginning 1-month posttransplant [23]. The same group has also shown preliminary evidence of the safety and efficacy of corticosteroid and calcineurin inhibitor-free immunosuppression in a relevant preclinical transplant model [24]. Induction immunosuppression was with intravenous basiliximab, anti-IL-2 receptor blockade, which has been used in clinical islet transplantation from non-heart-beating and living donors in our university instead of daclizumab [5, 6]. Maintenance immunosuppression was with everolimus, sirolimus analogue, and FTY 720. FTY 720 is a novel immunosuppressive agent that acts on lymphocyte homing and thus interferes with T-cell-antigen cognate interaction. The availability of FTY 720 for phase II clinical trials of islet transplantation is eagerly anticipated.

The use of lymphocyte-depleting agents during the induction period has been attempted with success in protocols based on tacrolimus-sirolimus association by the Minneapolis group. The use of anti-thymocyte globulin and the humanized anti-CD3 monoclonal antibody (mAb) hOKT3γ1 (ala-ala), lacking Fc-receptor-binding properties (and thus avoiding massive cytokine release by cross-linked macrophages) and with reduced immunogenicity, has resulted in high rates of insulin independence after single donor islet transplantation [25]. The Edmonton group is currently testing humanized mAb alemtuzumab (Campath-1H) in a group of islet transplant recipients [45]. This compound targets the CD52 molecule, located on the cell surface of lymphocytes and monocytes, resulting in the lasting and profound depletion of these lineages. Alemtuzumab has demonstrated considerable success in maintaining the function of renal allografts in patients [46]. Initial trials with almetuzumab and sirolimus in a small number of islet recipients in Edmonton did not show a superior outcome to standard tacrolimus-sirolimus-based therapy [47].

Perspectives for the Near Future

New Drug Development by Protein Transduction Technology

An important mechanism whereby calcineurin promotes T-cell activation and cytokine gene induction is largely attributed to a family of transcriptional regulators referred to as the nuclear factor of activated T cells (NFAT). Immunosuppressants cyclosporine A and FK506 inhibit the activity of calcineurin phosphatase on all its protein substrates, including NFAT [48, 49]. These drugs have revolutionized transplant therapy; however, the inhibition of calcineurin outside the immune system has a number of side effects, such as hyperglycemia, progressive loss of renal function, hypertension, neurotoxicity and increased risk of malignancy [50-53]. Even when drug levels are kept low, significant side effects may develop. The Edmonton group has reported that patients with underlying impaired renal function can experience accelerated nephrotoxicity even when low doses of tacrolimus are used [22]. Moreover, the use of FK506 and cyclosporine A in human organ transplantation has been associated with a 10−30% incidence of diabetes [54].

In the search for safer drugs, we developed a cell-permeable inhibitor of NFAT using the protein transduction system [29, 55-63]. The NFAT inhibitor peptide, VIVIT, was developed based on the conserved calcineurin docking site of the NFAT family [64]. The peptide interferes selectively with calcineurin-NFAT interaction without affecting any of calcineurin's other targets. Therefore, VIVIT might be useful as a therapeutic agent that is less toxic than current drugs. The NFAT inhibitory peptide was covalently linked at its C terminus to a short stretch of arginine residues (11R-VIVIT). Polyarginine facilitates the uptake of peptides and protein into cells with high efficiency [29, 56-60]. This peptide specifically and significantly inhibited NFAT function in a T-cell line, and appeared stable enough to survive in the circulation of a mouse model. Using a mouse model of diabetes, we investigated whether 11R–VIVIT could prevent transplant rejection. Following the transplantation of islet cells from fully mismatched mice, treatment with the peptide prolonged graft survival, and the transplanted islet cells were still producing insulin 50 days later. Moreover, insulin secretion did not change at any concentration of 11R-VIVIT, whereas FK506 inhibited insulin secretion, and the amount secreted decreased significantly. These results show that the NFAT inhibitor peptide is less toxic than calcineurin inhibitors with regard to insulin secretion [29]. The peptide also prevents pressure-overload cardiac hypertrophy [65], and has been used as an NFAT-specific inhibitor [66-68].

Recently, Choi et al. reported that intranasal delivery of the cytoplasmic domain of CTLA-4 using a novel protein transduction domain prevents allergic inflammation [30]. CTLA-4 is a negative regulator of T-cell activation, and its inhibitory effects can be accomplished either by competition with CD28 or by transmitting negative signals through its intracellular domain. They developed a cell-permeable protein of the cytoplasmic domain of CTLA-4 (Hph-1-ctCTLA-4) using the protein transduction system. After transduction into T-cells, Hph-1-ctCTLA-4 inhibited the production of IL-2, and downregulated CD69 and CD25. Intranasal administration of Hph-1-ctCTLA-4 resulted in markedly reduced infiltration of inflammatory cells, secretion of T helper type2 cytokines, serum IgE levels and airway hyper-responsiveness in a mouse model of allergic airway inflammation. These results indicated that Hph-1-ctCTLA-4 constitutes an effective immunosuppressive protein drug for potential use in the treatment of allergic asthma, via nasal administration. Cell-permeable protein may be useful for not only the treatment of allergic inflammation but also immunosuppressive agents to transplantation.

Although the peptide is a long way from clinical trials, the strategy is an interesting proof of concept as far as trying to make new immunosuppressive agents.

Tolerance Induction

Several experiments have been shown to induce tolerance in islet transplantation. Biological agents that block key T-cell costimulatory signals have demonstrated extraordinary promise in animal models. Blocking signaling through these molecules effectively prevents the activation and clonal expansion of T cells, forcing them into anergy and apoptosis [69, 70]. Both CD28 and CD154 molecules are located at the surface of CD4+ T-cells and deliver costimulatory signals. Two types of costimulatory blocking agents, CTLA4-Ig preventing CD28-CD80/86 interaction and anti-CD154 preventing CD40-CD154 interaction, have reached the preclinical stage. In a nonhuman primate model, LEA29Y, a mutant CTLA4-Ig molecule with increased binding activity, sirolimus, and anti-IL-2R regimen had significantly prolonged islet allograft survival [26]. Islet transplantation under the cover of anti-CD154 monotherapy consistently allows for allogeneic islet engraftment and long-term insulin independence in this highly relevant preclinical model [28]. From these studies, the concept of maintenance therapy with costimulatory blocking agents has emerged as a valid strategy for clinical islet transplantation. A clinical trial utilizing humanized anti-CD154 mAb in recipients of solitary islet transplants commenced in 1999; however, it was reported that unusual thromboembolic complications occurred in kidney transplant recipients receiving mAb in a concurrent trial [71, 72]. To circumvent this potential complication, an Emory University group developed a chimeric antibody targeting CD40 as an alternative to CD154. Anti-CD40 combined with LEA29Y dramatically facilitated long-term islet allograft survival [27].

In addition to the blockade of costimulation, T-cell depletion at the time of transplantation using potent lymphocyte-depleting agents is an effective strategy for facilitating tolerance. An anti-CD-3 diphtheria-based immunotoxin has been shown to facilitate long-term survival of islet xenografts [73, 74] and allografts [75] in primate models. This agent was most effective when combined with 15-deoxyspergualin (DSG) [73, 74].

Tolerance has been achieved clinically using mixed hematopoietic chimerism through donor-specific bone marrow transplantation. Attempts to induce clinical tolerance through mixed chimerism have been successful, with rare reports of bone marrow transplant recipients with established donor chimerism that have been able to accept a renal transplant from the same donor without further immunosuppression [76, 77, 78]. In islet transplantation, strategies to induce mixed chimerism may be of particular interest since it has the potential to prevent autoimmune recurrence by restoring self-tolerance through bone marrow transplantation, in addition to achieving permanent islet allograft acceptance. However, serious concerns regarding toxicity with recipient pre-conditioning and a risk of graft-versus-host disease have precluded more widespread clinical applications of this approach.

Islet Encapsulation

Encapsulation of pancreatic islets allows for transplantion in the absence of immunosuppression. The technology is based on the principle that transplanted tissue is protected for the host immune system by an artificial membrane. Encapsulation offers a solution to the shortage of donors in clinical islet transplantation because it allows animal islets or insulin-producing cells engineered from stem cells to be used. The encapsulation of islets in immunoprotective devices prior to implantation has been shown to enhance the survival of both allogeneic and xenogeneic islets [79-84]. However, the clinical application of these devices has been impeded by many important concerns, including adequate access of the encapsulated islets to blood supply and oxygen for survival, triggering of nonspecific foreign body reactions to biomaterials resulting in their destruction, practical concerns regarding the volume of infusion of an encapsulated preparation and graft loss from cytokine-mediated immunological responses. While the concept of protecting islets is enticing, developments in polymer biology are definitely required before this approach can be applied to patients.

Conclusions

Immunosuppression is critical in islet transplantation because islet grafts are prone to immune destruction not only by allorejection, but also by the recurrence of autoimmunity. Since it should be noted that, unlike other organ transplants, islet transplantation is disadvantaged because there is a lack of an effective predictive marker of early rejection, the immunosuppressive regimens used in islet transplantation currently err on the side of over-immunosuppression. New agents instead of calcineurin inhibitors should be developed with the aim of solving the diabetogenicity and nephrotoxicity problems. The next step should probably be the development of new agents instead of sirolimus to avoid the problematic side effects of the drug. Safer immune suppressors will have benefits not only for transplant patients but also patients with autoimmune diseases. If the degree of systemic immunosuppression could be reduced, ultimately towards tolerance, islet transplantation could be applied in the earliest stages of diabetes, including transplantation in children. The ultimate goal of islet transplantation is to completely restore glucose homeostasis and prevent long-term diabetic complications without the need to maintain immunosuppressive therapy.

Acknowledgements

We thank Dr. Shinichi Matsumoto (Diabetes Research Institute Japan, Fujita Health University) for valuable suggestions.

References

[1]   The Diabetes Control and Complications Trial Research Group (1993) The effect of intensive treatment of diabetes on the development and progression of long-term complications in insulin-dependent diabetes mellitus. *N. Engl. J. Med.* 329, 977-986.

[2]   UK Prospective Diabetes Study (UKPDS) Group (1998) Intensive blood-glucose control with sulphonylureas or insulin compared with conventional treatment and risk of complications in patients with type 2 diabetes (UKPDS 33). *Lancet.* 352, 837-853.

[3]   Ohkubo Y, Kishikawa H, Araki E, Miyata T, Isami S, Motoyoshi S, Kojima Y, Furuyoshi N, Shichiri M (1995) Intensive insulin therapy prevents the progression of diabetic microvascular complications in Japanese patients with non-insulin-dependent

diabetes mellitus: a randomized prospective 6-year study. *Diabetes Res. Clin. Pract.* 28, 103-117.

[4] Shapiro AM, Lakey JR, Ryan EA, Korbutt GS, Toth E, Warnock GL, Kneteman NM, Rajotte RV (2000) Islet transplantation in seven patients with type 1 diabetes mellitus using a glucocorticoid-free immunosuppressive regimen. *N. Engl. J. Med.* 343, 230-238.

[5] Matsumoto S, Okitsu T, Iwanaga Y, Noguchi H, Nagata H, Yonekawa Y, Yamada Y, Fukuda K, Tsukiyama K, Suzuki H, Kawasaki Y, Shimodaira M, Matsuoka K, Shibata T, Kasai Y, Maekawa T, Shapiro J, Tanaka K (2005) Insulin independence after living-donor distal pancreatectomy and islet allotransplantation. *Lancet.* 365, 1642-1644.

[6] Matsumoto S, Okitsu T, Iwanaga Y, Noguchi H, Nagata H, Yonekawa Y, Yamada Y, Fukuda K, Shibata T, Kasai Y, Maekawa T, Wada H, Nakamura T, Tanaka K (2006) Successful Islet Transplantation from Nonheartbeating Donor Pancreata Using Modified Ricordi Islet Isolation Method. *Transplantation.* 82, 460-465.

[7] Noguchi H, Ueda M, Nakai Y, Iwanaga Y, Okitsu T, Nagata H, Yonekawa Y, Kobayashi N, Nakamura T, Wada H, Matsumoto S (2006) Modified two-layer preservation method (M-Kyoto/PFC) improves islet yields in islet isolation. *Am. J. Transplant.* 6, 496-504.

[8] Noguchi H, Iwanaga Y, Okitsu T, Nagata H, Yonekawa Y, Matsumoto S (2006) Evaluation of islet transplantation from non-heart beating donors. *Am. J. Transplant.* 6, 2476-2482.

[9] Noguchi H, Matsumoto S, Matsushita M, Kobayashi N, Tanaka K, Matsui H, Tanaka N (2006) Immunosuppression for islet transplantation. *Acta. Med. Okayama.* 60, 71-76.

[10] Robertson RP (2004) Islet transplantation as a treatment for diabetes - a work in progress. *N. Engl. J. Med.* 350, 694-705.

[11] Najarian JS, Sutherland DE, Matas AJ, Steffes MW, Simmons RL, Goetz FC (1977) Human islet transplantation: a preliminary report. *Transplant. Proc.* 9, 233-236.

[12] Ricordi C, Lacy PE, Finke EH, Olack BJ, Scharp DW (1988) Automated method for isolation of human pancreatic islets. *Diabetes.* 37, 413-420.

[13] Scharp DW, Lacy PE, Santiago JV, McCullough CS, Weide LG, Falqui L, Marchetti P, Gingerich RL, Jaffe AS, Cryer PE (1990) Insulin independence after islet transplantation into type I diabetic patient. *Diabetes.* 39, 515-518.

[14] Ricordi C, Tzakis AG, Carroll PB, Zeng YJ, Rilo HL, Alejandro R, Shapiro A, Fung JJ, Demetris AJ, Mintz DH (1992) Human islet isolation and allotransplantation in 22 consecutive cases. *Transplantation.* 53, 407-414.

[15] Oberholzer J, Triponez F, Mage R, Andereggen E, Buhler L, Cretin N, Fournier B, Goumaz C, Lou J, Philippe J, Morel P (2000) Human islet transplantation: lessons from 13 autologous and 13 allogeneic transplantations. *Transplantation.* 69, 1115-1123.

[16] Oberholzer J, Toso C, Triponez F, Ris F, Bucher P, Demirag A, Lou J, Majno P, Buehler L, Philippe J, Morel P (2002) Human islet allotransplantation with Basiliximab in type I diabetic patients with end-stage renal failure. *Transplant. Proc.* 34, 823-825.

[17] Benhamou PY, Oberholzer J, Toso C, Kessler L, Penfornis A, Bayle F, Thivolet C, Martin X, Ris F, Badet L, Colin C, Morel P (2001) GRAGIL consortium: Human islet transplantation network for the treatment of Type I diabetes: first data from the Swiss-

French GRAGIL consortium (1999-2000). Groupe de Recherche Rhin Rhjne Alpes Geneve pour la transplantation d'Ilots de Langerhans. *Diabetologia.* 44, 859-864.

[18] Hering BJ, Bretzel RG, Hopt UT, Brandhorst H, Brandhorst D, Bollen CC, Raptis G, Helf F, Grossmann R, Mellert J (1994) New protocol toward prevention of early human islet allograft failure. *Transplant. Proc.* 26, 570-571.

[19] Bretzel RG, Brandhorst D, Brandhorst H, Eckhard M, Ernst W, Friemann S, Rau W, Weimar B, Rauber K, Hering BJ, Brendel MD (1999) Improved survival of intraportal pancreatic islet cell allografts in patients with type-1 diabetes mellitus by refined peritransplant management. *J. Mol. Med.* 77, 140-143.

[20] Secchi A, Socci C, Maffi P, Taglietti MV, Falqui L, Bertuzzi F, De Nittis P, Piemonti L, Scopsi L, Di Carlo V, Pozza G (1997) Islet transplantation in IDDM patients. *Diabetologia.* 40, 225-231.

[21] Ryan EA, Lakey JR, Rajotte RV, Korbutt GS, Kin T, Imes S, Rabinovitch A, Elliott JF, Bigam D, Kneteman NM, Warnock GL, Larsen I, Shapiro AM (2001) Clinical outcomes and insulin secretion after islet transplantation with the Edmonton protocol. *Diabetes.* 50, 710-719.

[22] Ryan EA, Lakey JR, Paty BW, Imes S, Korbutt GS, Kneteman NM, Bigam D, Rajotte RV, Shapiro AM (2002) Successful islet transplantation: continued insulin reserve provides long-term glycemic control. *Diabetes.* 51, 2148-2157.

[23] Hering BJ, Kandaswamy R, Ansite JD, Eckman PM, Nakano M, Sawada T, Matsumoto I, Ihm SH, Zhang HJ, Parkey J, Hunter DW, Sutherland DE (2005) Single-donor, marginal-dose islet transplantation in patients with type 1 diabetes. *JAMA.* 293, 830-835.

[24] Wijkstrom M, Kenyon NS, Kirchhof N, Kenyon NM, Mullon C, Lake P, Cottens S, Ricordi C, Hering BJ (2004) Islet allograft survival in nonhuman primates immunosuppressed with basiliximab, RAD, and FTY720. *Transplantation.* 77, 827-835.

[25] Hering BJ, Kandaswamy R, Harmon JV, Ansite JD, Clemmings SM, Sakai T, Paraskevas S, Eckman PM, Sageshima J, Nakano M, Sawada T, Matsumoto I, Zhang HJ, Sutherland DE, Bluestone JA (2004) Transplantation of cultured islets from two-layer preserved pancreases in type 1 diabetes with anti-CD3 antibody. *Am. J. Transplant.* 4, 390-401.

[26] Adams AB, Shirasugi N, Durham MM, Strobert E, Anderson D, Rees P, Cowan S, Xu H, Blinder Y, Cheung M, Hollenbaugh D, Kenyon NS, Pearson TC, Larsen CP (2002) Calcineurin inhibitor-free CD28 blockade-based protocol protects allogeneic islets in nonhuman primates. *Diabetes.* 51, 265-270.

[27] Adams AB, Shirasugi N, Jones TR, Durham MM, Strobert EA, Cowan S, Rees P, Hendrix R, Price K, Kenyon NS, Hagerty D, Townsend R, Hollenbaugh D, Pearson TC, Larsen CP (2005) Development of a chimeric anti-CD40 monoclonal antibody that synergizes with LEA29Y to prolong islet allograft survival. *J. Immunol.* 174, 542-550.

[28] Kenyon NS, Chatzipetrou M, Masetti M, Ranuncoli A, Oliveira M, Wagner JL, Kirk AD, Harlan DM, Burkly LC, Ricordi C (1999) Long-term survival and function of intrahepatic islet allografts in rhesus monkeys treated with humanized anti-CD154. *Proc. Natl. Acad. Sci. U S A.* 96, 8132-8137.

[29] Noguchi H, Matsushita M, Okitsu T, Moriwaki A, Tomizawa K, Kang S, Li ST, Kobayashi N, Matsumoto S, Tanaka K, Tanaka N, Matsui H (2004) A new cell-permeable peptide allows successful allogeneic islet transplantation in mice. *Nat. Med.* 10, 305-309.

[30] Choi JM, Ahn MH, Chae WJ, Jung YG, Park JC, Song HM, Kim YE, Shin JA, Park CS, Park JW, Park TK, Lee JH, Seo BF, Kim KD, Kim ES, Lee DH, Lee SK, Lee SK (2006) Intranasal delivery of the cytoplasmic domain of CTLA-4 using a novel protein transduction domain prevents allergic inflammation. *Nat. Med.* 12, 574-579.

[31] Kaufman DB, Baker MS, Chen X, Leventhal JR, Stuart FP (2002) Sequential kidney/islet transplantation using prednisone-free immunosuppression. *Am. J. Transplant.* 2, 674-677.

[32] Morel P, Kaufman DB, Field MJ, Lloveras JK, Matas AJ, Sutherland DE (1992) Detrimental effect of prednisone on canine islet autograft function. *Transplant. Proc.* 24, 1048-1050.

[33] Paty BW, Harmon JS, Marsh CL, Robertson RP (2002) Inhibitory effects of immunosuppressive drugs on insulin secretion from HIT-T15 cells and Wistar rat islets. *Transplantation.* 73, 353-357.

[34] Ricordi C, Zeng YJ, Alejandro R, Tzakis A, Venkataramanan R, Fung J, Bereiter D, Mintz DH, Starzl TE (1991) In vivo effect of FK506 on human pancreatic islets. *Transplantation.* 52, 519-522.

[35] Alejandro R, Feldman EC, Bloom AD, Kenyon NS (1989) Effects of cyclosporin on insulin and C-peptide secretion in healthy beagles. *Diabetes.* 38, 698-703.

[36] Drachenberg CB, Klassen DK, Weir MR, Wiland A, Fink JC, Bartlett ST, Cangro CB, Blahut S, Papadimitriou JC (1999) Islet cell damage associated with tacrolimus and cyclosporine: morphological features in pancreas allograft biopsies and clinical correlation. *Transplantation.* 68, 396-402.

[37] Fabian MC, Lakey JR, Rajotte RV, Kneteman NM (1993) The efficacy and toxicity of rapamycin in murine islet transplantation. In vitro and in vivo studies. *Transplantation.* 56, 1137-1142.

[38] Kahan BD (1997) The synergistic effects of cyclosporine and sirolimus. *Transplantation.* 63, 170.

[39] Kahan BD, Julian BA, Pescovitz MD, Vanrenterghem Y, Neylan J (1999) Sirolimus reduces the incidence of acute rejection episodes despite lower cyclosporine doses in caucasian recipients of mismatched primary renal allografts: a phase II trial. Rapamune Study Group. *Transplantation.* 68, 1526-1532.

[40] Kahan BD (1992) Cyclosporin A, FK506, rapamycin: the use of a quantitative analytic tool to discriminate immunosuppressive drug interactions. *J. Am. Soc. Nephrol.* 2, S222-227.

[41] Chen H, Qi S, Xu D, Fitzsimmons WE, Bekersky I, Sehgal SN, Daloze P (1998) Combined effect of rapamycin and FK 506 in prolongation of small bowel graft survival in the mouse. *Transplant. Proc.* 30, 2579-2581.

[42] Vu MD, Qi S, Xu D, Wu J, Fitzsimmons WE, Sehgal SN, Dumont L, Busque S, Daloze P and Chen H (1997) Tacrolimus (FK506) and sirolimus (rapamycin) in combination

are not antagonistic but produce extended graft survival in cardiac transplantation in the rat. *Transplantation.* 64, 1853-1856.

[43] McAlister VC, Gao Z, Peltekian K, Domingues J, Mahalati K and MacDonald AS (2000) Sirolimus-tacrolimus combination immunosuppression. *Lancet.* 355, 376-377.

[44] Bell E, Cao X, Moibi JA, Greene SR, Young R, Trucco M, Gao Z, Matschinsky FM, Deng S, Markman JF, Naji A, Wolf BA (2003) Rapamycin has a deleterious effect on MIN-6 cells and rat and human islets. *Diabetes.* 52, 2731-2739.

[45] Berney T, Buhler LH, Majno P, Mentha G, Morel P (2004) Immunosuppression for pancreatic islet transplantation. *Transplant. Proc.* 36, 362S-366S.

[46] Calne R, Moffatt SD, Friend PJ, Jamieson NV, Bradley JA, Hale G, Firth J, Bradley J, Smith KG, Waldmann H (1999) Campath IH allows low-dose cyclosporine monotherapy in 31 cadaveric renal allograft recipients. *Transplantation.* 68, 1613-1616.

[47] Nanji SA, Shapiro AM (2006) Advances in pancreatic islet transplantation in humans. *Diabetes Obes. Metab.* 8, 15-25.

[48] Rao A, Luo C, Hogan PG (1997) Transcription factors of the NFAT family: regulation and function. *Annu. Rev. Immunol.* 15, 707–747.

[49] Crabtree G.R (1999) Generic signals and specific outcomes: signaling through Ca2+, calcineurin, and NF-AT. *Cell.* 96, 611–614.

[50] Sigal NH, Dumont F, Durette P, Siekierka JJ, Peterson L, Rich DH, Dunlap BE, Staruch MJ, Melino MR, Koprak SL (1991) Is cyclophilin involved in the immunosuppressive and nephrotoxic mechanism of action of cyclosporin A? *J. Exp. Med.* 173, 619-628.

[51] Platz KP, Mueller AR, Blumhardt G, Bachmann S, Bechstein WO, Kahl A, Neuhaus P (1994) Nephrotoxicity following orthotopic liver transplantation. A comparison between cyclosporine and FK506. *Transplantation.* 58, 170-178.

[52] Pascual M, Swinford RD, Ingelfinger JR, Williams WW, Cosimi AB, Tolkoff-Rubin N (1998) Chronic rejection and chronic cyclosporin toxicity in renal allografts. *Immunol. Today.* 19, 514-519.

[53] Hojo M, Morimoto T, Maluccio M, Asano T, Morimoto K, Lagman M, Shimbo T, Suthanthiran M (1999) Cyclosporine induces cancer progression by a cell-autonomous mechanism. *Nature.* 397, 530-534.

[54] Odocha O, McCauley J, Scantlebury V, Shapiro R, Carroll P, Jordan M, Vivas C, Fung JJ, Starzl TE (1993) Posttransplant diabetes mellitus in African Americans after renal transplantation under FK 506 immunosuppression. *Transplant. Proc.* 25, 2433-2434.

[55] Noguchi H, Kaneto H, Weir GC, Bonner-Weir S (2003) PDX-1 protein containing its own antennapedia-like protein transduction domain can transduce pancreatic duct and islet cells. *Diabetes.* 52, 1732-1737.

[56] Noguchi H, Matsushita M, Matsumoto S, Lu YF, Matsui H and Bonner-Weir S (2005) Mechanism of PDX-1 protein transduction. *Biochem. Biophys. Res. Commun.* 332, 68-74.

[57] Noguchi H, Matsumoto S, Okitsu T, Iwanaga Y, Yonekawa Y, Nagata H, Matsushita M, Wei FY, Matsui H, Minami K, Seino S, Masui Y, Futaki S, Tanaka K (2005) PDX-

1 protein is internalized by lipid raft-dependent macropinocytosis. *Cell Transplant.* 14, 637-645.

[58] Matsushita M, Noguchi H, Lu YF, Tomizawa K, Michiue H, Li ST, Hirose K, Bonner-Weir S, Matsui H (2004) Photo-acceleration of protein release from endosome in the protein transduction system. *FEBS Lett.* 572, 221-226.

[59] Noguchi H, Nakai Y, Matsumoto S, Kawaguchi M, Ueda M, Okitsu T, Iwanaga Y, Yonekawa Y, Nagata H, Minami K, Masui Y, Futaki S, Tanaka K (2005) Cell Permeable Peptide of JNK Inhibitor Prevents Islet Apoptosis Immediately After Isolation and Improves Islet Graft Function. *Am. J. Transplant.* 5, 1848-1855.

[60] Matsushita M, Tomizawa K, Moriwaki A, Li ST, Terada H and Matsui H (2001) A high-efficiency protein transduction system demonstrating the role of PKA in long-lasting long-term potentiation. *J. Neurosci.* 21, 6000-6007.

[61] Noguchi H, Bonner-Weir S, Wei FY, Matsushita M, Matsumoto S (2005) BETA2/NeuroD protein can be transduced into cells due to an arginine- and lysine-rich sequence. *Diabetes.* 54, 2859-2866.

[62] Noguchi H, Matsumoto S (2006) Protein transduction technology offers a novel therapeutic approach for diabetes. *J. Hepatobiliary Pancreat Surg.* 13, 306-13

[63] Noguchi H, Matsumoto S (2006) Protein transduction technology: a novel therapeutic perspective. *Acta Med. Okayama.* 60, 1-11.

[64] Aramburu J, Yaffe MB, Lopez-Rodriguez C, Cantley LC, Hogan PG and Rao A (1999) Affinity-driven peptide selection of an NFAT inhibitor more selective than cyclosporin A. *Science.* 285, 2129-2133.

[65] Kuriyama M, Matsushita M, Tateishi A, Moriwaki A, Tomizawa K, Ishino K, Sano S, Matsui H (2006) A cell-permeable NFAT inhibitor peptide prevents pressure-overload cardiac hypertrophy. *Chem. Biol. Drug Des.* 67, 238-243.

[66] Managlia EZ, Landay A, Al-Harthi L (2006) Interleukin-7 induces HIV replication in primary naive T cells through a nuclear factor of activated T cell (NFAT)-dependent pathway. *Virology.* 350, 443-452.

[67] Crotti TN, Flannery M, Walsh NC, Fleming JD, Goldring SR, McHugh KP (2006) NFATc1 regulation of the human beta3 integrin promoter in osteoclast differentiation. *Gene.* 372, 92-102.

[68] So T, Song J, Sugie K, Altman A, Croft M (2006) Signals from OX40 regulate nuclear factor of activated T cells c1 and T cell helper 2 lineage commitment. *Proc. Natl. Acad. Sci. U S A.* 103, 3740-3745.

[69] Lenschow DJ, Walunas TL, Bluestone JA (1996) CD28/B7 system of T cell costimulation. *Annu. Rev. Immunol.* 14, 233-258.

[70] Schwartz RH (1990) A cell culture model for T lymphocyte clonal anergy. *Science.* 248, 1349-1356.

[71] Kawai T, Andrews D, Colvin RB, Sachs DH, Cosimi AB (2000) Thromboembolic complications after treatment with monoclonal antibody against CD40 ligand. *Nat. Med.* 6, 114.

[72] Buhler L, Alwayn IP, Appel JZ 3rd, Robson SC, Cooper DK (2001) Anti-CD154 monoclonal antibody and thromboembolism. *Transplantation.* 71, 491.

[73] Contreras JL, Eckhoff DE, Cartner S, Bilbao G, Ricordi C, Neville DM Jr, Thomas FT, Thomas JM (2000) Long-term functional islet mass and metabolic function after xenoislet transplantation in primates. *Transplantation.* 69, 195-201.

[74] Thomas FT, Ricordi C, Contreras JL, Hubbard WJ, Jiang XL, Eckhoff DE, Cartner S, Bilbao G, Neville DM Jr, Thomas JM (1999) Reversal of naturally occuring diabetes in primates by unmodified islet xenografts without chronic immunosuppression. *Transplantation.* 67, 846-854.

[75] Thomas JM, Contreras JL, Smyth CA, Lobashevsky A, Jenkins S, Hubbard WJ, Eckhoff DE, Stavrou S, Neville DM Jr, Thomas FT (2001) Successful reversal of streptozotocin-induced diabetes with stable allogeneic islet function in a preclinical model of type 1 diabetes. *Diabetes.* 50, 1227-1236.

[76] Spitzer TR, Delmonico F, Tolkoff-Rubin N, McAfee S, Sackstein R, Saidman S, Colby C, Sykes M, Sachs DH, Cosimi AB (1999) Combined histocompatibility leukocyte antigen-matched donor bone marrow and renal transplantation for multiple myeloma with end stage renal disease: the induction of allograft tolerance through mixed lymphohematopoietic chimerism. *Transplantation.* 68, 480-484.

[77] Buhler LH, Spitzer TR, Sykes M, Sachs DH, Delmonico FL, Tolkoff-Rubin N, Saidman SL, Sackstein R, McAfee S, Dey B, Colby C, Cosimi AB (2002) Induction of kidney allograft tolerance after transient lymphohematopoietic chimerism in patients with multiple myeloma and end-stage renal disease. *Transplantation.* 74, 1405-1409.

[78] Sayegh MH, Fine NA, Smith JL, Rennke HG, Milford EL, Tilney NL (1991) Immunologic tolerance to renal allografts after bone marrow transplants from the same donors. *Ann. Intern. Med.* 114, 954-955.

[79] Orive G, Hernandez RM, Gascon AR, Calafiore R, Chang TM, De Vos P, Hortelano G, Hunkeler D, Lacik I, Shapiro AM, Pedraz JL (2003) Cell encapsulation: promise and progress. *Nat Med.* 9, 104-107.

[80] Miura S, Teramura Y, Iwata H (2006) Encapsulation of islets with ultra-thin polyion complex membrane through poly(ethylene glycol)-phospholipids anchored to cell membrane. *Biomaterials.* 27, 5828-5835.

[81] Omer A, Duvivier-Kali V, Fernandes J, Tchipashvili V, Colton CK, Weir GC (2005) Long-term normoglycemia in rats receiving transplants with encapsulated islets. *Transplantation.* 79, 52-58.

[82] Duvivier-Kali VF, Omer A, Lopez-Avalos MD, O'Neil JJ, Weir GC (2004) Survival of microencapsulated adult pig islets in mice in spite of an antibody response. *Am. J. Transplant.* 4, 1991-2000.

[83] Omer A, Duvivier-Kali VF, Trivedi N, Wilmot K, Bonner-Weir S, Weir GC (2003) Survival and maturation of microencapsulated porcine neonatal pancreatic cell clusters transplanted into immunocompetent diabetic mice. *Diabetes.* 52, 69-75.

[84] Duvivier-Kali VF, Omer A, Parent RJ, O'Neil JJ, Weir GC (2001) Complete protection of islets against allorejection and autoimmunity by a simple barium-alginate membrane. *Diabetes.* 50, 1698-1705.

Index

250 Index

J

K